Children's Speech and Literacy Difficulties: Book 2

Identification and Intervention

Children's Speech and Literacy Difficulties: Book 2

Identification and Intervention

Edited By

JOY STACKHOUSE PHD

and

BILL WELLS DPHIL

Department of Human Communication Sciences
University of Sheffield

Consulting Editor: *Professor Margaret Snowling*
University of York

W

WHURR PUBLISHERS

LONDON AND PHILADELPHIA

© 2001 Whurr Publishers
First published 2001 by
Whurr Publishers Ltd
19b Compton Terrace, London N1 2UN, England and
325 Chestnut Street, Philadelphia PA 19106, USA

Reprinted 2002, 2004 and 2005

British Library Cataloguing in Publication Data
A catalogue record for this book is available from the British
Library.

ISBN: 1 86156 131 8

Printed and bound in the UK by Athenaeum Press Ltd,
Gateshead, Tyne & Wear

In memory of our friend and colleague
Clare Tarplee (1962–1999)

Contents

Foreword

Literacy and effective communication skills are basic prerequisites for success in the modern world. Unfortunately, many individuals experience great difficulty developing competencies in these areas. During the last decade, relationships between literacy and phonological processing have been studied extensively. We know now that certain phonological tasks (e.g. phoneme manipulation) are significant predictors of literacy and also that phonological awareness skills can be trained. What has been lacking, however, has been a comprehensive approach that not only facilitates identification of communication and literacy deficiencies, but also provides a logical framework for making decisions regarding how best to intervene.

Children's Speech and Literacy Difficulties: Book 2 Identification and Intervention, edited by Joy Stackhouse and Bill Wells, does just that. Book 2 takes the next critical step expanding the psycholinguistic framework, which was explicated in their Book 1, to detail intervention planning. The process of determining treatment goals that are optimal for each individual is explained meticulously. Stackhouse and Wells and ten contributors skilfully take us through 21 case studies, exemplifying the many differential-diagnosis aspects that need to be considered. The thought-provoking exercises throughout the book provide a solid foundation for novices and veterans alike to develop the skills necessary to extrapolate from the theoretical underpinnings and begin implementing this approach in their own professional settings.

One of the unique contributions of the psycholinguistic approach presented in this book is the emphasis placed on representations and on input. Currently a number of popular treatment programmes in the speech-language profession focus almost exclusively on output and oral motor tasks. Another unique highlight of this book is the recognition of the importance of identifying each individual's strengths.

Book 2 provides a cohesive bridge between research and practice. The methods presented in this book have a solid foundation in science. Hypotheses are systematically developed and tested at every step. Stackhouse and Wells have included 'cutting edge' information about topics that currently are attracting a great deal of research interest (e.g. working memory). In addition, new applications (e.g. incorporation of technology such as electropalatography) are introduced in this treatise. Clearly, this approach is continuing to evolve.

Stackhouse and Wells have 'pushed the boundaries' for professionals involved with literacy and communication disorders, and we are in their debt. It is anticipated that their efforts will have a far-reaching impact. Ultimately, it is the individuals with communication and literacy difficulties who are expected to be the real winners.

Barbara Hodson PhD
Department of Communicative Disorders and Science
The Wichita State University
Kansas, U.S.A

Preface

In Book 1 (Stackhouse and Wells, 1997), we presented a framework for psycholinguistic assessment which combines a theoretical model of speech processing with a developmental phase model for speech and metaphonological awareness. In this sequel the same systematic hypothesis testing approach is applied to identification and intervention. The approach is not tied to any specific clinical entity but can be used with any child who presents with speech, lexical or literacy problems.

The broad aims of this second book are:

(a) to show how the psycholinguistic approach can be used as a basis for identification, intervention and evaluation;
(b) to extend the psycholinguistic assessment framework to incorporate new areas, e.g. word-finding and intonation;
(c) to demonstrate how the psycholinguistic approach links with the curriculum delivered in schools;
(d) to illustrate the connection between research and practice.

The book is intended for professionals and researchers working with children who are having difficulties with the development of speech and/or literacy skills. We hope that it will be of particular interest to speech and language pathologists and therapists, and we have assumed a level of background knowledge (for example in phonetics) that therapists can be expected to have. At the same time, we have attempted to make the book accessible to other interested readers, such as teachers and psychologists working with children who have speech and literacy difficulties. Some familiarity with the principles of the psycholinguistic approach is also assumed.

Chapter 1 (Joy Stackhouse) revises these basic principles and links the psycholinguistic approach to the curriculum taught at school. The findings of a longitudinal study of children's speech and literacy skills are reported; these have implications for how potential literacy problems might be identified. Chapters 2 and 3 (Rachel Rees) guide the reader through the necessary stages of planning intervention: from hypotheses to aims, and from aims to tasks. Chapter 2 summarizes principles of intervention and Chapter 3 demonstrates how to analyse and control the components of a task to ensure that intervention is being targeted appropriately.

These themes are developed further in Chapters 4 and 5 (Juliette Corrin), which detail the process of moving from a psycholinguistic assessment profile to an intervention programme. These two chapters will be of particular interest to readers already experienced in using the framework and who wish to develop their own case study research in this area. Chapter 6 (Daphne Waters) demonstrates how the psycholinguistic principles covered in Chapters 2–5, in particular the method of building on processing strengths to help remediate deficits, can be incorporated into the management of a child with speech difficulties. At the same time, the case study highlights the role of the child as a learner in the intervention process, and the importance of factors other than the child's cognitive profile.

Chapter 7 (Hilary Dent) illustrates further how the psycholinguistic approach is 'carried in the head of the user' (Book 1, p.49) and not in a case of specifically designed tasks. The instrumental technique of electropalatography can reveal finer detail about a child's speech production than are available to listeners, and thus can lead to a more precise diagnosis of the level of deficit underlying a speech disorder. In addition, it is shown to be an effective feedback device in the remediation of such speech difficulties. Research and practice also neatly come together in Chapter 8 (Liz Nathan and Sarah Simpson). The child who is the subject of their case study had been discharged from speech and language therapy but was identified on a research project as having residual difficulties which were interfering with the development of his literacy skills. The subsequent teaching programme builds on the psycholinguistic profile and addresses the demands of the school curriculum.

The next three chapters show how the original psycholinguistic framework has been extended. Chapter 9 (Jill Popple and Wendy Wellington) describes the introduction of the psycholinguistic approach into a special school setting and its impact – not only on the assessment and management of the children but also on the professionals themselves. Collaborative working was facilitated by the sharing of common terminology developed through adopting the psycholinguistic approach. Chapter 10 (Alison Constable) uses the psycholinguistic framework to shed light on the nature of word-finding difficulties in children and reviews the implications of this approach for intervention. The often neglected area of prosodic difficulties in children, which had been touched on briefly in Book 1, is treated more extensively in Chapter 11 (Bill Wells and Sue Peppé). The comparison of two cases shows how psycholinguistically motivated procedures can differentiate levels of prosodic difficulty and can contribute towards an intervention programme. Chapter 12 (Joy Stackhouse and Bill Wells) pulls together the themes across the chapters and discusses future directions for the psycholinguistic framework.

All the contributors are experienced users of the psycholinguistic framework and teachers of the approach. They bring together research and practice through their work in a range of different settings, e.g. clinics, mainstream schools, 'special' schools and centres. As in Book 1, each chapter includes paper and pencil activities, and a suggested key to each activity follows the chapter. These answers are not intended to be definitive in any sense, but are offered as a stimulus for reflection and discussion.

Joy Stackhouse and Bill Wells
June 2000

The Contributors

Alison Constable, MSc – Lecturer in the Department of Human Communication Science, University College London, and registered speech and language therapist.

Juliet Corrin, MSc – Department of Human Communication Science, University College London. Formerly principal speech and language therapist, Nuffield Hearing and Speech Centre, London.

Hilary Dent, MA – Formerly lecturer, Department of Human Communication Science, University College London. Registered speech and language therapist.

Liz Nathan, MSc – Lecturer/research fellow, Department of Human Communication Science, University College London. Registered speech and language therapist.

Sue Peppé, PhD – Research fellow, Queen Margaret University College, Edinburgh.

Jill Popple – Rowan School, Sheffield. Registered speech and language therapist.

Rachel Rees, MSc – Lecturer, Department of Human Communication Science, University College London. Registered speech and language therapist; qualified teacher of pupils with specific learning difficulties.

Sarah Simpson, MSc – Department of Human Communication Science, University College London. Registered speech and language therapist; qualified teacher of pupils with specific learning difficulties.

Joy Stackhouse, PhD – Professor of Human Communication Sciences, University of Sheffield. Formerly Professor of Speech and Literacy in the Department of Human Communication Science, University College London. Registered speech and language therapist; chartered psychologist; qualified teacher of pupils with specific learning difficulties.

Daphne Waters, PhD – Lecturer, Queen Margaret University College, Edinburgh. Registered speech and language therapist.

Wendy Wellington – Rowan School, Sheffield. Registered speech and language therapist.

Bill Wells, DPhil – ESRC Senior Research Fellow, University of Sheffield. Formerly Professor of Clinical Linguistics, University College London.

Conventions

TIE   spoken real word target/stimulus, as in real word repetition test, rhyme production test, spelling to dictation of real words; also used for picture target/stimulus, as in naming test, or silent rhyme detection.

/straɪ/   spoken nonword target, as in nonword repetition or discrimination test; spelling nonwords to dictation; also used for real word target when phonological information is required.

‹tie›   written target, as in a test of single word reading (real or nonword).

[taɪ]   spoken response, where phonetic information is required.

"tie"   spoken real word response, where phonetic information is not required.

‹tie›   written response, as in a test of spelling to dictation, or free writing.

→   'is realized as', e.g. /straɪ/ → [taɪ]; ‹tie› → 'tie' ; TIE → ‹die›.

For phonetic symbols and diacritics, see Book 1, Appendix 1.

Chapter 1
Identifying Children at Risk for Literacy Problems

JOY STACKHOUSE

Most children learn to speak, read and write perfectly well. They tackle the complexities of spoken and written language and often enjoy doing so. For some children, however, the mastery of speech and literacy skills is an insurmountable barrier. Being asked to read or spell at home or school becomes a painful experience leading to avoidance behaviour and low self-esteem. Early identification and understanding of the nature of a child's difficulties can help to limit not only the extent of the literacy difficulties but also the impact of the problem on the child's general well-being.

This chapter examines children's literacy development from a psycholinguistic perspective. It extends some of the central issues presented in Book 1 (Stackhouse and Wells, 1997) and applies them to the curriculum in schools. The findings from a longitudinal study of children's speech and literacy development are presented to show how the psycholinguistic framework might be used to identify children with speech processing difficulties and to predict their literacy performance at around 7 years of age. In particular, the role of phonological awareness in predicting and promoting literacy skills is evaluated.

The National Curriculum

In the UK, there is a national curriculum which children follow at school. In England and Wales, this curriculum in the primary school years (ages 5–11 years) is divided into two *Key Stages* (Department for Education (DFE), 1995c). The *National Curriculum's Key Stage 1 Programme of Study for English* (ages 5–7 years) integrates speech, language, visual and motor skills developed in the pre-school years and makes explicit the links between spoken and written language. One of the main aims of the *Reading and Writing Programme* at this stage is to help children 'crack the code' of their writing system; an essential step in achieving independence in written language development.

At *Key Stage 2* (ages 8–11 years), children are expected not only to use expressive language functionally within the school environment but also to reflect on different language styles, develop insights and express opinions, and have the organizational skills and language abilities to communicate complex ideas. Reading at Key Stage 2 has moved beyond cracking the code. Independent reading for interest, pleasure and information is a clear objective. Use of information technology-based reference materials, encyclopaedias, dictionaries and thesauruses is commonplace. Reading performance is extended beyond simple phoneme-to-grapheme (sound-to-letter) matching and includes proficiency with more complex graphemic patterns and irregularities. Exposure to complex narrative and figurative language requires powers of inference and deduction. Increasingly abstract vocabulary is necessary to grapple with more imaginative ideas.

Writing at Key Stage 2 becomes a means of organizing information as well as developing ideas. It is used to record succinct notes on a topic and work is expected to be planned, drafted, revised and proof-read. Punctuation needs to be used appropriately to mark morphological endings, grammatical chunks, and expressions. The spelling of complex multisyllabic words is tackled by using prior knowledge of meaning and word structure, and the conventions of English spelling along with its irregularities are taught.

The more advanced literacy skills at Key Stage 2 are therefore linked to the development of higher-level language skills as well as to the basic literacy skills developed at Key Stage 1. Activities at Key Stage 2 increase the demand on children's metalinguistic and metacognitive skills. There is a shift from using language for accessing literacy to using literacy for promoting further language development (e.g. expansion of vocabulary). Thus, language and literacy skills are much more integrated at this stage (see Popple and Wellington, this volume, for further discussion).

Children pass through these stages with varying degrees of ease and success. Compare the written performance of the following two children, both in their first term of Year 3 at school (age range 7–8 years) and at the beginning of Key Stage 2. One of the projects for this term is *The Egyptians*. Both are able children who have enjoyed this topic and can talk about it enthusiastically. However, as you will see, one of them has specific learning difficulties.

Laura, CA 7;11

In her half-term break, Laura chose to write her own book based on work done at school. It was entitled *Children's Egypt Book* and it comprised seven pages of information, each one presenting an illustrated topic: *Pyramids*; *Mummies*; *Jewellery*; *Eye make-up*; *The Nile*; *Hieroglyphics* and *Scales*. In addition, there was a contents page, and a front and back cover. Writing this book was an enjoyable experience for her and she was left with a great sense of achievement. See Figures 1.1 and 1.2 for sample pages from her book.

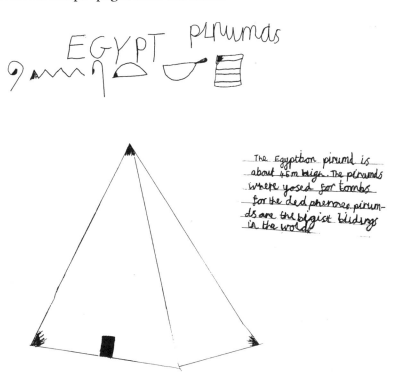

Figure 1.1: Laura's Egypt book: Pyramids. Text: The Egyptian pyramid is about 45m high. The pyramids were used for tombs for the dead Pharaohs. Pyramids are the biggest buildings in the world.

Edward, CA 7;7

Edward was equally knowledgeable about the Egyptians and was particularly interested in the construction of the pyramids. He knew the different types of pyramid and what they were like inside, for example the number of chambers and what was in them. He chose the topic of *pyramids* for a free writing exercise. However, his written performace bore no relationship to his knowledge of the subject. It took him a long time to write anything at all. He eventually wrote five isolated but semantically related words (see Figure 1.3): PYRAMIDS; ROCK; STEP-PYRAMID; CHAMBER; TREASURES. He then remembered a question from his Egypt project book: "HOW MANY ROOMS ARE THERE IN A PYRAMID?" which he added on the second line to expand his written work. In general, when writing at school he frequently dropped his pen on the floor and became disinterested and uncooperative. His behaviour and low self-esteem drew attention to his difficulties.

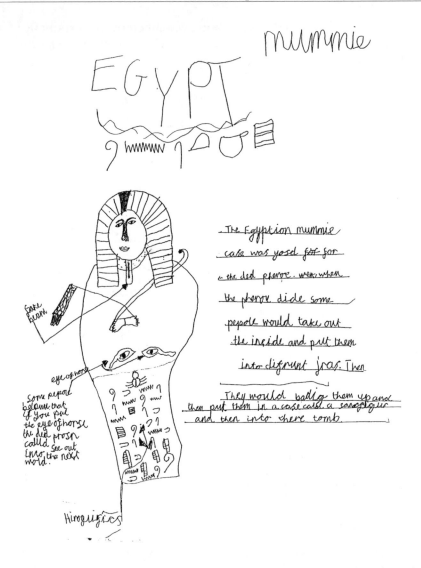

Text: The Egyptian Mummy case was used for the dead Pharaoh. When the Pharaoh died some people would take out the inside and put them into different jars. Then they would bandage them up and then put them in a case called a sarcophagus and then into their tomb.

Labelling of the Mummy from top to bottom:
(a) fake beard
(b) eye of Horus
(c) some people believed that if you put the eye of Horus the dead person could see out into the next world.
(d) hieroglyphics

Figure 1.2: Laura's Egypt book: Mummies.

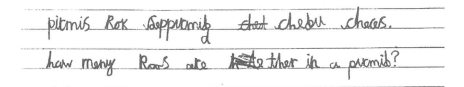

Figure 1.3: Edward's free writing: Pyramids. (CA 7;7)
Line 1: pyramids; rock; step-pyramid; chamber; treasures.
Line 2: How many rooms are there in a pyramid?

ACTIVITY 1.1

Aim: to assess free writing from children with and without difficulties and examine the findings in relation to the curriculum demands made on them.

1. Compare Laura's and Edward's written performance about the pyramids in Figures 1.1 and 1.3. Jot down your observations of their free writing. What additional information can you glean about Laura's writing skills from Figure 1.2?

2. With reference to Key Stage 2 outlined above, what conclusions might be drawn from your observations of their written language skills?

Check your response with Key to Activity 1.1 at the end of this chapter.

Edward is clearly in trouble as he starts Year 3 and the demands of Key Stage 2 are made. He still needs to work at the level introduced at Key Stage 1. He has not yet 'cracked the code' sufficiently to move on. He was unable to recite the alphabet in full. He was still learning letter names and had difficulty mapping letters on to sounds in words. His reading and spelling skills were about one year behind, as were his rhyme and blending skills. In contrast, his receptive vocabulary was just above age appropriate (55th percentile on *The British Picture Vocabulary Scales*, Dunn, Dunn, Whetton, et al., 1982) and his nonverbal skills were almost two years above age appropriate (95 percentile on *The Coloured Progressive Matrices*, Raven, 1984). Fortunately, his difficulties had been recognized by Year 2 when he had been at his school for only a few months, having moved from another area. Behaviour problems increased as Edward tried to avoid writing situations, and his handwriting decreased dramatically in size in an attempt to cover up his misspellings. Self-esteem also diminished. An individual 1 hour per week teaching session was carried out during his Year 3 at school. His teaching programme focused on alphabetic skills, phonological awareness, specific spelling rules, reading fluency, expressive spoken and written language (including word-finding skills), word recognition and spelling of common words and hand-writing. Edward also followed the *Phonological Awareness Training (PAT)* programme (Wilson, 1993–96) in a small group once a week. Progress was evident by the end of Year 3 when with help he was able to construct a short paragraph on a topic (see Figure 1.4). However, he was still performing less well at the end of Year 3 than would be predicted given his general abilities; he required further help with his literacy skills in Year 4.

In contrast, Laura had performed well in the end of Year 2 tests and was already tackling some of the demands of Key Stage 2. Before starting school, Laura had attended a nursey half-time for five terms where the emphasis was on play and interaction skills but not on literacy teaching explicitly. When Laura started school at the age of 4;11 she had well-developed language skills and intelligible speech. She knew her alphabet and enjoyed playing rhyme and sound games (e.g. I-spy). Listening and attention skills were good and in general she was an ideal candidate for literacy instruction. She had a firm foundation for her literacy development and was ready to learn from the teaching offered. By the second year of school (Year 1 in the UK system) Laura had confident phoneme–grapheme translation skills, though she still had a lot to learn about irregular spellings in English. Laura's literacy development had followed a normal route from spoken to written language.

From Speech to Literacy: Normal Development

In Book 1 (pp.13–14) we described Uta Frith's (1985) three-phase model of literacy development and mapped it on to a similar phase model of children's speech development (pp.330–332). In Frith's model, children move from an initial *logographic* or visual whole word recognition strategy of reading, on to an *alphabetic* phase utilizing phoneme–grapheme correspondences, and finally to an *orthographic* phase dependent on segmentation of larger units: morphemes.

In the first phase, children can recognize only words that they know and are not able to decode unfamiliar words. When spelling, they have some learnt programmes for familiar words (e.g. their own name) but, in general, spelling does not show phoneme–grapheme correspon-dences, e.g. ORANGE spelt as ‹oearasrie›. Breakthrough to the alphabetic

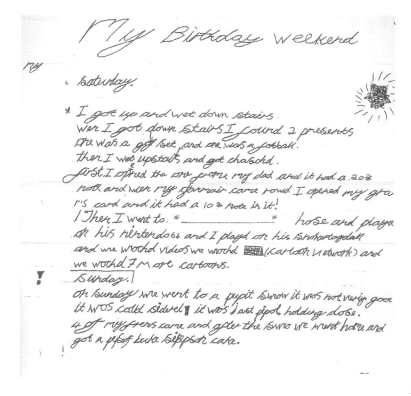

My Birthday Weekend

Saturday
I got up and went downstairs
when I got downstairs I found 2 presents
one was a golf set and one was a football.
then I went upstairs and got changed.
first I opened the one from my dad and it had a £20
note and when my grandma came round I opened my granm
r's card and it had a £10 note in it!
Then I went to [friend's name deleted] house and played
on his Nintendo and I played on his snooker table
and we watched videos we watched (cartoon network) and
we watched 7 more cartoons.

Sunday
On Sunday we went to a puppet show it was not very good
it was called Cinderella! it was just people holding dolls
4 of my friends came and after the show we went home and
got a piece of Bart Simpson cake.

Figure 1.4: Edward's free writing about his birthday weekend (CA 8;0).
(It took him two sessions to complete this)

stage occurs when a child can apply phoneme–grapheme rules to decode new words. Spelling becomes more logical: it demonstrates that the child is segmenting the word successfully and applying letter knowledge, but has not yet learned (or been taught) the conventions of English spelling, e.g. ORANGE spelt as ‹orinj›. Finally, in the orthographic stage, the child is able to recognize larger chunks of words such as prefixes and suffixes (e.g. ADDITION), and to read more efficiently by analogy with known words.

Thus, moving beyond the logographic phase of literacy development is dependent on understanding that spoken utterances can be segmented into smaller elements and that these elements can be represented via sound–letter correspondences. This is the key to cracking the alphabetic code (see Nathan and Simpson, this volume, for further discussion of models of literacy development).

ACTIVITY 1.2

Aim: to examine emerging spelling skills in a normally developing child.

Look at Laura's free writing of a popular nursery rhyme at age 6;1, shown in Figure 1.5.

(a) What is the nursery rhyme?
(b) What has been omitted?

Check your answer with Key to Activity 1.2 at the end of this chapter then continue with the activity.

(c) What do you notice about Laura's presentation of the rhyme compared to conventional text?
(d) Go through each word in the nursery rhyme and work out why Laura's spelling is as it is. Reflect on your own speech production when you say the words of the rhyme – this will give you a clue. What patterns of errors have you noticed?
(e) With reference to Uta Frith's phase model of literacy development outlined above, what can you conclude about Laura's spelling development?

Check your responses with Key to Activity 1.2 at the end of this chapter.

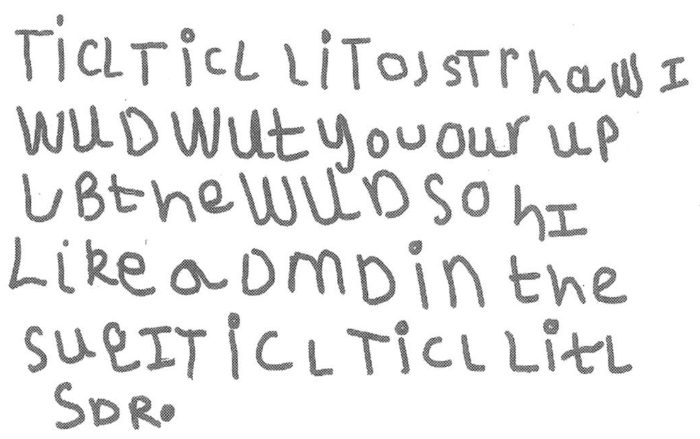

TicLTicL LiToJ sTrhaw I
WULD WUt youour uP
LBthe WULD SO hI
Likea DMDin the
SUEIT iCL TicL Litl
SDR.

Figure 1.5: Laura's free writing of a nursery rhyme (CA 6;1).

This activity shows clearly that normal spelling development is mapped in some way onto a speech foundation. Various studies have applied speech analysis skills to spelling and found similarities between speech and spelling development (Treiman, 1993; Stackhouse and Wells, 1993; McCormick, 1995; Clarke-Klein and Hodson, 1995). Young, normally developing children spell by linking their knowledge of the alphabet to their awareness of how it feels to produce speech sounds. They have not yet been taught the vagaries of English spelling but have learned how to convey meaning through print in an unconventional but logical way. This is typical of the alphabetic stage of literacy development.

Thus, consistent speech production is an important skill for the young child to bring when starting school. Children who begin school with delayed speech and language skills are disadvantaged in many ways, but particularly when tackling the first stages of a literacy programme. Such children may have delayed reading and spelling skills and move more slowly through the normal phases of literacy development compared to their peers. Children with specific speech difficulties may find cracking the code the biggest hurdle to get over, and develop dyslexic difficulties (see the cases of Michael and Caroline, who were both stuck at the logographic phase of literacy development at the age of 11 years, Book 1, pp.234–240).

Frith (1985) suggested that dyslexia occurs when a child fails to progress through the normal phases of literacy development. In particular, 'classic' developmental dyslexia is arrested development at the logographic phase because of a specific difficulty with acquiring alphabetic skills. The development of compensatory strategies is necessary for literacy to develop.

When seeing Laura's written nursery rhyme in Figure 1.5, one teacher expressed concern that there were not more 'correct' spellings, that could have resulted from whole word learning. Indeed, some children may be less speech-based than Laura and veer towards a more visual strategy; there is enormous variation in the so-called 'normal' population. However, if a child at this age produces a sample of written language which shows no attempt to link speech sounds with letters, this would suggest that the child is not developing phonological awareness skills or progressing to the alphabetic stage of literacy development.

What is Phonological Awareness?

Phonological awareness refers to the ability to reflect on and manipulate the structure of an utterance as distinct from its meaning (see Book 1, p.53). Popular phonological awareness tasks include rhyme, syllable and sound segmentation, blending and spoonerisms. Children need to develop this awareness in order to make sense of an alphabetic script, such as English, when learning to read and to spell. For example, children have to learn that the segments (the consonants and vowels) in a word can be represented by a written form – letters. When spelling a new word, children have to be able to segment (divide) the word into its segments before they can attach the appropriate letters. When reading an unfamiliar word, they have to be able to decode the printed letters back to segments and blend them together to form the word. Thus, it is not surprising that phonological awareness skill is said to be a strong predictor of literacy development (Goswami and Bryant, 1990) and is included in programmes for pre-school children (e.g. Bradley and Bryant, 1983; Layton, Deeney and Upton, 1997) as well as being in the National Curriculum for school-age children.

If speech, language and phonological awareness skills are so important for the development of literacy skills then it follows that early identification of children with difficulties in these areas could alert us to those at risk of literacy problems. Targeted intervention during Key Stage 1 (ages 5–7 years) is important; intervention may not 'cure' children's literacy problems but can reduce the full impact of them. If basic literacy skills are not set up at Key Stage 1, children will not be able to develop the more advanced literacy skills of Key Stage 2, which in turn will inhibit their development of higher-level language skills. For some children, behaviour problems may also ensue and many suffer from low self-esteem. Edward, described above, is typical.

How early and through what procedures can we predict a child's literacy outcome? Adopting a psycholinguistic approach to the profiling of children's speech processing and language skills may help to answer this question.

What is a Psycholinguistic Approach to Identifying Children's Speech and Literacy Difficulties?

The essence of the psycholinguistic approach is the assumption that the child receives information of different kinds (e.g. auditory, visual) about a spoken utterance or written form, remembers it and stores it in a variety of *lexical representations* (a means for keeping information about words) within the *lexicon* (a store of words), then selects and produces spoken and written words. Figure 1.6 illustrates the basic structure of a psycholinguistic model of speech processing.

On the left there is a channel for the input of information via the ear and on the right a channel for the output of information through the mouth. At the top of the model there are the lexical representations which store previously processed information, while at the bottom there is no such store. In psycholinguistic terms, *top-down* processing refers to an activity whereby previously stored information (i.e. in the

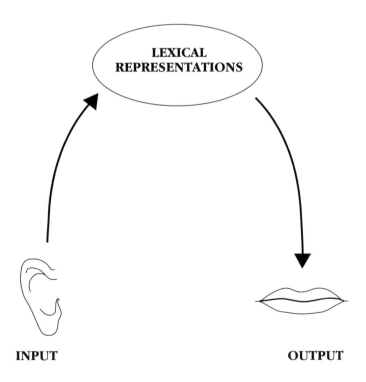

Figure 1.6: The basic structure of a psycholinguistic model of speech processing (from Stackhouse and Wells, 1997, p. 9).

lexical representations) is helpful and used. A *bottom-up* processing activity requires no such prior knowledge and can be completed without accessing stored linguistic knowledge from the lexical representations. Thus, there are two dimensions to the model (see Figure 1.7).

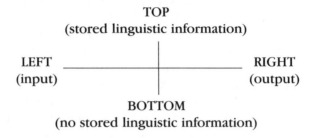

TOP
(stored linguistic information)

LEFT   RIGHT
(input)   (output)

BOTTOM
(no stored linguistic information)

Figure 1.7: The two dimensions of the speech processing model (from Stackhouse and Wells, 1997, p. 8).

In Book 1 we argued that this speech processing system was not only the basis for speech development but also the foundation for literacy development; 'written language' being an extension of 'spoken language'. Both top-down and bottom-up speech and language skills are necessary for literacy to develop satisfactorily (see Book 1, Chapter 1; Activity 1.4, p.20). Further, our analysis of popular phonological awareness tasks within a simple psycholinguistic model (see Book 1, Chapter 3) showed that phonological awareness is not a separate area of children's development but rather a product of their speech processing skills. As a consequence, any difficulty children have in their basic speech processing system will result not only in spoken difficulties but also in problematic phonological awareness development, which in turn will impact on their literacy performance. The precise nature of the speech and literacy problems, however, will depend on the location of the deficit(s) in the speech processing system (Snowling, Stackhouse and Rack, 1986). Figure 1.8 illustrates the relationship between speech, literacy and phonological awareness and how all three behaviours are dependent on the speech processing system depicted in Figure 1.6.

In Book 1 (Activity 1.2, pp.9–10) we examined the content of the lexical representations at the top of the model by discussing what an adult knows about the word CAT. Very often the first thing that comes to mind is what the word means *(semantic representation)* e.g. small furry domestic animal with whiskers. It may be classified along with similar domestic animals, e.g. DOG or with other members of the cat species e.g. LION. The spoken word can also be discriminated from other similarly sounding words, e.g. CAT vs CAP and speech errors made in a word can be detected, e.g. "tat" for CAT. This is because there is a *phonological representation* for CAT, which stores enough information

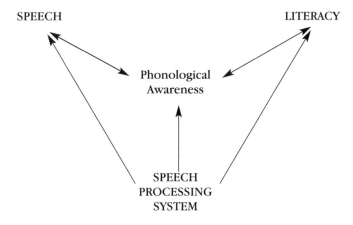

Figure 1.8: The relationship between speech, iteracy and phonological awareness (from Stackhouse and Wells, 1997, p. 58).

to allow a word to be identified on the basis of auditory and visual (e.g. lip reading) cues. The unimpaired adult can also produce the word CAT automatically, i.e. without any conscious effort. This is because there is a stored set of instructions for the pronunciation of a word stored in its *motor program*. However, words are rarely produced in isolation. More often they are put into a sentence structure, e.g. "Have you fed the CAT?". We therefore also know that the word CAT belongs to a certain class of word (i.e. nouns), which can be used in some positions in the sentence but not in others, and which has a plural form CATS that can be derived by rule. Such knowledge is stored in the *grammatical representation* for the word CAT. Finally, the printed form of the word CAT can be recognized and skilled spellers do not have to assemble letters one by one to spell it. There is therefore also stored information about what a word looks like in its printed form and this is held in the *orthographic representation*. In summary, information about a word is stored in the following representations within the lexicon:

(a) semantic representation;
(b) phonological representation;
(c) motor program;
(d) grammatical representation;
(e) orthographic representation.

Ideally, as in the case of Laura described above, when a child starts school around 5 years of age s/he should have an intact speech processing system in order to deal with spoken language. The child should be able to listen, attend and discriminate between similar sounding words. S/he should also be able to produce intelligible speech, even if not identical to the adult form. S/he should have semantic, phonological and grammatical representations for common words, together with stored motor programs for producing them. A main aim for the teacher is to develop the orthographic representations, i.e. to teach children about the printed word, ensuring that the right orthographic representation is linked with the other representations of the target word. Put like this it does not sound too onerous a task! In reality of course it is one of the most challenging jobs teachers have to face, not least because many of the children they are working with do not have a well-developed and stable foundation of spoken language.

The aim of the psycholinguistic approach is to find out exactly where on the speech processing model presented in Figure 1.6 a child's speech processing skills are breaking down and how this might affect their speech and literacy development. Thus, a psycholinguistic assessment investigates a child's underlying processing skills. In Book 1, a number of popular auditory, lexical, phonological awareness and speech output tasks were analysed from a psycholinguistic perspective (see Book 1, Chapters 2 and 3). This led to the development of a psycholinguistic framework which classifies tasks along the two dimensions presented in Figure 1.7 (see Book 1, Chapter 4).

First, tasks were classified according to the degree in which they are dependent on stored linguistic information in the lexical representations: top vs bottom. Second, tasks were classified as either input or output (left vs right). This led to a clustering of tasks at different levels on the speech processing model (see Figure 1.9).

Finally, we were able to pose an assessment question at each of the levels related to the processing demands made by these tasks. This provided the basis for a profile sheet (see Figure 1.10) which could be used to summarize a child's speech processing strengths and weaknesses (see Book 1, Chapter 5 on how to profile children's speech processing skills). On this speech processing profile sheet questions A–F on the left-hand side of the sheet relate to input processing. Question A is at the level of the ear and includes basic auditory perceptual skills as well as hearing acuity. Questions G–K on the right-hand side of the sheet relate to output processing, question K being at the level of the mouth. Tasks used to answer questions nearer the top of the profile require the child to access stored linguistic information (top-down), while those tasks used to answer questions lower down on the profile do not require access to as much stored information. Question L represents the link between output and input skills and taps a child's monitoring of his/her own speech.

A series of ticks (✓) and crosses (×) are used on the sheet to record a child's performance. Sometimes these are based on clinical or teaching

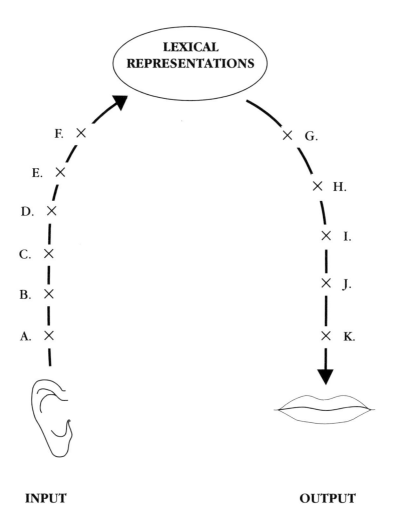

Figure 1.9: Crosses on the simple speech processing model to mark the levels at which tests cluster.

experience and judgement. However, where there is standardized information about a child's performance (i.e. a comparison with normal controls) the ticks and crosses can be used more objectively. For example, ticks on the speech processing profile show that performance is no different from normal controls, i.e. within 1 standard deviation (SD) from the mean. Crosses show where performance is significantly poorer than the controls. The number of crosses marks the degree of severity, i.e. $\times$ = −1 SD; $\times\times$ = −2 SD; $\times\times\times$ = −3 SD. Thus, this format

SPEECH PROCESSING PROFILE

Name   Comments:

Age

Date

Profiler

INPUT	OUTPUT

F

Is the child aware of the internal structure of phonological representations?

G

Can the child access accurate motor programs?

E

Are the child's phonological representations accurate?

H

Can the child manipulate phonological units?

D

Can the child discriminate between real words?

I

Can the child articulate real words accurately?

C

Does the child have language-specific representations of word structures?

J

Can the child articulate speech without reference to lexical representations?

B

Can the child discriminate speech sounds without reference to lexical representations?

A

Does the child have adequate auditory perception?

K

Does the child have adequate sound production skills?

L

Does the child reject his/her own erroneous forms?

Figure 1.10: A speech processing profile sheet (from Stackhouse and Wells, 1997).

allows a systematic collation of test results and gives a quick visual impression of a child's input vs output skills as well as top-down vs bottom-up speech processing skills.

ACTIVITY 1.3

Aim: to interpret a speech processing profile sheet.

Compare the following information on two children (reported in Stackhouse, 2000), both of whom have nonverbal IQ within normal limits:

Zara, CA 4;3

Zara presented as a chatty little girl in spite of her obvious speech difficulties. On a standardized speech assessment (*The Edinburgh Articulation Test*, Anthony, Bogle, Ingram, et al., 1971) she had a Standard Score of 80 (a score of 85 and above is classed as within normal limits) and an Articulation Age level of 3 years. However, her language skills were age appropriate on tests of verbal comprehension, receptive and expressive vocabulary, expressive language (both on information and grammar) and she was able to make herself understood to the listener most of the time.

Tom, CA 4;0

Tom initiated little language and was very difficult to understand. He seemed unable to use strategies to help himself when not understood; he would simply repeat what he had said with increasing frustration. On *The Edinburgh Articulation Test* (Anthony Bogle, Ingram, et al., 1971), he achieved a standard score of 60 which gave him an age equivalent below the baseline of the test (less than 3 years). His performance was also below average on both verbal comprehension and expressive language tests.

Compare Zara and Tom's speech processing profiles presented in Figures 1.11 and 1.12. Write down the similarities and differences between them. Who has the most severe difficulties and how is this manifested on the profiles?

Check your answer against Key to Activity 1.3 at the end of this chapter then read the following.

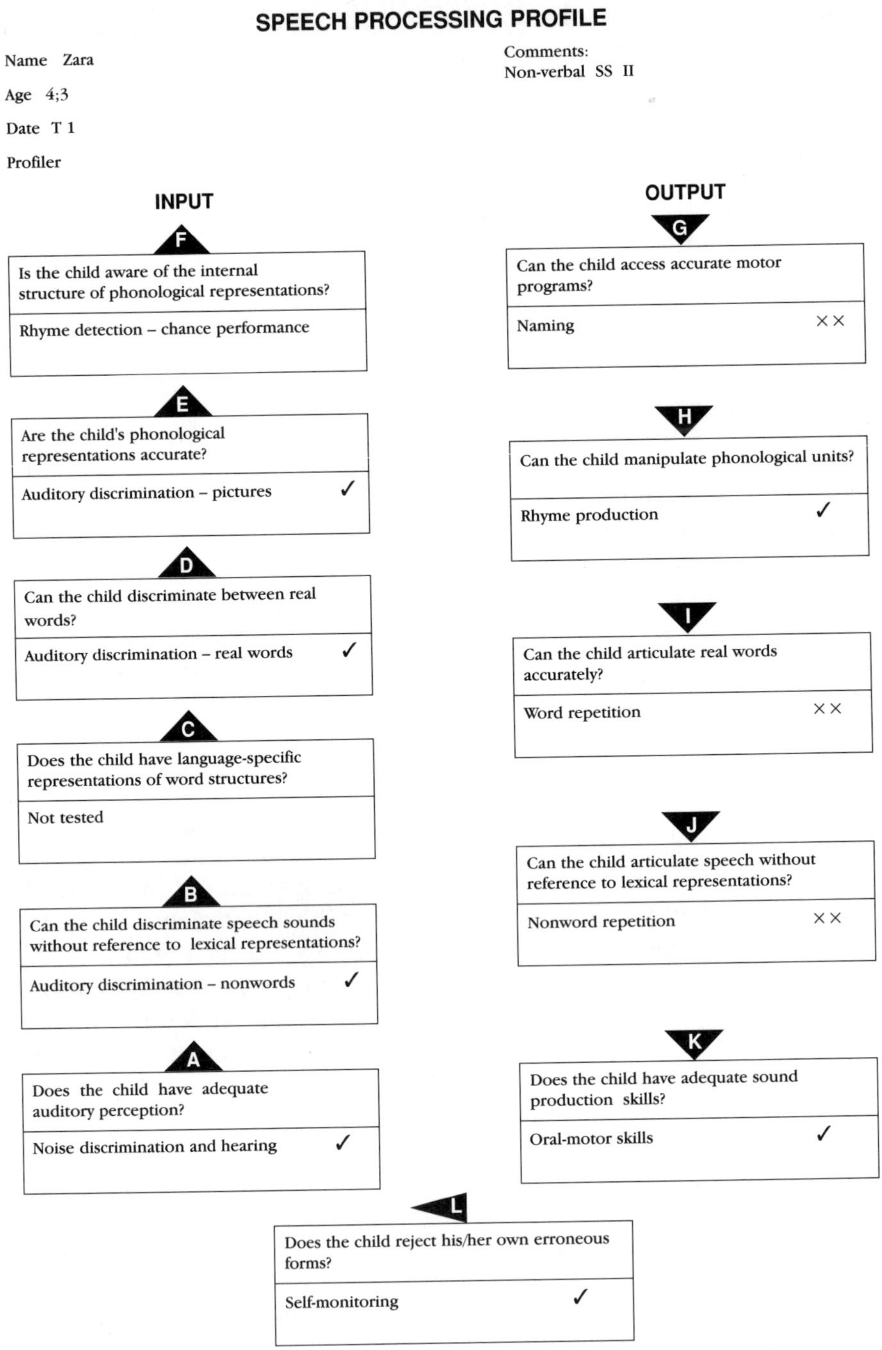

SPEECH PROCESSING PROFILE

Name   Zara

Age   4;3

Date   T 1

Profiler

Comments:
Non-verbal SS II

INPUT	OUTPUT
F	**G**
Is the child aware of the internal structure of phonological representations?	Can the child access accurate motor programs?
Rhyme detection – chance performance	Naming × ×
E	**H**
Are the child's phonological representations accurate?	Can the child manipulate phonological units?
Auditory discrimination – pictures ✓	Rhyme production ✓
D	**I**
Can the child discriminate between real words?	Can the child articulate real words accurately?
Auditory discrimination – real words ✓	Word repetition × ×
C	**J**
Does the child have language-specific representations of word structures?	Can the child articulate speech without reference to lexical representations?
Not tested	Nonword repetition × ×
B	**K**
Can the child discriminate speech sounds without reference to lexical representations?	Does the child have adequate sound production skills?
Auditory discrimination – nonwords ✓	Oral-motor skills ✓
A	
Does the child have adequate auditory perception?	
Noise discrimination and hearing ✓	

L

Does the child reject his/her own erroneous forms?

Self-monitoring   ✓

Figure 1.11: Zara's speech processing profile at CA 4;3 (from Stackhouse, 2000).

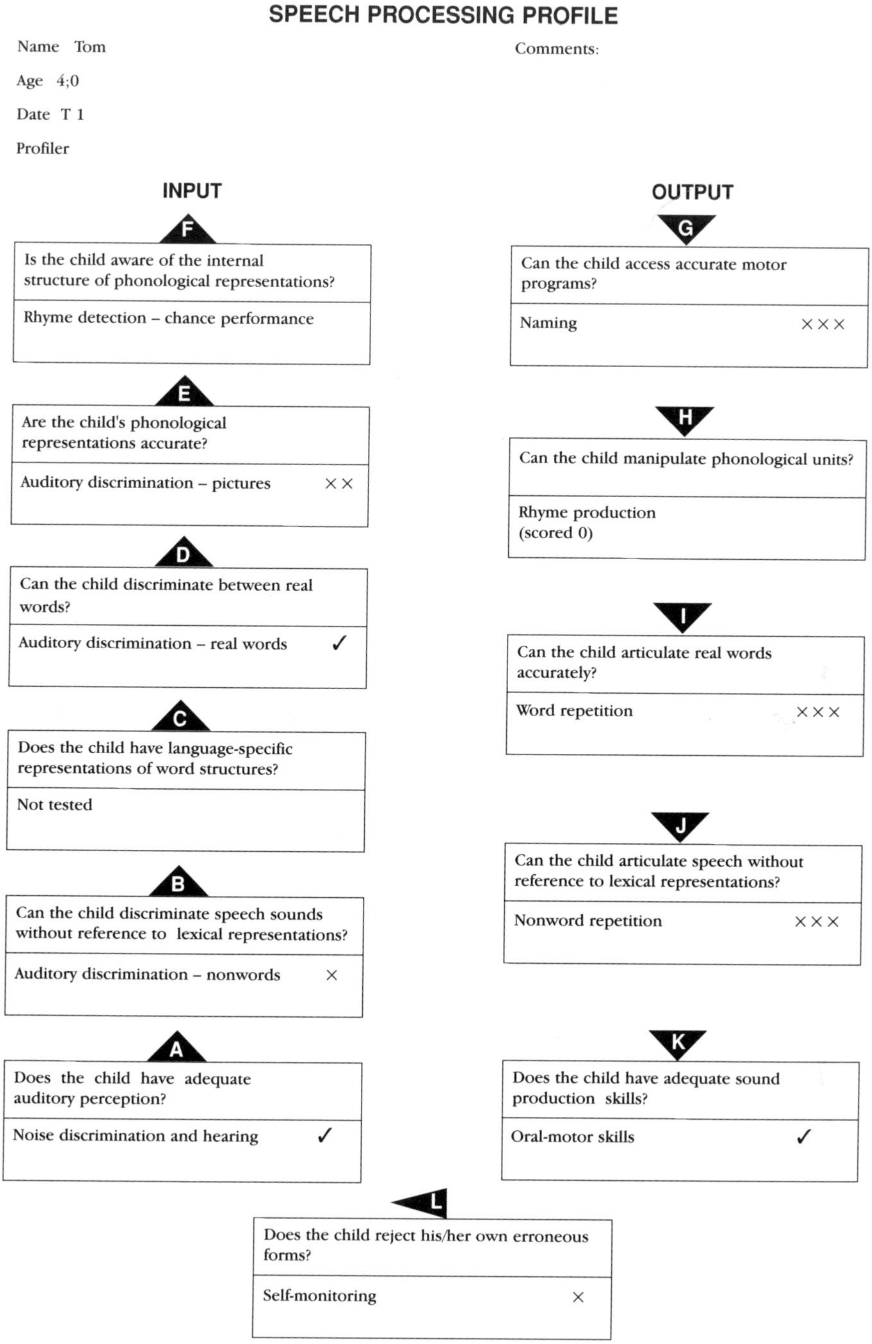

SPEECH PROCESSING PROFILE

Name Tom

Comments:

Age 4;0

Date T 1

Profiler

INPUT	OUTPUT

F

Is the child aware of the internal structure of phonological representations?

Rhyme detection – chance performance

G

Can the child access accurate motor programs?

Naming   × × ×

E

Are the child's phonological representations accurate?

Auditory discrimination – pictures   × ×

H

Can the child manipulate phonological units?

Rhyme production (scored 0)

D

Can the child discriminate between real words?

Auditory discrimination – real words   ✓

I

Can the child articulate real words accurately?

Word repetition   × × ×

C

Does the child have language-specific representations of word structures?

Not tested

J

Can the child articulate speech without reference to lexical representations?

Nonword repetition   × × ×

B

Can the child discriminate speech sounds without reference to lexical representations?

Auditory discrimination – nonwords   ×

A

Does the child have adequate auditory perception?

Noise discrimination and hearing   ✓

K

Does the child have adequate sound production skills?

Oral-motor skills   ✓

L

Does the child reject his/her own erroneous forms?

Self-monitoring   ×

Figure 1.12: Tom's speech processing profile at CA 4;0 (from Stackhouse, 2000.

Zara's speech processing profile at CA 4;3 revealed that she had no input processing difficulties. She performed as well as controls on auditory discrimination and input phonological awareness tasks such as rhyme detection. However, she had specific speech output difficulties on naming, word and nonword repetition. By CA 5;3 her speech problem had resolved and her speech processing profile was no different from controls on either input or output tasks. This suggested that she had no residual underlying speech processing problems that would affect her reading and spelling development. In fact, she progressed well with her literacy without any additional help. At age 6;3 she had a reading age of 7;11 (percentile rank 92) on the *British Ability Scales (BAS)* single word reading test (Elliott, Murray and Pearson, 1983). On an animal picture spelling test where she was asked to write down the name of each picture (without it being spoken by the tester) she scored 7/12 correct, which was well above average performance for her age. Errors revealed that she had good sound segmentation skills and could assign letters to sounds even if she did not yet know how to spell the words in a conventional way, e.g. CROCODILE → ‹crocerdieh›, GORILLA → ‹gerriler›.

In contrast, Tom's speech processing profile at CA 4;0 showed difficulties on both the input and output sides of the profile. Apart from the obvious speech output difficulties, he also performed poorly on a nonword auditory discrimination task and an auditory discrimination task involving pictures. This suggested that he had impaired ability to discriminate between unfamiliar words and that his phonological representations were inaccurately or incompletely stored. Unlike Zara, Tom's speech difficulties were still apparent a year later at CA 5;2. He also had persisting problems with processing speech input, on real and nonword auditory discrimination and auditory discrimination picture tasks, and speech output. Although he performed as well as controls on rhyme detection and production, he scored poorly on phonological awareness tasks that focus on the phoneme, i.e. alliteration fluency and phoneme completion. Letter knowledge was also 2 SD below the mean. Thus, Tom's speech processing deficits were much more pervasive and persistent than Zara's, and a poor foundation on which to build his literacy skills.

At age 6;2 he scored 0 on the *BAS* single word reading test (Elliott, Murray and Pearson, 1983) which gave him an age equivalent of less than 5 years (percentile rank 7). None of his spelling responses were correct on the animal picture spelling test. Further, his errors did not resemble the target words. For example, he had difficulty marking the correct number of syllables (e.g. ELEPHANT → ‹m›) and did not transcribe the beginning or end of test items correctly (e.g. SPIDER → ‹olxlm›). His choice of letters appears random, showing a difficulty with developing phoneme-to-grapheme correspondence.

Profiling children's speech processing skills and monitoring their language and alphabetic skills in this way, provides a systematic record of speech and literacy skills over time. The use of the psycholinguistic approach for identifying children's actual and potential literacy problems has been put to the test in a 4-year longitudinal study of the speech and literacy development of children with and without speech and language difficulties, (Stackhouse, Nathan, Goulandris, et al., 1999).

Predicting Literacy Performance: A Longitudinal Study

A number of studies have attempted to identify predictors of literacy outcome in children with speech and language difficulties. These studies have had interesting but sometimes conflicting results. Some report that syntax performance is a particularly good predictor of literacy outcome (e.g. Bishop and Adams, 1990; Magnusson and Naucler, 1990), while others have emphasized aspects of speech production as being the strongest predictor (e.g. Bird, Bishop and Freeman, 1995; Webster and Plante, 1992; Larrivee and Catts, 1999). Combined speech and language problems may also put children at risk for literacy difficulties (Leitao, Hogben and Fletcher, 1997). However, what all these studies have in common is that phonological awareness skills are particularly difficult for children with speech, language and literacy problems.

The basic premiss of our own longitudinal study was that the skills necessary for successful phonological awareness and literacy development arise from an intact speech processing system. The hypothesis was that, compared to matched controls, children with specific speech difficulties would have a deficit at one or more points in the speech processing system and that this deficit (or cluster of deficits) would manifest not only in speech difficulty but also affect performance on phonological awareness and later literacy tasks. The children with speech difficulties and their matched controls were assessed at three points in time (T1, T2 and T3) at ages around 4;6 (T1), 5;8 (T2) and 6;8 (T3).

Speech and language therapists in London were asked to refer children to the study who met the following criteria:

1. Chronological age 4–5 years.
2. Obvious speech difficulties but no evident physical cause (e.g. not cases with cleft lip and palate, or cerebral palsy).
3. No hearing impairment.
4. No associated medical condition (e.g. epilepsy, a named syndrome).
5. No severe receptive or pragmatic language difficulties.
6. Monolingual English speakers.

From 80 referrals, 47 children who met the following additional criteria were chosen for the main cohort (some of the other children not in the main cohort were followed up separately, see Stackhouse, 2000; and Nathan and Simpson, this volume):

1. Significant speech difficulties (more than 1 SD below the mean) on *The Edinburgh Articulation Test* (Anthony, Bogle, Ingram, et al., 1971).
2. Nonverbal IQ within normal limits, on two subtests of the WPSSI-R: Block Design and Picture Completion (Wechsler, 1992).
3. Nonreaders (raw score of 0) or beginning readers (scoring below 60th centile) on the *BAS* single word reading test (Elliott, Murray and Pearson, 1983).

Each child with speech difficulties was matched to a normally developing control child on the basis of chronological age (within a 6 months range), gender and nonverbal IQ (within 2 points on the averaged standard score of *Block Design* and *Picture Completion*, Wechsler, 1992). In 25 of the pairs, the control attended the same nursery or school as the matched child with speech difficulties in order to control for teaching environment. Where this was not possible, the control was taken from the same pool of nurseries/schools. All of the control children were monolingual English speakers and none had a history of speech, language or hearing difficulties. They were nonreaders (i.e. raw score of 0 on the *BAS*, $n=36$) or beginning readers (i.e. scoring below 60th centile on the *BAS*, $n=11$).

The test battery

A range of speech and language tests were selected to investigate: receptive and expressive language; speech input skills; precision of lexical representations; speech output skills; input and output phonological awareness; and letter knowledge. This test battery included both standardized tests and tests devised for the psycholinguistic framework. Table 1.1 lists the tests used at T1 when the children were aged around 4;6.

ACTIVITY 1.4

Aim: to analyse the processing requirements of different psycholinguistic profiling tasks.

Consider the processing demands of tasks numbers 5–14 presented in Table 1.1 and locate which level on the speech processing profile each one taps, i.e. which question (from A to L) about a child's performance would each task allow you to answer. Write the number of each task

Table 1.1: Tests used at T1 (CA 4;6) of the longitudinal study (Stackhouse, Nathan, Goulandris, et al., 1999)

Receptive language
1. *Test of Reception of Grammar* (*TROG*, Bishop, 1989)
2. *British Picture Vocabulary Scales* (*BPVS*, Dunn, Dunn, Whetton, et al., 1982)

Expressive language
3. *Action Picture Test* (*RAPT*, Renfrew, 1989)
4. *The Bus Story* (Renfrew, 1991)

Psycholinguistic profiling tasks
5. *Naming Test* (after Snowling, van Wagtendonk and Stafford, 1988)
6. *Real word repetition*
   Single one-, two- and three-syllable words were presented for the child to repeat, e.g. BRUSH; TRACTOR; ELEPHANT
7. *Nonword repetition*
   Matched nonwords derived from the real words were presented for the child to repeat, e.g. BRISH; TREKTI; ALIPHONT
8. *Speech rate*
   Child is asked to repeat one real word and one nonword 10 times on three different occasions as fast and as well as they can
9. *Auditory discrimination picture task* (after Locke, 1980)
   Child sees picture of e.g. PLATE and has to respond "Yes" or "No" to the tester's correct and incorrect productions of the target picture, e.g. "PLATE"; "PATE"
10. *ABX auditory discrimination task*
    Child is introduced to two puppets, each one 'says' a nonword e.g. puppet 1 says "VESH"; puppet 2 says "FESH" , the child is then asked by the tester which puppet said, e.g. "VESH"
11. *Auditory discrimination same/different task* (after Bridgeman and Snowling, 1988)
    Child listens to pairs of real and nonwords and decides if each pair is the same or different. The stimuli are either CVC or CVCC, e.g. LOSS~LOT; LOST~LOTS; VOS~VOT; VOTS~VOST
12. *Rhyme production*
    Child is asked to produce as many rhymes as s/he can in 20 seconds to a given stimulus, e.g. DOG
13. *Rhyme detection — pictures*
    Three pictures are presented but not named by the tester. Child has to select which two rhyme. The third picture is either semantically related or is an alliteration of one of the rhyming words, e.g. DOG, FROG, BONE; KITE, LIGHT, CAKE
14. *Phoneme completion tasks* (Muter, Hulme and Snowling, 1997)
    A picture is presented but not named by the tester, e.g. GATE. Tester produces word without the coda, i.e. "ga_" and child is asked to produce what is missing, i.e. "t"

Literacy tests
Name and letter sound knowledge

---

underneath the appropriate question on the blank speech processing profile sheet in Figure 1.10. Appendix 2 of Book 1 may help you with this activity.

Check your response against Key to Activity 1.4 at the end of this chapter and then read on.

A longitudinal study poses many challenges to researchers. One of these is to devise tasks that will be sensitive throughout the study. For example, in our study it was necessary to make the speech repetition tasks progressively more challenging by adding complex words as the children got older. The same applies to phonological awareness: on rhyme tasks older children may perform at ceiling, getting virtually all the items right. If this happens, the test does not discriminate between clinical and control groups and more challenging, phoneme-based tasks are needed. In our study, literacy measures were also added as the children grew older and nonword spelling was introduced in the final round of testing. Table 1.2 presents the additions to the test battery when the children were around CA 5;8 and 6;8.

ACTIVITY 1.5

Aim: to complete the psycholinguistic analysis of the assessment battery used in the longitudinal study.

Add the phonological awareness tasks (numbers 7–9) and the speech task (number 12) from Table 1.2 at the appropriate level (A–L) in the speech processing profile in Figure 1.10.

Check your response with Key to Activity 1.5 at the end of this chapter, then read on.

At T3 (CA 6;8) the children with speech difficulties were divided into two groups on the basis of reading and spelling: typical (i.e. within the normal range) and delayed. Their concurrent and past speech and language processing skills were examined (Nathan, Stackhouse and Goulandris, 1999). Children were classified as 'delayed' reader/spellers if they scored below −1 SD on the BAS Word Reading and/or BAS Spelling Tests and as 'typical' reader/spellers if they scored above −1 SD on one of these tests. According to this criterion, 36.2 per cent of the children with speech difficulties had poor literacy skills for their age at T3, and 63.8 per cent of the group had age appropriate or above

Table 1.2: Additional tests at T2 (CA 5;8) and T3 (CA 6;8) of the longitudinal study (Stackhouse, Nathan, Goulandris, et al., 1999)

Literacy tests
1. *BAS Word Reading* (Elliott, Murray and Pearson, 1983)
2. *Neale Analysis of Reading Ability* (1989)
3. *Graded Nonword Reading Test* (Snowling, Stothard and McClean, 1996)
4. *BAS Spelling* (Elliott, Murray and Pearson, 1983)
5. *Spelling animal names from pictures*
6. *Nonword spelling* (T3 only)

Phonological awareness
7. *Alliterative fluency*
   Child is asked to produce as many words as s/he can beginning with e.g. 'k'
8. *Phoneme deletion*
   Child is asked to produce given words without their onsets, e.g. "Say WIND without the 'w'"
9. *Rhyme Oddity* (T3 only)
   Child is asked to identify which is the odd one out (i.e. does not rhyme) in a series of three spoken words (no pictures), e.g. "Which is the odd one out in these words: JOB, KNOCK, ROB"

Language measures
10. *Recalling sentences* (Semel, Wiig, and Secord, 1987)
11. *Semantic fluency*
    Child is asked to produce a string of semantically related words, e.g. "Tell me as many ANIMALS as you can"

Speech measures
12. *Low frequency word and nonword repetition*

---

literacy skills. Thus, the majority of the group appear to have developed appropriate speech processing skills, though it is too early to say if this progress will be maintained. Children with a history of specific speech difficulties may not present with literacy problems (in particular, spelling difficulties) until they are 8 years of age (Dodd, Russell and Oerlemans, 1993) or older (Stothard, Snowling, Bishop, et al., 1998). However, what we can do within our study is to look back at the children's speech processing profiles and related skills and establish:

(a) which speech processing tasks are best suited to the different ages (4, 5 and 6 years);
(b) if any of the speech processing tasks can predict children's emerging literacy skills; and if so
(c) how early this can be done.

ACTIVITY 1.6

Aim: to consider which skills best predict children's literacy performance.

Look at the list of assessment areas presented below and indicate with a
* which you feel would be the three best predictors of literacy development in young school-age children around the age of 5–6 years. Use the
information about the four children presented in this chapter (Laura,
Edward, Zara and Tom) to help you. Tom may give you the most clues.

1. Receptive language (e.g. *TROG*; *BPVS*).
2. Expressive language (e.g. *RAPT*; *The Bus Story*; naming test).
3. Speech (real word repetition; nonword repetition; speech rate).
4. Auditory discrimination (Bridgeman and Snowling; ABX).
5. Auditory discrimination picture task (e.g. picture presented of a
   PLATE, tester asks "is it a PLATE?; is it a PATE?").
6. Rhyme tasks (e.g. detection; production; oddity).
7. Phoneme tasks (e.g. phoneme completion, phoneme deletion, alliterative fluency).
8. Letter knowledge (names and sounds).

Now look at Key to Activity 1.6 at the end of the chapter for the assessments which differentiated between children with typical vs delayed
literacy development at T3 (6;8) in our longitudinal study. Then read
the following.

Three things are apparent about the tests that differentiated between
children with typical vs delayed literacy development at T3 (6;8)
presented in Key to Activity 1.6. First, in children as young as 4 years of
age there were no predictors of literacy outcome at CA 6;8. Performance
on speech output, grammar and auditory lexical decision narrowly
missed being significant signs of future literacy problems. It was only at
CA 5;8 and 6;8 that the typical and delayed reading/spelling groups were
differentiated statistically. Second, there is no one 'magic test' that will
predict children's literacy outcome. Third, the tasks that do predict
literacy outcome change over time. Let us examine these more closely.

Auditory tasks

The auditory lexical task was a useful assessment for the younger
children (CA 4;6). Unlike the ABX task, which the young children found
too difficult, the auditory lexical task was completed by all of the

children. It differentiated not only between the clinical group and controls but also within the clinical group: those who had more severe speech problems and associated language problems performed less well on this task than those with speech problems alone (Nathan, Stackhouse and Goulandris, 1998; Stackhouse, Nathan, Goulandris, et al., 1999). Although in itself not a predictor of literacy performance directly, the auditory lexical task did indicate which children were likely to have persisting speech difficulties, which in turn were associated with delayed literacy development at CA 6;8. However, as many of the children were at ceiling on this task by CA 5;8 (i.e. it was too easy for most of them) it was not a sensitive task as the children got older; it would pick up only the children with the most severe auditory processing problems and might miss those with more subtle difficulties.

From CA of around 5;8, the ABX and the cluster sequence auditory discrimination (Bridgeman and Snowling, 1988) differentiated the typical and delayed reader/speller groups at T2 (CA 5;8). At this age the floor effects on the ABX task present at T1 (CA 4;6) had disappeared (the ABX task had been too difficult for even the normally developing 4-year-olds and therefore was not a useful diagnostic procedure for these young children). At CA 5;8 these two auditory discrimination tasks therefore took over from the auditory lexical decision task as the most reliable tests to use with school-age children.

Speech and language tasks

Persisting speech difficulties at T2 (on real and nonword repetition) and at T3 (on naming and repetition of low frequency real and nonwords) were an important clue to potential literacy difficulties, as were delayed grammatical skills at T2 (*TROG* and *The Bus Story*) and at T3 (*RAPT*). This supports the Critical Age Hypothesis (Bishop and Adams, 1990) which suggests that if a child's speech and language difficulties persist beyond CA 5;6 then literacy problems are likely to ensue.

Phonological awareness tasks

These presented a perhaps surprising result. Although the children with speech difficulties in general performed less well than their controls on the rhyme detection and production tasks, rhyme itself did not feature as a predictor of literacy performance because it did not differentiate between the typical vs delayed reader/spellers. In fact, at T2 and T3 the delayed readers performed as well as the typical readers on rhyme tasks. It was the phonological awareness tasks that tapped the level of the phoneme (rather than the syllable, as in the case of rhyme) that were the best predictors. Performance on alliteration fluency at T2 and on phoneme deletion and completion at T3 were more closely associated with reading and spelling development.

The role of rhyme in literacy development is certainly controversial. Some believe that it is central to literacy development (e.g. Bryant, 1998; Goswami, 1999) while others argue that it does not predict literacy outcome (e.g. Nation and Hulme, 1997; Muter, Hulme, Snowling, et al., 1998). The findings from our longitudinal study suggest that practitioners should be cautious about how they interpret children's performance on rhyme tasks. First, many of the young normally developing children that we studied could not perform rhyme tasks at around CA 4;6 (Stackhouse, Nathan and Goulandris, 1999). Even so, these children still went on to have normal literacy development. The opposite was also true. Some of the children who developed literacy difficulties could perform the rhyme tasks perfectly well (e.g. Tom presented above; cf. also Luke, described by Nathan and Simpson, this volume). Perhaps the popularity of rhyme tasks in teaching and therapy and the focus on rhyme in the National Literacy Strategy has influenced this result.

Our findings support the traditional view that persisting difficulties with rhyme detection and/or production indicate a faulty speech processing system and are likely to be associated with serious literacy problems, as with children like Zoe (Book 1, Chapters 9 and 10) and Anna (Chapters 4 and 5, this volume). However, the corollary of this is not supported by our results: being able to perform well on rhyme tasks does not guarantee good literacy outcome. That said, there is still an important place for rhyme tasks in our teaching and therapy programmes.

Using Rhyme Tasks to Promote Literacy Development

Even though rhyme did not emerge as a *predictor* of literacy outcome in our longitudinal study, this does not detract from its central role in teaching and therapy activities. However, the teaching of phonological awareness skills in isolation from the printed word will not necessarily promote literacy development, particularly in children with difficulties. Letter knowledge is central to the development of literacy skills (Treiman, Tincoff, Rodriguez, et al., 1998b) and was a significant predictor of reading and spelling skills in our longitudinal study. Making explicit links between letters and sounds is essential when teaching (Foorman, Francis, Novy, et al., 1991; Hatcher, 1996) and a number of training studies have demonstrated the importance of linking phonological awareness and the printed word (e.g. Hatcher,

Hulme and Ellis, 1994; Hatcher and Hulme, 1999; and see Goswami and Bryant, 1990 Chapter 7 for a review of earlier studies). Some of these studies involved mulitsensory/cueing systems (e.g. Lindamood, Bell and Lindamood, 1997; Gillon and Dodd, 1997).

One of the first empirical training studies was by Bradley and Bryant in 1983. They studied 65 children who were nonreaders and below average on phonological awareness tasks when starting school. The children were divided into experimental and control groups. At the end of a 2-year period, during which 40 individual teaching sessions were carried out, the group who had received sound categorization training (including rhyme) was no different from a control group who had received semantic categorization training. In contrast, the children who had received sound categorization training specifically linked to orthography (by plastic letters) were significantly better than controls on reading and spelling measures. Similarly, Hatcher, Hulme and Ellis (1994) working with 7-year-old children with reading delay found that although training in phonological awareness resulted in improved phonological awareness skills, there was no carryover to reading performance. It was only the children who received both phonological awareness training and explicit reading instruction who made significantly more progress than controls on reading and spelling measures at the end of the study.

This linking of auditory and visual skills is captured in the *New Phonics* teaching approach which is 'based on theories about the importance of phonology in learning to read' (Bielby, 1994, p.173). It takes into account how children develop phonological awareness through recognizable phases and marks a move away from traditional phonics teaching which encourages children to sound out each letter in a word and blend the sounds together, e.g. "c-a-t" spells CAT. In new phonics a more 'chunking' approach, based on the natural division of syllables into onset and rimes e.g. "c-at" spells CAT, is used as a starting point.

Children begin to develop their rhyme knowledge through exposure to nursery rhymes and songs. This experience is then mapped on to increasing exposure to letters and the printed word. Having developed the ability to segment onsets from rimes, e.g.C/AT, M/AT, BR/AT, SPL/AT, children are in a good position to match what they see in the written form to what they hear spoken. Introducing traditional phonics at this point could be premature since children may not be ready to segment within the rime (A/T). Further, the ability to segment onset and rime in words facilitates reading and spelling by analogy with known words (Goswami, 1994; Muter, 1996). Without the understanding that syllables can be divided into an onset/rime structure, each word in the rhyme string CAT, MAT, HAT, FAT, SAT, RAT, BAT, FLAT, BRAT, SPLAT, SPRAT would have to be learned as a separate item, instead of being incorporated into an existing sound family of -AT words.

New phonics therefore not only links phonological awareness with letter knowledge but also facilitates reading and spelling by analogy through explicit demonstration of how analogies work. A number of teaching programmes adopt this approach (e.g. Wilson, 1993–96; Hatcher, 1994; Reason and Boote, 1994). Teaching at the rime rather than sound level is also a more satisfying way of dealing with the irregularities of English orthography.

Promoting phonological awareness and linking it with letters facilitate children's progress through the normal phases of literacy development outlined by Frith (1985). In particular, it allows them to 'crack the code' when reading and spelling, and facilitates functional alphabetic skills. For example, onset segmentation is essential for using dictionaries or encyclopaedias. All these skills are essential if children are to become independent readers and writers. The basic phonological awareness skills taught at Key Stage 1 (5–7 years) are necessary for the later teaching and learning of more complex morphophonological spelling rules, e.g. ELECTRIC / ELECTRICIAN / ELECTRICITY, multisyllabic words, irregularities and exceptions.

However, successful literacy development involves more than cracking the alphabetic code. Understanding print is crucial to its enjoyment and to facilitating independence when reading and writing. Much of the functioning at Key Stage 2 is dependent on higher-level language skills: linking phonology, grammar, semantics and meta-cognition in understanding puns, inferences and metaphors. Thus, for children with language and literacy difficulties, Key Stage 2 is where their problems become more obvious as they fail to cope with the increasing linguistic and emotional demands made by the curriculum.

Literacy Awareness and Motivation for Learning to Read and Write

Alongside the psycholinguistic profiling tasks used in our longitudinal study, we also collected information from parents, teachers and the children themselves. A questionnaire (after Francis, 1982) was given to the children through a structured interview to investigate the children's attitude towards literacy situations (see Nathan and Simpson, this volume, for further discussion of this assessment technique). If understanding the functions of literacy helps children to develop the motivation necessary for working on literacy tasks, then the responses from this interview may well go some way in predicting literacy outcome!

ACTIVITY 1.7

Aim: to identify children in need of further investigation on the basis of their attitude towards literacy.

Look at the following responses from six children in the age range of 6–7 years to the question:

"Do you think that reading and writing is useful to children of your age, and why?".

Tick which ones you would like to investigate further for possible literacy difficulties.

1. Yes, 'cos when they grow up they can't be what they want to be if they can't read – like a nurse or a doctor.
2. No, 'cos they'd rather watch TV instead.
3. Yes, 'cos when I get Goosebumps books, I don't have to pretend (to read) anymore. I just have to read on my own.
4. Yes, when they grow up, they can read long stories to other people like their children.
5. Yea. Say you're going really fast on a motorway – you're usually going quite fast aren't you? – and then you come to a normal road and you're still going really fast and it says, like KILL YOUR SPEED on a sign, and you're going really fast and you can't see out the window properly and you, like, crash into a wall .... so if you could read KILL YOUR SPEED you would be able to go slowly.
6. Yea, (writing is) good exercise for your hands.

Check your response against Key to Activity 1.7 at the end of this chapter.

Summary

The psycholinguistic approach makes explicit the relationship between spoken and written language development and difficulties. It allows us to differentiate between children in terms of their input, representation and output skills. Using this approach in a longitudinal investigation of children's speech and literacy development has shown that a child's speech processing profile provides a basis for predicting their literacy outcome as well as planning a systematic remediation programme involving appropriate materials and strategies (see Chapters 2 and 3, this volume). However, the 'at risk' signs are not constant: they change as the children get older.

The following points have been raised in this chapter:

- Children starting school with an intact speech processing system and age-appropriate spoken language skills are in a good position to learn and develop their written language.
- Children with poor spoken language skills are at risk for literacy difficulties and would benefit from support with the Key Stage 1 activities (age 5–7 years) as early as possible.
- Children who have not mastered the foundation skills required at Key Stage 1 may fall still further behind their peer group at Key Stage 2 (age 8–11 years).
- Some children will not reveal the extent of their literacy difficulties until they are confronted by a more challenging curriculum from around the age of 8 years.
- The psycholinguistic approach can uncover 'hidden' speech processing problems and ensure that appropriate remediation is implemented as early as possible.
- There is not one 'magic' test in a psycholinguistic test battery that can be used to predict literacy outcome.
- The predictors of literacy performance change over time.
- There are no clear predictors of later literacy performance in children as young as 4 years of age.
- The speech processing profile can be used to predict children's literacy performance from around the age of 5 years.
- Children with pervasive speech-processing problems involving both input and output sides of the profile are the most likely to have associated language problems and literacy difficulties.
- Auditory lexical decision is a useful test with young children and can be used to investigate phonological representations.
- Complex auditory discrimination and ABX tasks are useful for children over the age of 5 years and can be used to predict literacy performance at 6 years.
- Children with persisting and specific speech output difficulties beyond CA 5;6 are at risk for literacy problems, particularly when spelling.
- Performance on rhyme tests needs to be interpreted cautiously, particularly in young children.
- Early rhyme skill is not a predictor of children's literacy performance at CA 6;8.
- Rhyme is a useful teaching and therapy strategy if it is linked explicitly with letter knowledge.
- Letter knowledge at 5 and 6 years of age is a useful predictor of literacy performance.
- Children's reports of their attitude towards literacy are an important part of an assessment procedure.

KEY TO ACTIVITY 1.1

1. Laura is able to construct sentences in a style appropriate for imparting information about a given topic. She has insight into both the function and scale of the pyramids and has used appropriate vocabulary. She has organized the information well and used punctuation. She is still relying on her phoneme–grapheme correspondence rules (e.g. DEAD → ‹ded›) but is also showing knowledge of morphological endings (e.g. ‹tion› in EGYPTION, and ‹ed› in USED) and some whole word learning (e.g. WHERE, FOR, THE, ABOUT, TOMBS). She has also used a ruler not only to draw the pyramid but also to draw lines for her writing and is aware of presentation skills.

Edward was not able to construct a sentence about the pyramids. Some children find this hard because of specific expressive language difficulties and he was certainly more comfortable writing a memorized sentence. However, the discrepancy between his spoken and written language suggested that his problem was particularly in the written domain. He seemed inhibited and anxious about his inability to spell the words. He does have some phoneme–grapheme knowledge but this is at an earlier stage compared to Laura. He is still omitting the nasal in nasal clusters (e.g. CHAMBER → ‹chebu›, ROOMS → ‹roos›) and his spellings in line 1 are more difficult to decipher than Laura's. He has obviously learned new vocabulary through the project and he introduced punctuation marks (full stop and question mark) at the end of each of the two lines. His severely restricted written language does not allow him to develop different presentation styles (compare Laura's labelling of the diagram of the mummy in Figure 1.2, her use of headings, and the format of the text).

2. Laura is tackling Key Stage 2 work well. Edward is not yet ready to move on to Key Stage 2 work; he is still struggling with some of the basic concepts introduced in Key Stage 1.

KEY TO ACTIVITY 1.2

(a) *Twinkle Twinkle Little Star*
　　Twinkle twinkle little star,
　　How I wonder what you are.
　　Up above the world so high,
　　Like a diamond in the sky.
　　Twinkle twinkle little star,
　　How I wonder what you are.

(b) The last line.
(c) The rhyme is written as continuous text without the conventional line breaks. There is no punctuation apart from the full stop at the end of the last line. Upper and lower case are used interchangeably. Spaces between words are used inconsistently.
(d) The pattern of errors suggest the following:

(i) Cluster simplification
e.g. TWINKLE → ‹TICL›
It is very common for children to delete an element of a cluster (or blend) as in the above example: ‹tw› → ‹t›; ‹nk› → ‹c›. Why? Look in a mirror and say the onset (i.e. all sounds before the vowel) of TWINKLE, /tw/, but stop before you release it. Where is your tongue tip? What is the position of your lips? The tip of your tongue has gone up behind your front teeth to make the [t] sound but at the same time your lips are rounded and more forward in anticipation of the [w] sound. The cluster /tw/ is not in fact produced as a simple sequence of [t] + [w] as when you write it, because the spoken elements of the cluster overlap. However, the contact you feel the most is the [t] rather than the [w]. The normally developing child reflecting on their speech for spelling will therefore often write ‹t› for the spoken target /tw/.

Similarly, when spelling the target cluster /ŋk/, the least salient contact is dropped. Try saying the rime, INKLE /ɪŋkl/. What sound can you feel in your mouth the most? You are most likely to say [k] because you can feel the contact for that sound at the back of your mouth. Can you feel the nasal sound [ŋ]? Probably not, as this sound is being carried by the vowel, which becomes nasalized as air escapes through the nose instead of the mouth for that element of the cluster. It is therefore typical of young spellers to delete nasals in clusters as they are less salient than other elements in the cluster, e.g. BUMP → ‹bup›; TENT → ‹tet›. See also the target WONDER and WORLD; the same principles apply.

(ii)Vowels vs consonants
Given the importance of articulation for the transcription of sounds to letters, it is not surprising that vowels are more difficult than consonants for young spellers. Compare your own speech production of the sounds of the vowels A E I O U with the consonant sounds for B D G F S. Which can you feel the best? The vowels have an open but changing mouth posture with few if any contacts between the moving (active) and static (passive) articulators in the mouth. The consonants have more articulatory

contacts, which are easier to feel and to hold on to (cf. Dent, this volume). You can see this clearly in the word DIAMOND → ‹DMD›: the three articulatory contact points, i.e. the consonants of the word are represented but not the movement between them, i.e. the vowels.

(iii) Voicing in clusters
STAR → ‹SDR› may look odd but it reflects the phonetics of the English language. Say STAR without the /s/. What does the onset of what you said sound most like – a /t/ or a /d/? It sounds most like a /d/ because it is deaspirated, i.e. it does not have the puff of air which normally accompanies a voiceless stop (e.g. /p t k/) at the beginning of words. Now say the word TAR (as in what covers most roads) and compare your production of that word with your production of STAR without the /s/: if you are a native English speaker, they should sound different: /t/ vs /d/ . Thus, spelling STAR as ‹SDR› is a truer reflection of our speech production of that word than its conventional spelling.

Now look at SKY – did you spot that what has been written contains a letter reversal for the ‹g›. Her spelling is thus ‹sugi›. The same phonetic principle applies here as for STAR. Say SKY without the /s/ and you will produce a sound much closer to /g/ than /k/. These examples show the influence of speech production on children's spelling before they have been taught the conventions of English orthography.

(iv) Use of letter names
The spelling of STAR as ‹sTr› is another typical example of spelling from young children who do not know how to transcribe vowels in English. However, what they do know is letter names. The name of the letter R, pronounced 'ah' /ɑ/ in southern British English, is phonetically identical to the rime (AR) of the target STAR, pronounced /stɑ/. The letter name is therefore often used for the vowel sound by young spellers. See also the use of the letter name for I in HIGH and SKY.

(v) Assimilation
Without knowing how words are written it is not always clear where they begin and end when they are spoken; you may have experienced this when listening to a language that you do not know. It is a similar experience for the preliterate child listening to their own language. This is particularly the case when the end of a word is similar to the beginning of the next, as in ABOVE THE → ‹ubthe›. The sound at the end of ABOVE, [v], is acoutically very similar to [ð], the sound at the beginning of 'the'; in fact in London, target /ð/ is frequently realized as [v]. Laura clearly knows how to write the word THE and has used it

twice in this rhyme. However, in the above example she has 'lost' the /v/, which is masked by the following /ð/, and so the two words are run together in her spelling.

(vi) Confusion of similar sounding vowels

It is very common for vowels to be confused in beginner spellers e.g. HOW → ‹haw›, WHAT → ‹wut› because the differences between vowels can be quite subtle in terms of their articulatory postures. The spelling of ARE as ‹our› is a good example. There are no articulatory contacts in either of these words. Each word consists of a long vowel, which in the course of its pronunciation may undergo subtle changes in quality due to movements of tongue and lips: try saying them one after the other three times: ARE/OUR; ARE/OUR; ARE/OUR. For many speakers of British English, the vowels in the two words are more or less different, while for other speakers the two words are homophonous. These words are therefore quite hard to 'get hold of'. Laura has learned the spelling for one of them and is extending it with good phonetic motivation to a similar sounding word, even though the result happens to be orthographically incorrect.

(vii) Whole word learning

Laura has clearly learned the spellings of some common words: I; YOU; OUR; UP; THE; SO; LIKE; A; IN.

(e) Laura is developing her logographic skills (see (vii) above) but has clearly broken through to the alphabetic phase of literacy development. She shows good segmentation skills and is applying her letter knowledge. She has not yet learned the conventions of English spelling.

KEY TO ACTIVITY 1.3

Tom's speech difficulties are not only more severe than Zara's (as evident in the number of crosses) but he also has more pervasive speech processing problems; crosses are recorded on both input and output sides of the profile.

KEY TO ACTIVITY 1.4

See Figure 1.13 for the location on the speech processing profile of the tasks administered at T1 (CA 4;6) in the longitudinal study. (To complete the profile hearing had been tested (A) and none of the children had structural abnormalities or difficulties with oral movement (K). Any difficulties at L were noted).

KEY TO ACTIVITY 1.5

See Figure 1.14 for he location on the speech processing profile of the tasks administered at T2 (CA 5;8) and T3 (CA 6;8) in the longitudinal study.

KEY TO ACTIVITY 1.6

The areas tested at the three different CA (4;6, 5;8, 6;8) in the longitudinal study which differentiated between children with typical vs delayed literacy development at CA 6;8 were as follows:

CA	Tests
4;6	None
5;8	Auditory discrimination:(Bridgeman and Snowling, 1988; ABX) Speech output (real and nonword repetition) Grammar (*TROG* and *The Bus Story*) Alliteration fluency Letter names
6;8	Speech output (naming and low frequency repetition) Grammar (*RAPT*) Phoneme deletion and completion Letter names

SPEECH PROCESSING PROFILE

Name

Age

Date

Profiler

Comments:

INPUT

F

Is the child aware of the internal structure of phonological representations?

13.

E

Are the child's phonological representations accurate?

9.

D

Can the child discriminate between real words?

11. (real words)

C

Does the child have language-specific representations of word structures?

B

Can the child discriminate speech sounds without reference to lexical representations?

10.
11. (nonwords)

A

Does the child have adequate auditory perception?

OUTPUT

G

Can the child access accurate motor programs?

5.

H

Can the child manipulate phonological units?

12.
14.

I

Can the child articulate real words accurately?

6.
8. (real words)

J

Can the child articulate speech without reference to lexical representations?

7.
8. (nonwords)

K

Does the child have adequate sound production skills?

L

Does the child reject his/her own erroneous forms?

Figure 1.13: Key to Activity 1.4.

SPEECH PROCESSING PROFILE

Name   Comments:

Age

Date

Profiler

INPUT

F

Is the child aware of the internal
structure of phonological representations?

E

Are the child's phonological
representations accurate?

D

Can the child discriminate between real
words?

9.

C

Does the child have language-specific
representations of word structures?

B

Can the child discriminate speech sounds
without reference to lexical representations?

A

Does the child have adequate
auditory perception?

OUTPUT

G

Can the child access accurate motor
programs?

H

Can the child manipulate phonological units?

7.
8.

I

Can the child articulate real words
accurately?

12. (real words)

J

Can the child articulate speech without
reference to lexical representations?

12. (nonwords)

K

Does the child have adequate sound
production skills?

L

Does the child reject his/her own erroneous
forms?

Figure 1.14: Key to Activity 1.5.

KEY TO ACTIVITY 1.7

We ticked children 2, 3 and 6 as needing further investigation because, compared to 1, 4 and 5, they seemed to lack awareness about the functions of reading and spelling.

Chapter 2
Principles of Psycholinguistic Intervention

Rachel Rees

A comprehensive psycholinguistic assessment with reference to a theoretical model helps practitioners to plan intervention for a particular child (see Book 1, Stackhouse and Wells, 1997, Chapters 4–6). This chapter discusses rationale for intervention and provides guidelines for planning aims. Principles and procedures outlined in Book 1 are revised and applied to intervention. Explanations are illustrated through practical examples and case studies.

The first bridge from assessment to intervention is the setting of clear aims. This is not only an essential prerequisite to task selection but is necessary for evaluating the effectiveness of therapy or teaching tasks. When referring to therapy studies with adults with acquired aphasia, Byng (1995) noted that the difficulty many studies had in demonstrating the effects of therapy related to the lack of specificity about therapy aims. The more specific the aims of intervention, the easier it is to evaluate their achievement. Intervention aims are usually divided into long-term aims and short-term aims.

Long-term Aims for Intervention

Long-term therapy aims refer to where a child might be at the point of discharge (Bray, Ross and Todd, 1999). They are often drawn from aims of service delivery to wider groups. For example, in the UK, the Royal College of Speech and Language Therapists (RCSLT) gives professional guidelines and standards relevant to specific client groups and specific communication disorders (*Communicating Quality 2*, 1996). These include suggested aims of service delivery that are general and focus on functional communication. The first aim of service delivery suggested for children with developmental speech and language disorders is:

> ...To promote the child's communication skills in order that s/he may achieve optimally:
> in satisfying the child's/others' needs and desires;
> in exchanging information;

in using language creatively;
in initiating and maintaining social interaction;
in learning and in participating in education...

(RCSLT 1996, p.171)

For children in education, long-term aims often draw on the attainment targets set by the Revised National Curriculum, Department for Education (DfE, 1995a). These targets are also general and functional and do not specify a time span, although there are guidelines regarding the age by which targets should be attained (see Popple and Wellington, and Stackhouse, this volume). For example, most 7-year-old children should 'usually listen carefully and respond with increasing appropriateness to what others say' (DfE, 1995a, p.18).

Short-term Aims for Intervention

Short-term aims chunk the timescale of intervention into manageable pieces (Bray, Ross and Todd, 1999). They refer to a set period of time and are more specific than long-term aims. Short-term aims should be linked to short-term objectives, i.e. tangible outcomes that can be measured. Both need to be negotiated with the appropriate people, e.g. the client, the family and other professionals. For school-age children with special educational needs (SENs), short-term aims and objectives often form part of their individual education plans (IEPs). The *Code of Practice* (DfE, 1994) gives guidance to local education authorities and the governing bodies of all maintained schools on their responsibilities towards all children with SENs (see Popple and Wellington, this volume). The guidelines advise that all mainstream schools should designate a teacher to take the role of co-ordinating SEN services within the school. This SEN co-ordinator (SENCo) should follow a five-staged response in giving help to children with suspected SENs. At Stage 3 the SENCo should seek advice from other agencies and/or draw up a new IEP, including the involvement of support services. Therefore it is often at this stage that the SENCo will liaise with the speech and language therapist as well as other teachers to compile an IEP for a child. The plan should include 'targets to be achieved in a given time' (DfE, 1994, p.28). The child's progress from this time onwards is regularly monitored against these targets, which are modified or changed as necessary. Therefore, it is essential that the targets should be measurable and specify exactly what is to be achieved in the stated time period.

Short-term aims from hypotheses

It is important that short-term aims and objectives are based on hypotheses that concern the exact nature of a child's speech and language difficulties. Reference to a psycholinguistic framework helps us to look beyond linguistic symptoms and examine the underlying speech processing system. Identifying the specific speech processing skills that are causing difficulties will lead to aims that are more likely to form the basis for an appropriate selection of therapy tasks.

Aims and objectives based solely on observed 'symptoms' (e.g. problems in remembering instructions, difficulty in naming pictures, inaccurate repetition of words) do not take account of which speech processing skills and other skills are required by these tasks. For example, repeating real words accurately involves a number of speech processing skills. The psycholinguistic model presented in Book 1, enables us to analyse this task into its components.

ACTIVITY 2.1

Aim: to revise what speech processing skills, are necessary to complete a real word repetition tasks.

Read through the list of speech processing skills presented in Figure 2.1, that are based on the speech processing model presented in Book 1 (Chapter 6) and reproduced here in Appendix 2.

List the skills that are involved when repeating real words by referring to the appropriate letters: (a) to (j). For the purposes of this activity, you can presume that the child knows the target words, i.e. the words are in his/her receptive vocabulary and that s/he can spontaneously produce these words during a naming activity using a recognizable speech pattern that may or may not be accurate.

Try drawing the route(s) for real word repetition through the 'blank' model in Figure 2.2. See Keys to Activities in Book 1, Chapter 6, pp.173–187 for similar examples.

Check your answer against the Key to Activity 2.1 at the end of this chapter and then read the following.

The lexical route

As the child knows the words, this is the route that is most likely to be taken. Repeating real words involves *peripheral auditory processing* and *speech/nonspeech discrimination* since the stimuli are spoken. As the spoken words are familiar, *phonological recognition* is involved. Next, the child will probably scan the *phonological representations*

a. Peripheral auditory processing
b. Speech/nonspeech discrimination
c. Phonological recognition
d. Scanning of stored representations
e. Accessing stored phonological representations
f. Accessing stored semantic representations
g. Accessing stored motor programs
h. Creating a new phonological representation and a new motor program
i. Motor planning
j. Motor execution.

Figure 2.1: Speech processing skills.

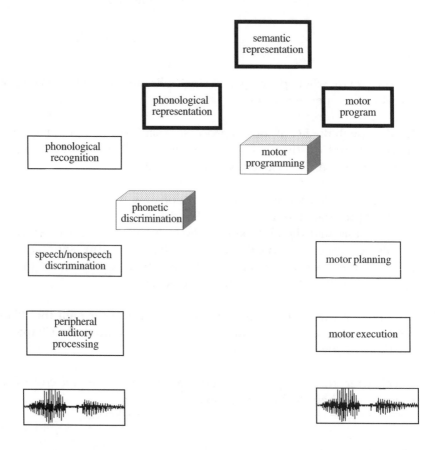

Figure 2.2: Blank speech processing model.

stored in the lexicon to establish whether the word exists. When the child has matched the word heard to a word in his/her lexicon by accessing the phonological representation and *semantic representation*, a pre-existing *motor program* can be used as the basis for speech production. This motor program is forwarded to *motor planning*, where further phonetic aspects of the utterance are planned, and instructions are sent to the articulators in *motor execution*.

The nonlexical route

There is a possibility that, even though the child knows the word, s/he will treat its repetition as an articulatory exercise and may not access the stored meaning of the word. Some children may access the meaning after the articulation; they suddenly realize which word they have said. In this case the route taken will be different after phonological recognition has taken place. Instead of searching the lexicon the child will create a new motor program as the basis for a spoken response. For this to be done accurately, the child has to create a new phonological representation against which subsequent repetitions can be checked. Once this new phonological representation has been made it is forwarded to motor programming, where the appropriate phonological units, with gestural targets encoded in them, are located and assembled into the correct sequence. This new motor program is forwarded to the motor planning stage and instructions are sent to the articulators in motor execution. This is the same route as for nonword repetition (cf. p.180, Book 1).

Having established which speech processing skills are involved in the repetition of real words it is possible to begin to analyse the 'symptom' of inaccurate repetition of real words. As real word repetition involves a large number of skills, difficulty with any of these skills or combinations of skills could lead to difficulty with the task.

To establish which speech processing skills are causing a child the most difficulty, it is necessary to compare the child's performance on real word repetition with other similar tasks that involve a slightly different subset of skills. Ideally, for a direct comparison to take place the word repetition task should be compared with other tasks that should contain identical or matched sets of stimuli. Thus, the effects of different stimuli can be minimized and stronger conclusions can be drawn from dissociations of performance across the tasks. When choosing words for repetition it is important to choose words that can be illustrated easily so that the same words can be used for a naming task. In this way the stimuli will be identical. When designing a nonword repetition task with similar stimuli derived from the real words, it is important that the nonwords should be phonologically legal in English. For example BLIK is an acceptable nonword and BNIK is not, because the combination of /b/ and /n/ is illegal. The nonwords should not be other real words in the child's lexicon or too similar to other real words (see Activity 11.7, p.318 in Book 1 for examples of how matched nonwords can be derived from real words). For further guidance on designing tests with matched stimuli see Chapter 11 in Book 1.

ACTIVITY 2.2

Aim: to identify the speech processing skills required to complete three assessment tasks with identical or matched stimuli.

Robert, a 7-year-old boy with mild cerebral palsy, has speech that is sometimes difficult to understand. He was asked to complete the following three tasks. His responses were tape-recorded and transcribed phonetically:

1. *Word repetition*
Robert was asked to repeat 20 words that he knew but had had difficulty repeating in the past, e.g. SNAKE; GUITAR; VAN.

2. *Naming*
Robert was asked to name pictures illustrating the same 20 words.

3. *Nonword repetition*
Robert was asked to repeat 20 nonwords that were matched to the real words, e.g. /snaɪk/, /gɛ'tɔ/ and /vɪn/.

Read through the speech processing skills again in Figure 2.1 and list the ones needed for each of these three tasks by referring to the letters (a) – (j). Refer to the model in Figure 2.2 to help you think of the routes.

Check your answer against the Key to Activity 2.2 at the end of this chapter and then read the following.

The speech processing skills needed for word repetition and the route that is taken have already been described in the Key to Activity 2.1. Naming does not involve auditory input skills. Processing begins with accessing the appropriate semantic representation for the picture presented. If a known word, the child can then access already established phonological representations and motor programs, which are forwarded to motor planning. There is no need to create new phonological representations or motor programs.

Repeating nonwords involves peripheral auditory processing and speech/nonspeech discrimination since the stimuli are spoken. As the stimuli conform to English phonological patterns, the route proceeds to phonological recognition and then the child will scan the phonological representations stored in the lexicon to establish whether the word exists. On finding no entries the child then has to assemble new motor programs. In order to do this the child has to create new phonological representations, which are forwarded to motor programming. New motor programs (without semantic representations) are then forwarded to the motor planning and motor execution stages. This task differs from word repetition and naming in that the child does not access semantic representations and therefore does not rely on established phonological representations and motor programs.

Robert's responses to these three tasks are presented in Table 2.1. On the word repetition tasks, Robert repeated each word once and made no attempt to change his attempts. As can be seen in the second column of Table 2.1, 11 of the words were repeated inaccurately. Robert named each picture without hesitation and made no attempt to change his productions. As can be seen by comparing the second and third columns in Table 2.1, the same 11 words were inaccurate during this task and their realizations corresponded almost exactly to his responses on the word repetition task. The matched nonword stimuli are presented in the fourth column of Table 2.1 and his responses to these in the fifth column. Fifteen of these were accurate. The remaining five nonwords that were repeated inaccurately contained speech errors that were evident in the naming and repetition tasks.

Table 2.1: Robert's responses on real word repetition, naming and nonword repetition tasks

Real word Stimuli	Real word repetition	Naming	Nonword Stimulus	Nonword repetition
SNAKE	sneɪç	sneɪç	snaɪk	snaɪk
GUITAR	ɪtˈɑ	ɪtˈɑ	gɛˈtɔ	gɛˈtɔ
VAN	væn	væn	vɪn	vɪn
PLATE	pjeɪʔ	pjeɪʔ	pləʊt	kəʊt
SAUSAGE	ˈsɒsɪʔz	ˈsɒsɪʔz	ˈsesədʒ	ˈsesəz
SLIPPER	ˈslɪpʰə	ˈslɪpʰə	ˈslɔpə	ˈslɔpə
ELEPHANT	ˈɛləfənʔt	ˈɛləfənt	ˈælɪfɒnt	ˈælɪfɒnt
UMBRELLA	ʌmˈbɛlə	ʌmˈbɛlə	æmˈbɹælɪ	æmˈbɹælɪ
BUTTERFLY	ˈbʌtəflaɪ	ˈbʌtəflaɪ	ˈbætəfləʊ	ˈbætəfləʊ
FISH	fɪs	fɪs	fɛs	fɪs
YELLOW	ˈlɛləʊ	ˈlɛləʊ	ˈjælɒɪ	ˈjælɒɪ
AEROPLANE	ˈɛəʊəpeɪn	ˈɛəʊəpeɪn	ˈɒɹəpləʊn	ˈɒɹəgen
TRACTOR	ˈtɹæktə	ˈtɹæktə	ˈtɹɛktɪ	ˈtɹɛktɪ
BRUSH	bjʌs	bjʌs	bɹɪʃ	bɹɪʔʃ
CATERPILLAR	ˈkætəpɪlə	ˈkætəpɪlə	ˈkɪtəpælə	ˈkɪtəpælə
SPIDER	ˈspaɪdə	ˈspaɪdə	ˈspeɪdɪ	ˈspeɪdɪ
PYJAMAS	pəˈdʒɑməz	pəˈdʒɑməz	pɪˈdʒɔmɪz	pɪˈdʒɔmɪz
SPONGE	spʌnz	spʌnz	spændʒ	spænz
TRAIN	tʋeɪn	tʋeɪn	tɪɒɪn	tɪɒɪn
GLOVE	dlʌv	dlʌv	glɛv	glɛv
Score	9/20	9/20		15/20

ACTIVITY 2.3

Aim: to interpret Robert's responses on the naming and repetition tasks in order to make hypotheses about which speech processing skills are underpinning his difficulties.

With reference to Table 2.1 and the description above, write out a list of hypotheses suggesting which speech processing skills are problematic for Robert, and which could form the basis for further investigation.

Check your hypotheses against the Key to Activity 2.3 at the end of this chapter and then read the following.

The finding that Robert's performance on the naming task was identical to his performance on the word repetition task suggests that he was using the lexical route for both. The lack of hesitation and struggle in both tests suggests that he was not having difficulty in accessing the representations in his lexicon. However, these representations may be inaccurate. Alternatively, he may have had difficulty with output processing skills. As naming does not involve input processing skills, but nonword repetition does, and as he is better at nonword repetition, it is clear that Robert's difficulties are not caused solely by auditory processing skills. Superior performance on nonword repetition, which does not involve accessing the stored representations, suggests that inaccurate lexical representations are at least partly responsible for the inaccurate real word repetitions and spontaneous productions. It also strengthens our hypothesis that auditory processing skills are probably intact as nonword repetition requires auditory processing skills.

All three tasks involve lower-level output skills. As Robert repeated 15 of the nonwords accurately, we can conclude that lower-level output skills were adequate for these stimuli. Two of the incorrect repetitions of nonwords could have been due to lexicalization. Robert may have interpreted /pləʊt/ as COAT and /ˈsesəd/ as SCISSORS. On the other hand, there were no examples of correct realizations of the following targets in any of the tests: syllable-initial /pl/ and syllable final /dʒ/ and /ndʒ/. This suggests that motor execution difficulties were at least partly responsible for the inaccurate realizations of these sounds. The only other explanation is that Robert had difficulty in discriminating these consonants from similar ones. Even though the naming task does not involve auditory processing skills, inaccurate representations of words containing these consonants could be a sign that a child has in the past had difficulty in discriminating them from other sounds.

One of the main reasons for using hypotheses is to have a principled starting point for intervention. Hypotheses can be modified in the light of what happens in therapy and teaching, and the intervention programme redirected accordingly. The validity of a hypothesis can be monitored during intervention rather than investigated specifically. For example, an assumption has been made that Robert is not having difficulty with *accessing* semantic representations. This could be checked during intervention by looking out for any signs of struggling to find the right word, such as long hesitations. If such signs were noted, then it would be necessary to modify the hypothesis and change the therapy programme as a result. Thus, it is not necessary to postpone intervention until every possible hypothesis has been formally assessed. Some hypotheses may need to be tested through further investigation, but this can be combined with intervention tasks as part of a management programme. For example, Robert's programme included auditory lexical decision activities in order to evaluate the following competing hypotheses:

> *Hypothesis* 1: Robert has established inaccurate phonological representations and motor programs for all or some of the 11 words that he was unable to repeat or name.
> *Hypothesis* 2: Robert has established accurate phonological representations for all or some of the 11 words that he was unable to repeat or name, but motor programs for these words are inaccurate.

Robert was asked to complete an auditory lexical decision task that incorporated the 11 target words that he had difficulty repeating and naming; the spoken stimuli were based on a phonetic transcription of his own realizations of these words. He was shown one stimulus picture at a time and, for each picture, was presented in a random order with five accurate productions of the target word and five examples of his inaccurate realizations of it. After each presentation, he had to indicate whether the production he had heard was correct or incorrect. For example, Robert looked at the picture of SNAKE and had to respond "yes" or "no" to questions: "Is this a snake?"; "Is this a [sneɪç] ?"; "Is this a [sneɪç]?"; "Is this a snake?" etc. The results of this task are shown in Table 2.2.

Table 2.2: Robert's performance on the auditory lexical decision task

Stimulus	Number of accurate presentations identified as correct	'Inaccurate' presentations	Number of 'inaccurate' presentations identified as correct
SNAKE	5/5	sneıç	1/5
GUITAR	5/5	ıt'ɑ	0/5
PLATE	5/5	pjeıʔ	4/5
SAUSAGE	5/5	'sɒsıʔz	1/5
UMBRELLA	5/5	ʌm'bɛlə	0/5
FISH	5/5	fıs	5/5
YELLOW	5/5	'lɛləʊ	0/5
AEROPLANE	5/5	'ɛəʊəpeın	4/5
BRUSH	5/5	bjʌs	5/5
SPONGE	5/5	spʌnz	1/5
GLOVE	5/5	dlʌv	5/5

ACTIVITY 2.4

Aim: To interpret the results of an auditory lexical decision task in order to form a hypothesis for planning intervention.

What light do the results presented in Table 2.2 cast on the accuracy of Robert's phonological representations and motor programs? Compare his performance on this auditory lexical decision task with his performance on the naming and repetition tasks presented in Table 2.1.

Check your answer against the Key to Activity 2.4 at the end of this chapter and then read the following.

This activity shows that the locus of the speech processing deficit underlying Robert's mispronunciations can vary from word to word. This is not uncommon (cf. Zoe, presented in Chapters 9 and 10 of Book 1; and Michael, discussed by Constable, this volume). Thus, it is important to separate out groups of words in this way as they will need to be treated differently during an intervention programme. For example, Robert's programme would need to include aims concerned with improving auditory discrimination of words such as FISH and GLOVE as his phonological representations of these words are inaccurate. For words such as SNAKE, GUITAR and SPONGE on the other hand, aims would focus on production skills. Before Robert could be expected to articulate SPONGE accurately, however, he would probably need some specific work on producing the cluster /ndʒ/.

Guidelines for setting short-term aims

Such a hypothesis-driven approach to intervention can lead naturally to the formation of precise and child-specific short-term aims. Short-term aims and objectives provide a basis for selecting tasks, for monitoring a child's progress and for evaluating the effectiveness of intervention methods, provided the following guidelines are adhered to:

1. Base aims on hypotheses that derive from a theoretical framework and address the exact nature of a child's speech and language difficulty .
2. Integrate aims and objectives with those set by other professionals involved in a child's management (e.g. teacher, speech and language therapist, physiotherapist). For children in school, aims could form part of a child's IEP (cf. Popple and Wellington, this volume).
3. Specify the time period by which the objectives should be achieved (e.g. one school term, 6-week block of therapy).
4. Ensure that the objectives are measurable. Having selected the speech processing skills to target, it is important to indicate exactly how much improvement is expected in the time set. This ensures that achievement can be evaluated at the end of that period. For example, assessment may have identified that a child had difficulty in manipulating and rearranging onset and rime units of words in order to produce rhyme strings. Expectations would depend on the degree of difficulty that the child was experiencing, abilities at other skills, and the time span specified. Objectives for the end of the block of intervention might be:
   (a) to produce one rhyming word for each of three stimulus words, or
   (b) to produce three rhyming words for each of 10 stimulus words.

Principles of Intervention

As well as specifying *what* to achieve and *how long* it will take, it is desirable to have a theoretical rationale that links aims and objectives to the method of intervention. Byng (1995) points out that, in studies of aphasia therapy, theoretical rationale is often not made explicit. She concludes:

> there seems to be a general assumption that therapy will
> just modify the language in some unspecified way. (p.7)

The psycholinguistic model provides a theoretical framework in which we can base a series of rationales for intervention. In working with children we need to consider developmental aspects, both in terms of stages of acquisition and processes that we believe facilitate the acquisition of spoken language. We also have to make some assumptions about the way in which we can strengthen speech processing skills.

This section presents a set of 11 principles based on theoretical rationale which can be used to link short-term aims and objectives with tasks chosen for intervention.

1. Work on the system

The psycholinguistic framework presented in Book 1 represents a system, not an unconnected series of levels of processing. Therefore, while we can identify weaknesses with specific levels and connections, it makes little sense to target these as if they occurred in isolation. Intervention can take advantage of the whole system; activating the relatively stronger levels of processing could help to strengthen the weaker ones. For example, if a child is having difficulty in discriminating a consonant contrast in a pair of nonwords, his/her ability to do this may be improved by feeling how these consonants are produced. The child can repeat and reflect on the articulation of the consonants in isolation and in nonwords before returning to the auditory discrimination exercises in the same session. The importance of feeling and hearing the correct production of targets simultaneously for self-monitoring is emphasized by Hodson and Paden (1991).

2. Strengthen links in the lexicon

Highlighting links between different forms of representation will help to strengthen these links in a child's system. For example, at 12 years of age, Jacob had an inaccurate motor program for the word METAL that resulted in him saying "netal" [nɛtəl]. This production happens to coincide with another word in English, NETTLE, which has its own separate semantic representation. Jacob had both words in his lexicon and so had separate semantic representations for METAL and NETTLE. As part of his intervention programme, these words were illustrated and he was asked to name them for the therapist to identify the correct picture. This helped him to realize that the listener was perceiving his attempt at METAL as NETTLE. This strengthened the links between the phonological representations and semantic representations for these words and motivated him to change his production of METAL from "nettle".

This approach is known as meaningful minimal contrast therapy (MMCT, Weiner, 1981) and has been used by therapists for many years. There is now a wealth of published intervention materials involving the use of meaningful minimal pairs (e.g. Connery, 1992; Howell and Dean, 1994). Minimal pair material can also be used for auditory training activities to strengthen links between phonological and semantic representations, provided the child's inaccurate representation has a real and separate meaning. For example, if a child is producing the word KEY as [ti], the child can be shown pictures of TEA and KEY and asked to point to the one that is named by the therapist/teacher. If a child is producing the word KEY as [gi] (i.e. a nonword in English), the child can be given an auditory-verbal lexical decision task: the child is shown a single picture illustrating KEY and asked to say whether the auditory stimuli /ki/ and /gi/ are correct or incorrect productions of the target picture. These activities help to strengthen and refine the phonological representation of the lexical item.

3. Familiarize

If a child is unable to distinguish between a sound contrast in nonwords or words, s/he will probably need a period of familiarization to this contrast before s/he can learn to distinguish one sound from another. For example, at the age of 4 years, Janie could not hear the difference between /st/ and /ts/ in nonword pairs such as /VOST/ ~ /VOTS/. Learning to do this was chosen as a short-term aim because the skills required to perform this task are necessary for learning and classifying new words, as well as understanding morphological endings such as plurals. Initially, Janie's intervention programme involved giving her opportunities to hear that contrast without being expected to demonstrate an ability to discriminate. One activity involved the use of a puppet who was asked to tell the therapist whether pairs of stimuli such as KEST ~ KETS; KEST ~ KEST; and KETS ~ KETS were the same or different. Janie was involved in the activity by giving rewards to the puppet when she was told to do so, but she did not have to make the same/different judgement for herself. In this way she could concentrate solely on listening to the contrast.

If a child is unable to produce a sound solely due to lower-level output difficulties, s/he may learn to produce it quickly with some teaching. However s/he may also need to hear that sound many more times before s/he can learn to repeat it and integrate it into his/her phonology. Ingram (1986) studied the early phonological development of five children, each learning a different language, and found that the first speech sounds that the children produced in words were not only dependent on articulatory constraints but also on the frequency with which the sounds occurred in the language that the child was exposed to. This and other findings are the basis for the auditory bombardment technique advocated by Hodson and Paden (1991). This technique involves giving the child opportunities to hear many examples of a sound targeted for therapy while s/he is engaged in a play activity. Flynn and Lancaster (1996) provide useful resource materials for this technique.

The case of Robert illustrates how the technique of auditory bombardment can be used. Robert was unable to link the written letters he was
being taught in class to parts of spoken words. He had been taught the
names and sounds of several letters but was unable to think of words
beginning with those letters or recognize when one of these letters
occurred at the beginning of a spoken word. The hypothesis was that
Robert had no awareness of the internal structure of his representations.
One of the short-term aims of his intervention programme during a
school term was therefore for him to identify the first sound of spoken
words beginning with /m/, /d/ and /s/ by pointing to the corresponding
written letter (when all three written letters were presented). These three
sounds had been chosen because they are not too similar acoustically and
Robert already knew the names of the corresponding letters. The first
stage of the programme involved auditory bombardment. Robert was
asked to colour in a large outline of one of the letters while he listened
to the therapist saying lists of nonwords or words beginning with the
corresponding sound. During one of these sessions, while he was
colouring in 'M', the therapist switched from words to nonwords, saying
'Now I'm going to say some silly words that are not real words'.
Nonwords beginning with /m/ were called out while Robert seemed very
engrossed in his colouring-in activity. One of the words was "MOG";
Robert lifted his head and remarked "No, Mog is Meg's cat!". This was
evidence that he was paying attention to the auditory stimuli even though
he was not asked to respond to them. During the same activity in the next
session he began to offer a few words beginning with /m/. When the
therapist had called out five words beginning with /m/ (MONEY, MORE,
MONKEY, MAN, ME), he added "and Mike!". This initial stage of auditory
bombardment allowed Robert to listen to the target sounds without the
pressure of having to respond as in discrimination tasks. This seemed to
help him to segment and identify the initial sound of the words he heard.

4. Include nonword stimuli

The use of nonword stimuli in therapy for adults with aphasia has been
criticized for being too far removed from functional language. For
children, however, dealing with nonwords is an important skill,
because they are constantly having to deal with and learn *new* words.
Thus, using nonwords in intervention programmes with children is
functional. It also mirrors the process of phonological acquisition:
children first hear sounds in words that are unfamiliar to them. An
unfamiliar word is at first a 'nonword' for the child because at that
point the word has no semantic representation. Thus in the auditory
bombardment task described in the previous section, the therapist used
nonwords as well as real words because children have to learn to
segment unfamiliar as well as familiar words.

5. Mirror normal phonological development

Knowledge of aspects of normal development, such as the order of acquisition of sounds and the presence of simplification processes, can guide intervention. This is particularly important for the younger child. A detailed speech assessment and reference to developmental charts such as the developmental assessment from the *Phonological Assessment of Child Speech* (Grunwell, 1985), will help to ensure that sounds, contrasts and words chosen as targets are in line with developmental stages. This developmental stage approach can be integrated with an approach that considers the whole of a child's speech processing system. For example, if a child is realizing most fricatives as homorganic plosives, e.g. FOUR is realized as [p̪ɔ] and SUN is realized as [tʌn], while most other aspects of a child's phonology are more advanced, a therapist guided by the pattern of normal phonological development may choose 'the suppression of stopping' as a target for therapy. However, before planning therapy, it would be important to have more information about why the child was realizing words with fricatives in this way. The following questions need to be addressed:

(a) Does the child have difficulty in discriminating plosive ~ fricative contrasts?
(b) Does the child have inaccurate phonological representations for all or some of the words containing fricatives?
(c) Does the child have inaccurate motor programs for all or some of the words containing fricatives?
(d) Does the child have difficulty with the physical production of fricatives?

It would be important to have provisional answers to these questions before planning the details of intervention. The psycholinguistic approach presented in Book 1 provides a framework for answering these questions.

6. Design stimuli that reflect patterns of errors

A child's ability to process speech will depend on various factors. These factors may be quite general, e.g. the number of syllables in the word; or the number of consonants in a cluster. There may also be more specific factors, e.g. difficulties with all words containing /str/ and /skr/; or with a particular group of words. Often processing ability may depend on a combination of factors, some of which are more specific than others.

It is important to identify these factors through a detailed psycholinguistic assessment. The errors made by the child on a naming test often form a good basis for further investigation, as illustrated in Robert's case. When targeting a specific speech processing skill, it is important to focus on the patterns or specific words that the child has found difficult. For example, Robert has difficulty producing particular consonant clusters in words and nonwords, i.e. syllable initial /pl/ and syllable final /dʒ/ and /ndʒ/. It is likely that his difficulty with these particular patterns applies to all or most words containing these consonants and clusters. This hypothesis can be tested by asking him to name pictures of other words with these sounds. If the hypothesis is supported, intervention should target a range of words with syllable initial /pl/ and syllable /dʒ/ and /ndʒ/. As we saw in the auditory lexical decision task in Activity 2.4, Robert's ability to process speech varied from one group of words to another. When he was presented with his own speech errors for all the words that he had originally produced incorrectly, his performance varied from word to word. For six of the words, he identified his errors as being incorrect. Therefore, it would not be necessary to include auditory discrimination tasks for these words in his intervention programme. However, for the words PLATE, FISH, AEROPLANE, BRUSH and GLOVE, he usually identified his own erroneous production as the correct version of the target word. Thus, Robert's programme would need to include auditory discrimination tasks for these particular words.

7. Confront the child with his/her own speech errors

A child's own speech errors may be used to raise awareness and so trigger change. If a child has inaccurate phonological representations for particular words and these words are targeted in an intervention programme, it is often necessary to use the child's inaccurate productions of these words in auditory training tasks. Using other erroneous realizations of the target word as a contrast may have no effect, as the child may easily be able to distinguish them from the correct pronunciation. For example, Robert was not able to distinguish between his own incorrect productions and correct pronunciations of the following words: PLATE, FISH, AEROPLANE, BRUSH and GLOVE. However, when presented with other variants of these words, e.g. VISH for FISH, he identified them as being incorrect. In Robert's case it would be important to work on discriminating the target words specifically from his own erroneous productions, e.g. FISH vs FIS [fɪs], rather than on discriminating the target words from other incorrect variants (e.g. FISH vs VISH). If a child's inaccurate production of a word corresponds to another real word in the child's lexicon then MMCT can be used both for input and output tasks, as discussed under Principle 2 above.

8. Supplement weak auditory processing skills

Weak auditory processing skills can be strengthened by supplementing the auditory input with simultaneous visual information. If a child is having difficulty in discriminating two different auditory patterns such as the /s/ ~ /t/ contrast in minimal pairs, or a level vs falling intonation on single words, the contrast can be illustrated visually as the words are spoken. This may help the child to be aware of the difference illustrated and may eventually help him/her to hear the contrast when the visual cues are removed. For example, at 5 years of age, Harry was unable to hear the difference between /s/ and /t/ in syllable initial position in words. The therapist presented Harry with minimal pairs such as SEA ~ TEA and asked him to point to the word in the pair that she had just said. Instead of just saying the word, which would have made the task extremely difficult for him, the therapist accompanied the initial consonants with two different hand signs used in *Cued Articulation* (Passy, 1993a). In this system each hand sign represents a different phoneme and the features of each phoneme are illustrated by the position, shape or movement of the sign. This made the task simpler for Harry, drawing his attention to the difference between the two words. At a later stage he was able to complete the task successfully without needing the visual cues.

Similarly, Michelle, a 10-year-old girl with a severe hearing loss, was unable to distinguish between a spoken word produced in a monotone and the same word said with a falling intonation. The therapist used a laryngograph (Abberton, Hu and Fourcin, 1998) to illustrate these two intonation patterns as she modelled the two versions of the word. The laryngograph includes a display of fundamental frequency, which is closely correlated with the pitch of the voice. This fundamental frequency contour is displayed against time and so, as the pitch of the speaker's voice changes, a line, travelling across the screen, moves upwards and downwards, reflecting these pitch changes simultaneously. Familiarization with the two auditory patterns plus the simultaneous presentation of their visual patterns, drew Michelle's attention to the difference. At a later stage in therapy she was able to complete the task without the support of the laryngograph display.

9. Provide the child with experience of producing new speech patterns

Many children with speech difficulties have very little experience of producing certain sounds or words in the correct way. Even though they hear others produce these speech patterns they have had no experience of the simultaneous auditory and kinaesthetic feedback that results from accurate production. Normal self-monitoring of speech is dependent on this combination of feedback, both forms supporting each other. New speech patterns can often be elicited in therapy by using one or more of the following techniques.

Verbal instruction

The child is told how to position his/her articulators and how to make a particular sound. This may be a necessary first step if the child has never produced the sound before. These descriptions could be accompanied by modelling, copying models with a mirror and, for the older child, drawings or diagrams of the articulators. For example, at the age of 5 years, Donna did not have [f] in her repertoire of sounds. She was asked to gently bite her bottom lip and blow. The therapist demonstrated this while she and Donna sat side by side looking into a large mirror. While Donna was carrying out the instructions she was also looking at and listening to the therapist's model.

Tactile feedback

The child can be encouraged to feel how a sound is produced. For example Saju was a 6-year-old profoundly deaf child who did not have [m] in his repertoire of sounds. He was asked to feel the nasal resonance of this sound; while the therapist produced a long [m] sound she placed the fingers of Saju's right hand on the side of her nose. She then placed his fingers on the side of his own nose while he imitated this sound. This technique often enables a deaf child to imitate [m] for the first time and provides them with kinaesthetic feedback to supplement the limited auditory feedback they receive while making the sound.

Visual aids

When discussing Principle 7 it was suggested that visual aids could be used to supplement auditory input. They can also be used to aid a child's production of speech and thus give more experience of producing accurate speech patterns. Some visual aids illustrate an aspect of speech, e.g. pitch change and place of articulation, and provide visual displays that occur simultaneously with speech. These include the laryngograph (Abberton, Hu and Fourcin, 1998) and electropalatography (Dent, this volume). Receiving simultaneous visual feedback about an aspect of his/her speech that is inaccurate can help the child experiment and modify their production until the target pattern is achieved. For example, Michelle, who produced many of her spoken words on a monotone, attempted to use a falling intonation on the word NO. The teacher had modelled the target for her using the laryngograph so that she could see on the monitor the shape of the pitch contour she was trying to achieve. While Michelle experimented with different productions of the word, she could see the line on the screen moving up and down as her pitch rose and fell. She experimented until she produced a pitch contour that was similar to the original model.

Other visual aids serve as reference symbols to remind the child to produce a speech pattern in a particular way, even though these aids do not display simultaneous feedback of aspects of a child's speech pattern. The aid may employ symbols that encode phonological features. For instance, there are sets of plastic letters that use one colour for consonants and another for vowels (cf. *Taskmaster*; *Edith Norrie Lettercase*). Further instances of this type of aid are the positions of the hand signals in *Cued Articulation* (Passy, 1993a) which vary according to place of articulation, and the use of coloured bricks to mark segments in words (Lindamood, Bell and Lindamood, 1997). Donna had recently learnt to imitate /f/ in isolation and was now trying to use it in syllable-initial position when naming illustrations of words such as FIRE and FISH. She had accurate phonological representations of these words, but because the corresponding motor programs for these words were still inaccurate, she usually produced them as [paɪə] and [pɪʃ]. She had been taught to recognize the cued articulation hand signs for /p/ and /f/. The hand sign for /p/ involves the index finger separating from the thumb to correspond to the stop and release of this plosive, while the hand sign for /f/ involves a forward and downward movement to correspond to the continuous airflow of this fricative (see Figure 2.3).

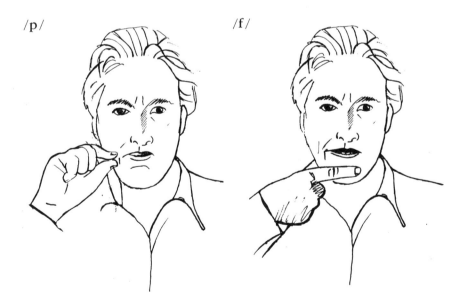

Figure 2.3: Cued articulation symbols for /p/ and /f/.

If Donna produced a target word with an initial [p], the therapist modelled the target word with the hand sign for /f/. Seeing the forward and downward movement of the sign reminded her of the continuous nature of the initial sound, which she was capable of producing, and she was reminded to repeat the target word correctly. Through repeated experience of correctly articulating the words beginning with /f/, accurate motor programs were established.

Many therapy and teaching programmes, systems and activity books give suggestions on how to use such techniques. For example, Lancaster and Pope (1989, Chapter 5) review different approaches and give a comprehensive description of techniques and activities. It is usually suggested that techniques are used in a graded programme. For example, they may be used initially to elicit single consonants or vowels and then in sound combinations with favourable phonetic contexts and then moving on to a wider range of words and connected speech. Even though such approaches are removed from the natural context of spontaneous conversations, they do give a child experience of articulating, hearing and feeling words simultaneously. As well as helping speech output problems, this should indirectly strengthen the whole speech processing system, including the phonological representations.

10. Promote generalization

By working on, and thereby strengthening, the whole speech processing system, including input and output skills and accuracy of representations, in relation to a particular pattern or words, generalization of that pattern or word to a variety of contexts should be facilitated. If, for example, the motor program for the correct production of a word is strengthened to such an extent that it replaces the child's previous inaccurate motor program, then the child's ability to say that word correctly should become more automatic. This automatization may lead to relatively effortless production of the word or speech pattern in a variety of contexts. However, if generalization does not occur, or happens very slowly, then it may be necessary to use generalization techniques to facilitate it.

Michelle had successfully added [k] to her repertoire of consonants and could use it when naming illustrations of words that include this consonant. However, she still did not use [k] in more spontaneous speaking situations: she usually reverted to realizing /k/ as [t]. The therapist and teacher asked her to complete a survey on how the children in the class came to school. They gave Michelle a card with four columns headed WALK, BUS, CAR and BIKE, and asked her to interview each child in the class. Michelle was to keep a count of how many children used each form of transport. First, Michelle rehearsed the interview with the therapist and teacher, who encouraged her to use [k] in all the targeted words (e.g. COME; SCHOOL; WALK; CAR; BIKE) and revised any errors she made. Once she could do this accurately in the rehearsal, the teacher observed her completing the survey. For a description of different kinds of generalization and further examples of activities, see Lancaster and Pope (1989), Chapter 6.

11. Make explicit links with literacy

Activities aiming to improve phonological awareness will not promote literacy skills unless specific links are made (Hatcher, Hulme and Ellis, 1994; Stackhouse, this volume). Therapists and teachers often provide reference symbols either to increase a child's awareness of sound patterns or as a reminder to use them. If written letters are used, e.g. as part of these symbols, then links with literacy will be strengthened. For example, most of the picture symbols representing phonemes in the *Nuffield Dyspraxia Programme* (Connery, 1992) depict objects that begin with a corresponding grapheme, e.g. /b/ is represented by the picture of a BALL and /z/ is represented by the picture of a ZIP (for further illustration, see Chapter 5, this volume). Picture symbols that include the written letter are also available so that children can make links between phonemes and graphemes, e.g. *Jolly Phonics* (Lloyd, 1992) and *Letterland*.

Summary

This chapter has stressed the importance of setting clear aims and objectives for intervention and has provided a theoretical rationale for how these can be linked to tasks. This should ensure that the tasks designed, selected or adapted for a child's programme of work are appropriate. Long-term aims are concerned with functional communication and are often quite general, e.g. to improve communicative competence in social situations. Short-term aims and objectives, on the other hand, are more specific and should:

- be based on hypotheses derived from a speech processing profile for an individual child
- be integrated with aims and objectives set by other professionals
- specify targets to be achieved in a given time
- be measurable

When aims and objectives are set, a theoretical rationale leads to the following principles for task selection:

- work on the system.
- strengthen links in the lexicon
- familiarize
- include nonword stimuli

- mirror normal phonological development
- design stimuli that reflect patterns of errors
- confront the child with his/her own speech errors
- supplement weak auditory processing skills
- provide the child with experience of producing new speech patterns
- promote generalisation
- make links with literacy explicit.

KEY TO ACTIVITY 2.1

There are two ways of repeating real words: lexical and nonlexical. The child will probably take a lexical route involving the speech processing skills: a – g, i and j. If a nonlexical route is taken the speech processing skills: a – c and h – j will be involved.

The accompanying figures illustrate these two routes through the model.

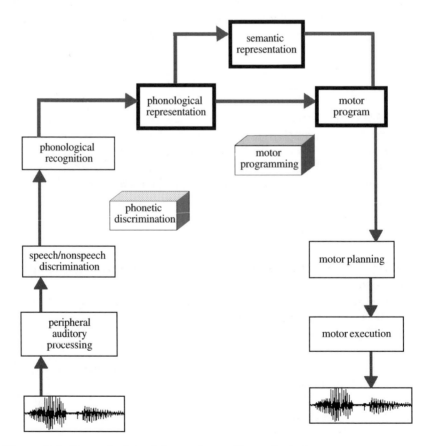

Figure 2.4: Key to Activity 2.1: word repetition – lexical route.

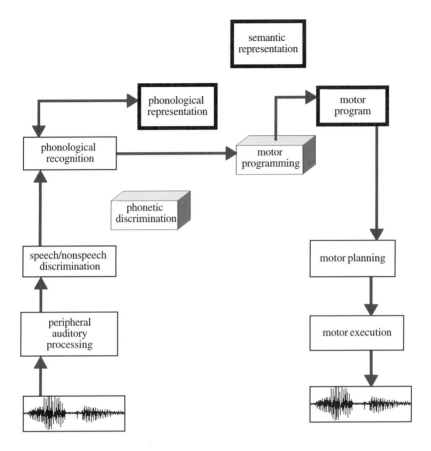

Figure 2.5: Key to Activity 2.1: word repetition – nonlexical route.

KEY TO ACTIVITY 2.2

1. Word repetition: a lexical route is most likely, involving a – g, i and j (see Figure 2.4 for route through model).
2. Naming: f, g, i, j (see Figure 2.6, (from Book 1, p.179) for route through model).
3. Nonword repetition: a nonlexical route is most likely, involving a – e, h – j (see Figure 2.5 above).

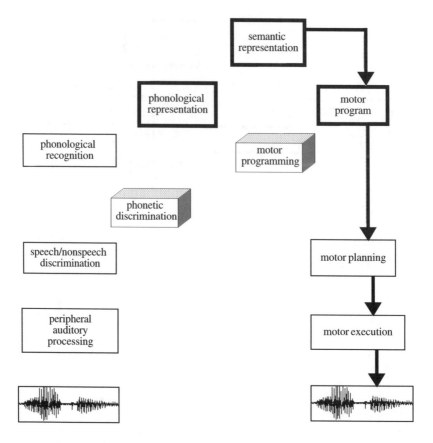

Figure 2.6: Key to Activity 2.2: naming.

KEY TO ACTIVITY 2.3

Useful hypotheses about Robert's performance on the naming and repetition tasks are:

1. Robert has established inaccurate phonological representations and motor programs for all or some of the 11 words that he was unable to repeat or name.
2. Robert has established accurate phonological representations for all or some of the 11 words that he was unable to repeat or name, but motor programs for these words are inaccurate.
3. There is no difficulty in accessing these representations.
4. Robert has additional motor execution difficulties concerning the production of the following sounds: syllable-initial /pl/ and syllable final /dʒ/ and /ndʒ/.
5. Auditory processing skills are intact.

6. Robert has some difficulty with auditory discrimination including tasks involving syllable-initial /pl/ and syllable final /dʒ/ and /ndʒ/.

KEY TO ACTIVITY 2.4

For five of the stimuli (PLATE, FISH, AEROPLANE, BRUSH, GLOVE), Robert identified the inaccurate presentations as accurate all or most of the time. Therefore, for these words, Hypothesis 1 is supported (Robert has inaccurate phonological representations and inaccurate motor programs). In the nonword repetition test Robert was able to produce syllable initial /gl/ when he repeated the nonword matched to GLOVE and was able to produce syllable initial /br/ and syllable final /ʃ/ when repeating the nonword matched to BRUSH Therefore, for the words GLOVE, BRUSH and FISH, Robert has inaccurate phonological representations and motor programs but does not seem to have any additional difficulties in executing the consonants and consonant clusters required for these words. However, there are no examples of accurate realizations of syllable initial /pl/ in the nonword repetition test. Therefore, for the words PLATE and AEROPLANE, Robert may have an additional difficulty in articulating /pl/.

For the remaining stimuli (SNAKE, GUITAR, SAUSAGE, UMBRELLA, YELLOW, SPONGE), Robert was able to identify the inaccurate presentations as incorrect all or most of the time. Therefore, for these words, Hypothesis 2 is supported (Robert has accurate phonological representations but inaccurate motor programs). The results of the nonword repetition test indicate no difficulties with the motor execution of the nonwords matching SNAKE, GUITAR, UMBRELLA and YELLOW. Therefore it is likely that, for these words, Robert has inaccurate motor programs but no particular difficulty in executing the consonants and consonant clusters required for the words. However, the results of the nonword repetition test indicate difficulties with the syllable final /dʒ/ and /ndʒ/ in SAUSAGE and SPONGE respectively. Therefore, for these words, output processing problems include motor execution difficulties with these consonant clusters.

Chapter 3
What Do Tasks Really Tap?

RACHEL REES

Chapter 2 of this book discussed the planning phase of intervention by discussing the following progression:

Assessment → Hypotheses → Aims.

This chapter deals with what happens after aims have been set and focuses in particular on the psycholinguistic properties of tasks. It therefore tackles the next step in intervention:

Aims → Tasks.

In order to select suitable intervention materials, potential tasks have to be analysed from a psycholinguistic viewpoint. There is no 'box' of psycholinguistic tests. Rather, as stated in Book 1 (Stackhouse and Wells, 1997):

> Psycholinguistic assessment is an approach carried in the head of the user and not in a case of tests. (p.49)

Similarly, there are no specially designed psycholinguistic materials for intervention. Almost all teaching and therapy material can be used in a psycholinguistic way.

A psycholinguistic approach to intervention is derived from a way of thinking. Just as it is important to analyse what tests are really testing in an assessment (see Book 1, Chapters 2 and 3), it is also necessary to analyse what tasks are really tapping when they are being used in therapy or teaching. This helps the user to select tasks that are well suited to the intervention aims, and modify the tasks in an appropriate way based on a child's performance. Practice in working in this way should also help practitioners and researchers who want to design their own tasks for principled intervention.

Speech and language therapists and teachers use a wide variety of tasks designed to improve children's auditory discrimination, speech and phonological awareness. There is a wealth of published material for such tasks, some of which include equipment such as pictures, audio-tapes and board games. Most of this material can be useful if it is used with the right child at the right time. This chapter offers a particular method for analysing tasks in a psycholinguistic way. First let us try to define what is meant by a task.

What is a Task?

A 'task' includes any materials used for intervention, the procedure followed (including any instructions), the feedback given to the child and any technique used to support speech processing, such as *Cued Articulation* (Passy, 1993a). This can be summarized by the following formula:

$$\text{TASK} = \text{Materials} + \text{Procedure} + \text{Feedback} \pm \text{Technique.}$$

Altering any one of these four components, even minimally, can change the psycholinguistic nature of the task. Later activities in this chapter will involve 'fine tuning' one or more of these four components of the task in order to achieve a different aim, as well as analysing the psycholinguistic properties and other features of some familiar tasks. In part, these activities parallel those presented in the chapters on 'What Do Tests Really Test' in Book 1. The tasks will be analysed using the set of questions presented in Figure 3.1. The purpose of these questions is:

(a) to investigate the psycholinguistic properties of intervention tasks;
(b) to aid the selection or modification of tasks that will target intervention aims for a particular child.

This will be illustrated by taking each question in Figure 3.1 in turn.

1. Does the child have to use his/her lexical representations to complete the task? If not, how likely is it that representations may be accessed?

If a child has lexical representations for the stimuli used in the task, for example if they are familiar words, it is very likely that they will be accessed during the task. However, it may not be necessary to do this in order to complete the task. For example, if the child is asked to listen to familiar spoken words beginning with /t/ or /k/ and decide which consonant each word begins with by pointing to the corresponding written letter, the child will probably access the representations for these words. However, the representations do not *have to* be accessed to complete the task successfully. It is the first consonant of the word that has to be segmented from the remainder and matched to a written

1. Does the child have to use his/her lexical representations to complete the task? If not, how likely is it that representations may be accessed?
2. Does the task target the input channel, the output channel or both?
3. Does the task target a specific level (or levels) of speech processing? If so, which level/s are targeted?
4. Metaphonological skills:
   (a) Does the child have to reflect on his/her speech production?
   (b) Does the child have to show awareness of the internal structure of phonological representations or of spoken stimuli?
   (c) If so, what kind of segmentation is required?
   (d) Does the child have to manipulate phonological units?
5. What demands are made on the child's memory in order to make responses during the task?
6. What are the task demands? Can all or parts of the task be demonstrated?
7. Is any technique being used to support the child with the task? If so, how is the technique providing support?

Figure 3.1: Task analysis questions.

letter; this could be done regardless of whether the word presented is in the child's lexicon.

2. Does the task target the input channel, the output channel or both?

Many tasks involve both the input and output channel, but it is important to decide which channel is being targeted in the intervention. For example, a child may be asked to respond with the words 'same' or 'different' after judging whether two spoken words presented were identical or not. Although the child has to produce speech as part of the task, the response could equally be nonverbal, e.g. pointing to symbols representing 'same' and 'different'. The purpose of the task is to give the child practice in making an *auditory* judgement about the stimuli. Therefore this task is targeting only the input channel.

3. Does the task target a specific level (or levels) of speech processing? If so, which level/s are targeted?

In the same way as *channels* may need to be targeted specifically (Question 2 above), many tasks also involve different *levels* of processing, and it is important to decide if any of these need to be targeted specifically. For example, naming tasks involve all the speech processing levels on the output side of the speech processing model presented in Book 1 (see Appendix 4), but certain naming tasks, because of their exact design and place in a structured programme, are targeting one or more levels specifically.

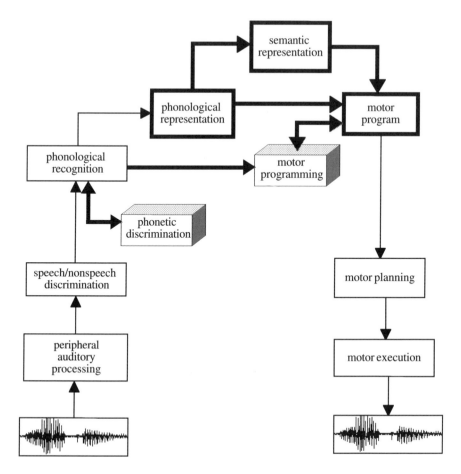

Figure 3.2: Speech processing model.

ACTIVITY 3.1

Aim: to identify which level of processing is being targeted in a given naming task.

Marcio is 5 years old and was referred to speech and language therapy because of his speech difficulties. When he started therapy, Marcio pronounced words beginning with /f/ incorrectly, realizing the initial /f/ as [p]. After three months, he could imitate these words correctly but his spontaneous production of the words varied; sometimes he remembered to say them correctly and sometimes he reverted to realizing the initial /f/ as [p]. Consider the following task designed for Marcio and decide which level of speech processing in the model presented in Figure 3.2 is being targeted.

The task

Materials: A series of 10 squares (see Figure 3.3) was presented. In the first nine squares there are pictures that illustrate words beginning with /f/ e.g. FIRE, which Marcio used to pronounce incorrectly. The last square is empty. The remaining materials are a red counter and a sticker of a red star.

Procedure: Marcio was asked to name each picture in the series. If he named a picture correctly, he could place the counter on the relevant square. When he had named all pictures correctly he could stick the red star in the last square.

Feedback: When Marcio named a picture correctly, the therapist rewarded him verbally and allowed him to place a counter on the square. If he named a picture incorrectly, realizing the initial /f/ as [p], the therapist did not allow him to move the counter on to that square and said 'Can you say that word in the new way?'. If he still had difficulty, the therapist asked him to imitate the word, which he was able to do without much difficulty as this had been covered in the previous stage of therapy.

Check your answer against the Key to Activity 3.1 at the end of this chapter and then read the following.

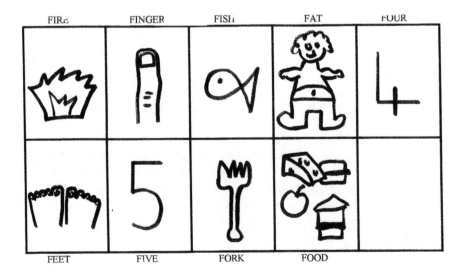

Figure 3.3: Pictures for task with Marcio.

This naming task included a set of words that Marcio had previously practised repeating, using an updated motor program. He was immediately rewarded for using the updated motor programs to name the pictures spontaneously. Thus, motor programming and making links between the updated motor program and the semantic representation were being specifically targeted by the task. In addition, Marcio had to use all the other lower levels of speech processing on the output side.

Some tasks are specifically designed to target awareness or manipulation of the internal structure of representations, rather than a specific level of speech processing. For example, a syllable segmentation task, where a child has to count the number of syllables in a written word by tapping out the syllables, is aiming to increase the child's awareness of the internal syllabic structure of the word. Although specific levels of speech processing are not the target of the task, its successful completion relies on the integrity of the underlying system. This is explained and illustrated in Chapter 3 of Book 1.

4. Metaphonological skills

It may be helpful to think of the awareness of the structure of spoken words as a continuum from tacit to explicit, as described by Stackhouse (1997) (also Book 1, p.55). Early in their development, children have a tacit awareness; this may be demonstrated, for example, by the child's exaggerating a consonant or vowel in a word in a playful way or in a fondness for rhymes. Later in development they can use their knowledge of 'language about language', including the names of letters, to demonstrate a more explicit understanding of how words are structured.

Some tasks encourage children to reflect on their own speech production by confronting them with a discrepancy between their intended meaning and the meaning understood by the listener. This technique is used in meaningful minimal contrast therapy (MMCT), as described by Weiner (1981), who successfully used this method to reduce the frequency of three phonological simplifying processes in the speech of two children with phonological disability. MMCT involves selecting pairs of words, where one member of the pair corresponds to the child's intended meaning, e.g. KEY, and the other corresponds to the child's mispronunciation of the word, e.g. TEA (see also Rees, Chapter 2, this volume). If the child asks an adult to point to a picture of the KEY but mispronounces the word as [ti], then the adult will point to the picture of the TEA. This confronts the child with a discrepancy between the meaning intended and the meaning understood. In some cases, this confrontation may merely confuse the child or lead them to assign the fault of the communication breakdown to the listener. However, children with more advanced metalinguistic skills will reflect on their own speech production and will recognize the need to alter their pronunciation to eliminate the ambiguity. Note that this therapy is appropriate only if the child is easily able to alter his/her pronunciation pattern once s/he has recognized the need to do so (Stackhouse, 1984).

Reflecting on speech production and recognizing the need to alter pronunciation do not necessarily require the child to segment a spoken utterance or word into constituents. To realize that two words such as KEY and TEA are different, a child does not have to segment the words into phonemes but could just recognize that one whole word is different from the other whole word. Altering pronunciation of the word from "tea" [ti] to "key" [ki], through imitation of the whole word, could also be done without segmenting the words in any way.

Some therapy and teaching programmes advocate using activities that are designed to develop a more explicit understanding of the structure of utterances or words, so that the child's acquisition of metaphonological skills can be accelerated in order to improve speech and/or literacy skills. Dean, Howell, Waters, et al. (1995) describe a therapy approach, known as *Metaphon*, which is based on the theory that the most effective way to help children make required changes in their speech is to combine the MMCT approach with providing children with specific information about the nature of the target contrasts using a shared vocabulary that is built up in therapy. Examples of shared vocabulary that may be used in therapy are 'long' and 'short' to denote the fricative and plosive properties of individual consonants such as /f/ and /p/. In order to use and benefit from this kind of information, the child needs to segment the phoneme concerned from the rest of the word. Children who have little awareness of the internal structure of words will be unlikely to benefit from an approach that gives them detailed information about properties of individual phonemes. Although Dean, Howell, Waters, et al. (1995) describe the successful use of Metaphon in efficacy studies, this success could be due to the MMCT approach itself and not necessarily to the extra information given regarding properties of individual phonemes through specially taught vocabulary (Grundy, 1995). This is why it is important first to decide whether a task involves segmentation and then to relate this to our knowledge of an individual child's awareness of the internal structure of words. It is also important to know what kind of segmentation the task involves.

Awareness of how one phoneme can be segmented from the rest of the word is just one kind of segmentation. The term 'phonological awareness' refers to the metaphonological skill of reflecting on the sound structure of an utterance rather than its meaning, and covers a range of different kinds of segmentation (see Book 1, Chapter 3, p.53). It is important to consider this range and the developmental order in which awareness of different kinds of segmentation occurs.

Word segmentation

Awareness of words in an utterance as separate linguistic entities begins very early in development due to their strong link with separate meanings. This awareness grows gradually; although many word boundaries understood by a young child may coincide with adult word boundaries, others may not do so until later or when literacy draws the child's attention to the discrepancies (Broomfield and Combley, 1997). For example, a child may understand LADYBIRD as two words, JUMBLE SALE as one, or A KNIFE as AN IFE, and this may be reflected in the child's early attempts at writing (see Figure 1.3 in Chapter 1).

Syllable segmentation

Awareness of syllables does not require any understanding of word meanings. It is possible for adults to tap out the syllables of an utterance spoken in a language unknown to them. Pre-school children can easily be trained to indicate the syllables in a word by, for example, tapping them out (Layton, Deeny and Upton, 1997).

Onset-rime segmentation

The syllable can be divided into its onset (the initial consonant or consonant cluster) and its rime (the remainder of the syllable), e.g. P/AT; SP/AT; SPL/AT. Goswami and Bryant (1990) describe a child's awareness of this division as falling between sensitivity to syllables and sensitivity to phonemes. As discussed and illustrated in Chapter 2 of Book 1, awareness of this division facilitates learning to read and spell by analogy with other words. For example, if a child is aware of the onset/rime division in words such as LIGHT and FIGHT, s/he can start to associate the rime with its letters IGHT. Storing this association will then help the child to read and spell other words with rimes spelt in the same way, e.g. NIGHT and RIGHT.

Phoneme segmentation

Very young children can recognize a change from one phoneme to another and how this can alter meaning (e.g. MORE ~ DOOR). They can also make many of these fine distinctions in speech to express their desired meaning. However, a more conscious analysis of phoneme segmentation is a sophisticated metaphonological skill that is often not mastered until much later. Hatcher (1996) explains that an awareness of phonemes begins with the child's ability to segment at the onset/rime division (e.g. M/AN), but the ability to segment final and medial sounds (e.g. M/A/N) emerges later. Children's difficulties with conscious phoneme segmentation are often reflected in their early spelling errors e.g. STREET spelt as ‹set› (see Activity 1.1 in Stackhouse, this volume). Goswami and Bryant (1990) argue that, although syllable segmentation and onset/rime segmentation are possible before the onset of literacy, more thorough phonemic segmentation occurs as a result of exposure to alphabetic script. Whether or not knowledge of letters is *essential* for phonemic segmentation, this kind of segmentation seems to be the last to be mastered and is aided by alphabetic knowledge. Effective phonological awareness training programmes reflect the developmental order of different kinds of awareness of segmentation and closely combine phonological awareness tasks with training in reading (e.g. *Sound Linkage*, Hatcher, 1994; and *Sound Awareness*, Layton, Deeney and Upton, 1997).

There is a range of published material available for phonological awareness training and MMCT, including resource materials that accompany Metaphon (Dean, Howell, Hill, et al., 1990) and the *Nuffield Dyspraxia Programme* (Connery, 1992). Tasks taken from these resources may be useful if they are well matched to an individual child's level of metaphonological awareness and intervention needs. This is why it is so important to assess the metaphonological demands of a task. Here are the three questions for analysing a potential task in this way:

4(a). Does the child have to reflect on his/her speech production?

4(b). Does the child have to show awareness of the internal structure of phonological representations or of spoken stimuli ?

4(c). If so, what kind of segmentation is required?

Some tasks are designed to encourage the child to reflect on his/her speech production, but not all of these require segmentation skills.

ACTIVITY 3.2

Aim: to distinguish between two tasks that require a child to reflect on his/her speech production, by deciding which task requires segmentation skills and which does not.

Consider Task A and Task B. Answer questions 4(a)–4(c) above for each task. Decide which of the tasks requires the child to be aware of how the stimuli are segmented.

Task A

Jimmy is 8 years old and has been receiving individual help with his speech for six months. The following task was presented to him:

Materials: Five picture cards of simple words beginning with /t/: TAP, TEA, TALK, TALL and TOAST.
Five picture cards of simple words beginning with /k/: KING, KISS, KEY, KITE and KICK.
Two posting boxes, one labelled 't' and one labelled 'k'.

Procedure: The picture cards were shuffled and placed picture side downwards on the table in front of Jimmy. Both posting boxes were within his reach. He had to pick up each picture in turn, name it aloud, decide whether the word started with /t/ or /k/, match this choice to the label on one of the boxes and post the card in the appropriate box.

Feedback: When Jimmy named the picture correctly and chose the correct box, the therapist rewarded him verbally. If he was not sure which box to choose or started moving a picture towards the wrong box the therapist asked him to say the word again and asked him what sound the word starts with. If Jimmy was unable to respond, she repeated the first consonant and then asked him to choose one of the labels. If Jimmy was still unable to choose, or chose incorrectly, the therapist repeated the consonant and pointed to the corresponding letter simultaneously and then asked him to post the picture.

Task B

Suzie is 4 years old and has been receiving individual help with her speech for five weeks. The following task was presented to her:

Materials: Three picture cards of each of the following words (making 12 cards in total): TEA, KEY, TAP, CAP.
One posting box.

Procedure: The picture cards were shuffled and placed picture side up in front of Suzie. She had to name each one in turn. After each one was named the therapist picked up the appropriate card, asked Suzie whether it was the correct one and, if it was, posted it in the box.

Feedback: When Suzie named the picture correctly the therapist picked the appropriate card and posted it in the box. If Suzie looked at a picture and named it using its minimal pair (e.g. looked at the picture of KEY and said "tea"), the therapist picked up the picture of TEA and said 'this is what I heard' and encouraged her to change her pronunciation to match the word she had intended to say. If Suzie said "key" the therapist picked up the picture of KEY and said something like 'now I clearly heard that one' and posted the picture in the box. Check your answers against the Key to Activity 3.2 at the end of this chapter and then read the following.

Task A and Task B both required the children to reflect on their speech. To carry out Task A successfully, Jimmy had to segment the first consonant from the rest of the word; this involved onset/rime segmentation. It would have been impossible to do the task without this skill as Jimmy had to match this segmented consonant to a symbol on the posting box. Moreover, some words had the competing consonant in coda position, e.g. TALK; KITE, which makes the task more difficult.

To carry out Task B successfully, Suzie could use the strategy of segmentation to remind herself which consonant she should use. However, segmentation is not *necessary* to complete the task. When Suzie was encouraged to use a different pronunciation, due to the nature of the task, she could experiment with a 'whole word' type approach until she produced the correct pronunciation. Many young children, or older children with a speech delay, have [t] and [k] in their repertoire of sounds but fail to use them contrastively to convey meaning. Such children could easily experiment with different pronunciations of the whole word until the therapist indicated that they had produced the correct label.

There is one more question under (4) that is concerned with metaphonological skills:

4(d). Does the child have to manipulate phonological units?

Even though Task A required Jimmy to be aware of the internal structure of the words he spoke, he did not have to manipulate these structures by rearranging the phonological units in any way by, for example, generating phonologically similar words. If, however, he had to carry out a follow-on task that involved thinking of other words beginning with /t/ or /k/, then he would either have to select such words from a network of lexical representations organized appropriately and choose ones that had different rimes, or else he would need to use a mechanical slot filling routine where /t/ and /k/ are joined to different rimes and compared with the lexicon (see Book 1, pp.93–94). Both strategies involve the manipulation of phonological units. Other tasks that involve a manipulation of phonological units as well as an awareness of internal structure include rhyme string production (see Book 1, pp.64–65) and spoonerisms (see Book 1, pp.68–69).

Questions 4 (a)–(d) can be answered regardless of whether the words that the child is listening to or producing are already in his/her lexicon. This variable is dealt with separately by Question 1. The purpose of Questions 4 (a)–(d) is to assess what metaphonological skills are required by tasks, irrespective of whether the tasks involve words the child already knows, new words for the child, or nonwords.

5. What demands are made on the child's memory in order to make responses during the task?

Question 5 refers to the demands made on working memory by the individual speech processing tasks presented to the child. The task in its entirety, which may include game rules or other procedures, may make its own memory demands, which will be considered under Question 6. However, first complete the following activity, which demonstrates how different tasks aiming to strengthen the system in the same way may make different memory demands.

ACTIVITY 3.3

Aim: to identify which level of processing is being targeted in two tasks and to compare the memory demands made by these tasks.

Consider Task A and Task B. Refer to Figure 3.2 and identify which aspect of the speech processing system they are aiming to strengthen. Compare the memory demands each task makes on working memory.

Task A – Odd One Out

Philip is 6 years old. He has normal hearing but has some difficulty with speech discrimination, including the /s/~/t/ contrast in words and nonwords. The following task was presented to him:

Materials: Three small cuddly toys representing three different animals. List of items consisting of groups of three nonwords.

Each nonword consists of a Consonant Vowel (CV) or Consonant Vowel Consonant (CVC) sequence and begins with /s/ or /t/. In each group two of the nonwords are identical and begin with /s/ or /t/ and the third begins with the other consonant; all three have the same rime, e.g. SAF, TAF, SAF. The order of the stimuli varies randomly across items. The items are as follows:

SEG, SEG, TEG

TOOG, SOOG, TOOG

SIG, TIG, SIG

SUL, TUL, TUL

TATCH, TATCH, SATCH

SAF, SAF, TAF

TOOG, TOOG, SOOG

TIG, SIG, SIG

SEG, TEG, SEG

TAF, SAF, TAF

TUL, SUL, SUL

SATCH, TATCH, TATCH.

Procedure: The three cuddly toys were placed in front of Philip. The therapist said, 'Each of these toys is going to say something. One of them is going to say something different from the other two. We are going to pat the head of the one that says something different'. The therapist then read out the first group of nonwords (SEG, SEG, TEG). As she said each nonword she pointed to each toy in turn. The therapist then patted the head of the toy that had 'said' TEG. She then repeated this part of the procedure for the next group of nonwords. As the activity progressed she encouraged Philip to join her in patting the head of the toy who had 'said' the different stimulus. When Philip did this confidently she asked him to pat the head of the chosen toy.

Feedback: When Philip patted the head of the appropriate toy he was rewarded verbally. If he did not choose the appropriate toy, he was asked to listen carefully to the three stimuli again. If Philip's second attempt was also incorrect the stimuli were repeated again.

Task B – Same/Different

Adam is 5 years old. Like Philip, he has normal hearing but has some difficulty with speech discrimination, including the /s/~/t / contrast in words and nonwords. The following task was presented to him:

Materials: Small coloured counting blocks that join together.
           A list of items consisting of pairs of nonwords.

Each nonword consists of a CV or CVC sequence and begins with /s/ or /t/. Some items consist of pairs of identical words e.g. SAF / SAF, TOOG / TOOG; others are minimal pairs, e.g. TEG / SEG, SIG / TIG. The order of identical vs non-identical stimuli varies randomly. The stimuli are as follows:

SAF, SAF

TEG, SEG

TOOG, TOOG

SATCH, SATCH

SUL, TUL

TOOG, SOOG

SIG, TIG

SEG, SEG

TAF, TAF

TUL, SUL

TATCH, TATCH

SIG, TIG.

Procedure: The blocks were placed in front of the child. The therapist explained that she would say two silly words and then they would decide if they were the same or different. She read out the first few pairs and told Adam whether they were the same or different, encouraging him to join her in making the decision. When he felt confident that he would like to make the decision, she told him that he could join two blocks together if he was right.

Feedback: When Adam said "same" or "different" appropriately, the therapist rewarded him verbally and allowed him to join another block to the string of blocks. If he made an inappropriate response, the therapist did not allow him to reach for another block and asked him to listen carefully to the stimuli again. Any second response was right due to the chance factor.

Check your answer against the Key to Activity 3.3 at the end of this chapter and then read the following.

Both tasks encourage the child to notice the difference between a nonword beginning with /t/ and a nonword beginning with /s/. The child does not have to compare the stimuli to items in his/her lexicon to complete the task. No spoken response is required. Both tasks are therefore targeting *phonological recognition*.

Task A required the child to hold three one-syllable stimuli in his/her working memory, compare them and detect which one is different (an ABX detection task). Task B required the child to hold two one-syllable stimuli, compare them and judge whether they were identical or not (an AB judgement task). Therefore, Task A has a slightly greater memory load.

6. What are the task demands? Can any part of the task be demonstrated?

Task demands include vocabulary and grammatical structures that the child is expected to know, e.g. in the instructions, and the amount the child is expected to remember at any one time. These can be greatly reduced if parts or all of the task can be demonstrated. It is important to consider these demands when choosing a task. Often it is easier for a child to concentrate on the aspect of speech processing targeted if the other demands of the task are minimal. This particularly applies to younger children or children with a limited memory span, a limited comprehension of vocabulary or of grammatical structures. However, other children may be motivated to concentrate if the activity is made more interesting and demanding. Some games designed for intervention have complicated rules which would be confusing for some children but may motivate an older or more able child to participate.

7. Is any technique being used to support the child with the task? If so, how is the technique providing support?

A technique involves providing extra information for the child that illustrates some aspect of speech in order to help the child with the task. This information is usually visual. As explained in Chapter 2, visual information can be used to supplement the auditory input or to aid a child's production of speech. Various aspects of speech can be represented, such as pitch contour, voicing or particular consonants. These representations can take different forms, such as patterns on a screen, colour coding or hand signals. In answering this question it is important to determine what form the technique takes, which aspect of speech it is illustrating, and whether it is being used to supplement auditory input or to aid a child's production of speech.

Analysing a task with the questions presented in Figure 3.1 should lead to a greater awareness of its psycholinguistic properties and suitability for a particular child. The next three activities provide an opportunity to analyse the psycholinguistic properties of popular tasks and to examine how these properties can be manipulated when designing intervention tasks.

ACTIVITY 3.4

Aims:
1. To analyse the psycholinguistic properties of a task using the task analysis questions.
2. To identify how the task's psycholinguistic properties change if one aspect of it is changed.

Read through the description of the task.
Answer all the task analysis questions presented in Figure 3.1.
Note the change to the task, and the effects of the change on the psycholinguistic properties of the task.

Task 3.4
The following task was presented to Imogen when she was 5 years of age:

Materials: Two cuddly toys.
          A list of items comprising groups of three nonwords.

Each nonword consists of one syllable and has /s/ or /st/ as its onset. In each group of three, the first two stimuli are a minimal pair (e.g. SEG / STEG) and the third stimulus is identical to the first or second stimulus. The order of the stimuli is varied randomly across items. The stimuli are as follows:

> STIM, SIM, SIM
> SEG, STEG, STEG
> STOF, SOF, STOF
> STOOK, SOOK, SOOK
> SIM, STIM, SIM
> SOF, STOF, STOF
> SOOK, STOOK, SOOK
> STEG, SEG, STEG
> SOF, STOF, STOF
> SIM, STIM, SIM
> STOOK, STOOK, SOOK
> STEG, SEG, STEG.

Procedure: The two cuddly toys were placed in front of Imogen. The teacher said 'Each of these toys is going to say a silly word'. She demonstrated by pointing to the first toy and reading out the first nonword in the first group and then pointing to the second toy and reading out the second nonword. She then said, 'We have to decide which one said this'. Lastly she read out the third stimulus in the group and pointed to the appropriate toy. As the activity progressed she encouraged Imogen to join her in pointing to the toy that had 'said' the third stimulus. When Imogen did this confidently, the teacher asked her to point to the chosen toy on her own.

Feedback: When Imogen pointed to the appropriate toy the teacher rewarded her verbally. If she did not choose the appropriate toy, the teacher asked her to listen carefully to the third stimulus again. Any second attempt was correct due to the chance factor.

Change to Task 3.4

The stimuli are changed from nonwords to words. An example of a group of three words would be: SAY, STAY, STAY.

Check your answer against the Key to Activity 3.4 at the end of this chapter and then read the following.

---

1. Does the child have to use his/her lexical representations to complete the task? If not, how likely is it that representations may be accessed?
Imogen did not have to access her lexical representations as the stimuli were nonwords. She could have accessed her lexical representations for this task and may have done so if she had compared the stimuli to similar words (e.g. compare STEG to STEGOSAURUS).

2. Does the task target the input channel, the output channel, or both?
The task was targeting input only. Imogen was not required to produce a verbal response. The aim of the task was to give Imogen experience in hearing the difference between initial /s/ and initial /st/ in nonwords.

3. Does the task target a specific level (or levels) of speech processing? If so, which level/s are targeted?
In order to point to the appropriate toy in this task, Imogen had to compare and differentiate between nonwords beginning with /s/ and /st/. Therefore she needed to hear the speech and compare the sound patterns of each whole stimulus. She did not need to recognize non-English sound types or phonetic sequences and therefore phonetic discrimination was not involved. As discussed in the answer to Question 1, she did not have to compare the stimuli to words in her lexicon, so phonological representations were not necessarily involved. The level of processing targeted in this task was phonological recognition. This involves the process of recognizing English phonological patterns.

4.   Metaphonological skills
4(a) Does the child have to reflect on his/her speech production?
No speech production was required for this task.

4(b) Does the child have to show awareness of the internal structure of phonological representations or of spoken stimuli?
As discussed under Question 3, Imogen could have completed this task by comparing the sound patterns of each whole stimulus. She did not have to segment any of the nonwords to achieve success in the task.

4(c) Does the child have to manipulate phonological units?
No again, as no speech production was required.

5. *What demands are made on the child's memory in order to make responses during the task?*
Imogen had to hold an item consisting of three monosyllabic stimuli in her working memory in order to make the comparisons necessary to complete the task.

6. *What are the task demands? Can all or parts of the task be demonstrated?*
For this task Imogen had to understand that the toys 'say' the stimuli. Most of the task can be demonstrated clearly. Demands on vocabulary and grammar comprehension are minimal.

7. *Is any technique being used to support the child with the task? If so, how is the technique providing support?*
The materials helped to motivate Imogen to complete the task, but no technique was used to support the speech processing skills being targeted.

Effects of changing the task

Referring to Question 1, if the stimuli are real words Imogen could still complete the task successfully without accessing her lexicon. However, for all the words she knows, she would have the possibility of accessing her representations and so would be much more likely to do so. As phonological representations are not essential to complete the task, it would still be targeting phonological recognition (Question 3). The answers to the other questions would remain the same. Therefore, by changing one of the materials (the spoken stimuli), from nonwords to real words, Imogen would be more likely to use her representations to complete the task.

ACTIVITY 3.5

Aims:
1. To analyse the psycholinguistic properties of a task using the task analysis questions.
2. To identify how the task's psycholinguistic properties change if one aspect of it is changed.

Read through the description of the task.
Answer all the task analysis questions presented in Figure 3.1.

Note the change to the task, and the effects of the change on the psycholinguistic properties of the task.

Task 3.5

The following task, taken from the *Nuffield Dyspraxia Programme (NDP)* (Connery, 1992), was presented to Alex when he was 6 years of age:

Materials: A set of cards as depicted in Figure 3.4. The pictures below the written words are symbols used in the *NDP*; they represent the consonants at the beginning of each syllable of the target word in the picture above the written word. For example, under the picture of BARBECUE, the picture of the BALL represents /b/ to cue the onset of the first two syllables (BAR-BE) and the picture of the CAMERA represents /k/ to cue the onset of the third syllable (-CUE). These symbols had been used in previous sessions with Alex. He could easily produce the consonants in isolation when he saw the symbols and could also use them to remind himself to say CVC words such as BALL and BIKE. The words on the cards were known to Alex, but when he attempted to say them in spontaneous conversation, he often misarticulated them (e.g. CARDIGAN was realized as "gardidan" ['gɑdɪdən].

Procedure: The cards were placed face down in front of Alex. He was asked to turn each one over in turn and name the picture. He was encouraged to use the symbols to help him articulate the consonants in the right order.

Feedback: Alex was encouraged to use the symbols to make as many attempts at the word as he wished until he produced a version that he thought was correct. If this version was correct, he was rewarded verbally. If he misarticulated the word, e.g. realized MOTORBIKE as ['məʊtəkaɪʔ], the therapist said 'You need to try that one again', and encouraged him to pay more attention to the symbols and their order when she repeated the word. The therapist allowed Alex to produce the word several times in this way. If he articulated it correctly after a few more attempts he was rewarded verbally, and if he persisted in having difficulty the therapist asked him to move on to the next card.

Change to Task 3.5

If Alex misarticulated the word, the therapist would produce the correct version of the word for him to imitate. If Alex's imitation was incorrect, the therapist would model the word again. If he produced several consecutive incorrect repetitions, the therapist would ask him to move on to the next card.

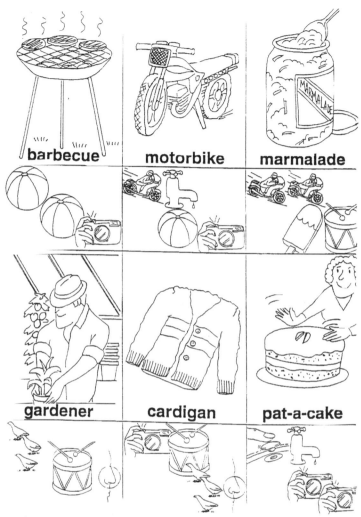

Figure 3.4: Pictures for task with Alex from Nuffield Dyspraxia Programme (Connery, 1992).

Check your answer against the Key to Activity 3.5 at the end of this chapter and then read the following.

---

1. Does the child have to use his/her lexical representations to complete the task? If not, how likely is it that representations may be accessed?

As Alex was naming pictures he had to access his own representations.

2. Does the task target the input channel, the output channel or both?

As no spoken models were provided, the task was targeting output only.

3. Does the task target a specific level (or levels) of speech processing? If so, which level/s are targeted?

Alex could already use the symbols to help him articulate CV and CVC words accurately and consistently. Therefore it was assumed that he did not have difficulty with the motor execution of the consonants represented by the symbols in simple contexts. It was also presumed that Alex had accurate phonological representations of these longer words and so could discriminate between his incorrect productions and the correct versions in an auditory lexical task, and that he had accurate semantic representations of the words. This task helped him to articulate words that he often mispronounced, despite having the individual consonants and vowels in his repertoire of sounds. Therefore the task was targeting Alex's motor programs for these words, as they were inaccurate or unstable. It was also targeting motor programming skills, as Alex needed to use these to revise an inaccurate program and construct a more accurate one. Using the symbols to remind himself about the correct sequence of consonants in a word and practising its correct production many times helped him to establish a more accurate and stable motor program for the word.

4. Metaphonological skills
4(a). Does the child have to reflect on his/her speech production?
If Alex misarticulated a word, he usually realized that he needed to make another attempt. If he did not display this awareness, then the therapist encouraged him to reflect on his speech production by telling him that he would need to say the word again.

4(b). Does the child have to show awareness of the internal structure of phonological representations or of spoken stimuli?
In order to revise a misarticulated word by making use of symbols, Alex had to have some awareness of how the word was structured.

4(c). If so, what kind of segmentation is required?
Awareness of onsets would not be adequate for this task as Alex had to use symbols to remind himself about syllable-final consonants as well as syllable-initial consonants. More detailed phoneme segmentation was therefore required.

4(d). Does the child have to manipulate phonological units?
Using symbols to remind himself to use particular consonants in a particular order was evidence of Alex manipulating phonological units.

5. What demands are made on the child's memory in order to make responses during the task?
Each response involved looking at one picture, accessing representations

for the appropriate word and articulating it. Therefore minimal demands were made on Alex's memory.

6. *What are the task demands? Can all or parts of the task be demonstrated?*

When naming pictures, Alex had to remember to use the symbols to guide his articulation. He had already learnt which consonants they represent and therefore he did not need to remember these associations. He had to remember to turn over the next card when he had successfully named the previous one. This aspect of the task could easily be demonstrated.

7. *Is any technique being used to support the child with the task? If so, how is the technique providing support?*

The *NDP* symbols were used as a technique to help Alex revise his motor programs. The symbols, which were already familiar to him, reminded him which consonants he had to produce and their correct sequence. They were a support for his motor programming skills when he needed to produce a more accurate version of the word.

Effects of changing the task

If Alex correctly named the picture on his first attempt, the psycholinguistic properties of the task would remain the same. However, if he failed to do this and then imitated the spoken model, he would have the possibility of bypassing the lexical route. If he did this, he would still be using motor programming skills but would not be referring to his motor programs, which are stored in his lexicon. Also, if he relied heavily on the spoken models, he would be less likely to use the symbols to help him construct a revised motor program. Therefore this change to the feedback given would alter the psycholinguistic properties of the task.

ACTIVITY 3.6

Aims:
1. To analyse the psycholinguistic properties of a task using the task analysis questions.
2. To identify how the task's psycholinguistic properties change if one aspect of it is changed.

Read through the details of the task.
Answer all the task analysis questions presented in Figure 3.1.
Note the change to the task, and the effects of the change on the psycholinguistic properties of the task.

Task 3.6

The following task was presented to Jade when she was 8 years of age:
Materials: A set of plastic letters.

Procedure: Plastic letters that spell the rime OCK were placed in the
correct order in front of Jade. The following letters were placed above
the rime in a semi-circle in the order indicated: ‹b, l, g, r, s, y› (see Figure
3.5). Jade was asked to place each of these letters in turn in front of the
rime OCK. Each time a letter was joined to the rime she had to read the
pattern aloud and answer the question 'Is that a real word?'. If the
answer was 'yes' she was asked to describe the meaning of the word.

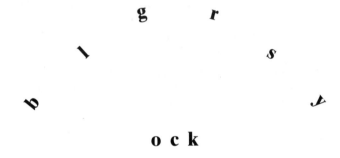

Figure 3.5: Arangement of plastic letters for task with Jade.

Feedback: If Jade read the joined letters accurately, made the correct
decision about whether they formed a real word and defined the real
word adequately, she was rewarded verbally. If she misread the letters,
the teacher encouraged her to sound out the onset and rime separately
and then blend them together. If this failed as a strategy to help Jade
read the stimulus accurately, the teacher blended the onset and rime as
a model for her to imitate. If she identified a nonword, such as BOCK, as
a real word she was asked to explain its meaning. At this point she
sometimes realized that the word had no meaning. If Jade offered a
meaning to another word, such as 'thing you use for building', the
teacher tried to suggest another word that matched this meaning, such
as BLOCK, pointing out that that word is said and spelt differently. If Jade
identified a word as a nonword, such as LOCK, the teacher checked to
see if the word was known to her. If it was not, he taught her about the
word, using strategies such as drawing and offering definitions and
examples of how the word is used.

Change to Task 3.6

When Jade had read aloud the group of letters she would *not* be asked
'Is that a real word?'. If she had difficulty with reading, the teacher

would provide the feedback in the same way but there would be no discussion about word meaning.

Check your answer against the Key to Activity 3.6 at the end of this chapter and then read the following.

---

1. Does the child have to use his/her lexical representations to complete the task? If not, how likely is it that representations may be accessed?
In order to recognize whether the combination of the onset and rime made a real word Jade had to access her lexical representations.

2. Does the task target the input channel, the output channel or both?
The teacher did not provide any spoken models before Jade made a judgement about whether the letters formed a real word. Therefore Jade could successfully complete the task without processing speech input.

3. Does the task target a specific level (or levels) of speech processing? If so, which level/s are targeted?
In order to judge whether the letters form a real word, Jade had to match the orthographic patterns of the onset and the rime with their phonological patterns, join these phonological segments together and compare this whole to phonological representations of words in her lexicon. Therefore, in terms of speech processing, the task was targeting her ability to access phonological representations and their internal structures.

4. Metaphonological skills
4(a). Does the child have to reflect on his/her speech production?
Although Jade did not have to judge the accuracy of her articulation, she did have to decide whether the spoken syllable was a real word.

4(b). Does the child have to show awareness of the internal structure of phonological representations or of spoken stimuli?
As stated in answer to Question 3, Jade had to access segments of her phonological representations.

4(c). If so, what kind of segmentation is required?
The orthographic patterns corresponded to onset and rime, so Jade had to be aware of how some of her phonological representations are segmented into onset and rime.

4(d). Does the child have to manipulate phonological units?

Even though Jade was physically manipulating the plastic letters, each group of letters had to be read only once. She did not have to manipulate the phonological patterns of each letter group in order to complete the task successfully.

5. *What demands are made on the child's memory in order to make responses during the task?*
The task required one syllable to be held in working memory while Jade made a judgement on it.

6. *What are the task demands? Can all or parts of the task be demonstrated?*
The first parts of this task could be demonstrated physically. Jade had to understand the concept of a 'real word' in order to respond to the last part of the task.

7. *Is any technique being used to support the child with the task? If so, how is the technique providing support?*
In this task, the plastic letters were primarily being used to help Jade link orthographic and phonological patterns rather than to support speech processing on its own. However, these visual stimuli may have helped Jade to segment her phonological representations into onsets and rimes.

Effects of changing the task

If Jade were no longer required to decide whether or not a word is real, she would still have to match orthographic patterns with phonological patterns, but would not have to compare any of the separate phonological patterns to words that she has already stored in her lexicon. Therefore this change to the procedure would alter the psycholinguistic nature of the task in an important way.

Summary

This chapter has provided a set of task analysis questions that provide a structured format for examining the psycholinguistic properties of intervention tasks. Each question has been explained and the full set of questions has been answered in relation to three different tasks. For each task, the effect of changing one aspect of either the materials, procedure or feedback has been examined. The purpose of analysing and discussing how the various aspects of a task are related to psycholinguistic properties is to help the reader to select and modify tasks that will target intervention aims for a particular child.

- Principles of the psycholinguistic framework can be used to analyse intervention tasks in the same way as assessment tasks were analysed in Book 1 (see Chapters 2 and 3).
- There are no specially designed materials for 'psycholinguistic intervention'; almost all teaching and therapy material can be used in a psycholinguistic way.
- An intervention task comprises materials, a procedure, feedback and ± technique(s).
- The psycholinguistic nature of a task is changed if any one or more of these components are changed.
- Answering the task analysis questions presented in Figure 3.1 reveal the demands a task makes on a child's processing system.
- Recognizing the demands made by a task in this way helps the teacher/therapist to modify the task appropriately in the light of a child's response, i.e. make it easier or more challenging.
- Psycholinguistic analysis of tasks facilitates principled intervention.

KEY TO ACTIVITY 3.1

The speech processing skills being targeted specifically in the task with Marcio are:

(a) motor programming, and
(b) making links between updated motor programs and their semantic representations.

KEY TO ACTIVITY 3.2

Task A with Jimmy
Q4(a). Does the child have to reflect on his/her speech production?
A: Yes.

Q4(b). Does the child have to show awareness of the internal structure of phonological representations/spoken stimuli?
A: Yes.

Q4(c). If yes, what kind of segmentation is required?
A: onset/rime.

Task B with Suzie
Q4(a). Does the child have to reflect on his/her speech production?
A: Yes.

Q4(b). Does the child have to show awareness of the internal structure of phonological representations/spoken stimuli?

A: No.

Therefore, only Task A requires segmentation.

KEY TO ACTIVITY 3.3

Task A with Philip and Task B with Adam are targeting phonological recognition.
Task A makes more demand on working memory than Task B; Philip has to hold one more item in his working memory compared to Adam.

KEY TO ACTIVITY 3.4

Task presented to Imogen (CA 5;0)

Q1. Does the child have to use his/her lexical representations to complete the task? If not, how likely is it that representations may be accessed?

A: No. May access representations if comparing nonwords to words.

Q2. Does the task target the input channel, the output channel or both?

A: Input.

Q3. Does the task target a specific level (or levels) of speech processing? If so, which level/s are targeted?

A: Phonological recognition.

4.   Metaphonological skills
Q4(a). Does the child have to reflect on his/her speech production?
A: No.

Q4(b). Does the child have to show awareness of the internal structure of phonological representations or of spoken stimuli?
A: No.

Q4(c). Does the child have to manipulate phonological units?
A: No.

Q5. What demands are made on the child's memory in order to make responses during the task?
A: Holding three one-syllable stimuli in working memory.

Q6. What are the task demands? Can all or parts of the task be demonstrated?
A: Appreciating symbolism and using imagination. Most of the task can be demonstrated.

Q7. Is any technique being used to support the child with the task? If so, how is the technique providing support?
A: No.

Effects of changing the task
More likely to use her phonological representations to complete the task.

KEY TO ACTIVITY 3.5

Task presented to Alex (CA: 6;0)
Q1. Does the child have to use his/her lexical representations to complete the task? If not, how likely is it that representations may be accessed?
A: Yes.

Q2. Does the task target the input channel, the output channel or both?
A: Output.

Q3. Does the task target a specific level (or levels) of speech processing? If so, which level/s are targeted?
A: Motor programs; motor programming.

4. Metaphonological skills
Q4(a). Does the child have to reflect on his/her speech production?
A: Yes.

Q4(b). Does the child have to show awareness of the internal structure of phonological representations or of spoken stimuli?
A: Yes.

Q4(c). If so, what kind of segmentation is required?
A: Phoneme segmentation.

Q4(d). Does the child have to manipulate phonological units?
A: Yes.

Q5. What demands are made on the child's memory in order to make responses during the task?
A: Minimal demands.

*Q6. What are the task demands? Can all or parts of the task be demon-
strated?*
A: Remembering to use symbols; remembering to turn over next card.
Task can be demonstrated.

*Q7. Is any technique being used to support the child with the task? If
so, how is the technique providing support?*
A: The *NDP* symbols.

Effects of changing the task
By providing a spoken model, the task can be completed without
accessing the lexical representations.

KEY TO ACTIVITY 3.6

Task presented to Jade (CA 8;0)

*Q1. Does the child have to use his/her lexical representations to
complete the task? If not, how likely is it that representations may
be accessed?*
A: Yes.

Q2. Does the task target the input channel, the output channel or both?
A: Output.

*Q3. Does the task target a specific level (or levels) of speech processing?
If so, which level/s are targeted?*
A: Accessing phonological representations and their internal structure.

4. Metaphonological skills
Q4(a). Does the child have to reflect on his/ her speech production?
A: Yes.

*Q4(b). Does the child have to show awareness of the internal structure
of phonological representations or of spoken stimuli?*
A: Yes.

Q4(c). If so, what kind of segmentation is required?
A: Onset-rime.

Q4(d). Does the child have to manipulate phonological units?
A: No.

Q5. What demands are made on the child's memory in order to make responses during the task?
A: Holding one syllable in working memory.

Q6. What are the task demands? Can all or parts of the task be demonstrated?
A: Understanding the concept of a real word. The first part of the task can be demonstrated.

Q7. Is any technique being used to support the child with the task? If so, how is the technique providing support?
A: Yes.

Effects of changing the task
Jade would not need to access her lexicon.

Chapter 4
From Profile to
Programme: Steps 1–2

JULIETTE CORRIN

A professional encounter with a single child can sometimes prove revolutionary; and so it was with Anna. It was her case that set our speech and language therapy department on the road to psycholinguistic practice with children with speech disorders. Furthermore, it was by grappling with her case that I discovered a meeting point between research and clinical practice. This chapter and the one that follows offer a practical guide to bridging the gap between assessment and intervention: the Profile to Programme methodology. The steps involved will be illustrated through a case study.

Anna

At CA 3;2, Anna was referred by her local speech and language therapist to the Nuffield Hearing and Speech Centre in London. She presented as a sociable child who was comprehending language well, beginning to produce two-word combinations, but whose speech was grossly unintelligible. She had a husky, poorly co-ordinated voice stream, a highly reduced range of consonants and vowels, and a pattern of consonant omission and glottal stop substitution. A programme of intervention began at CA 3;11 based on the diagnostic hypothesis of oral and speech dyspraxia. The aim was to build foundation skills in breath control, voice production, oral movements, speech discrimination and motor patterns for consonant and vowel production. Progress was slow and by CA 4;8 it was evident that Anna's speech difficulties would have educational implications. Furthermore, assessment by our occupational therapist revealed that Anna was experiencing sensori-motor integration difficulties; her dyspraxic difficulties seemed widespread. It was also evident that her language skills had reached a plateau and were a further area of risk. After a formal application, her special educational needs were officially recognized by her education authority and from the age of 6 years she received extra learning support in her mainstream class. Intervention had continued throughout this time, but Anna's increasing overlay of behaviour difficulties obstructed the programme. Both in school and in clinic sessions, Anna was now a girl who had adopted the role of clown as a

96

strategy for task avoidance, with laughter easily spilling over into aggression.

My own involvement with Anna began at CA 7;4. Clearly she had come a long way, albeit slowly. Her speech was now mainly intelligible. She was able to make herself understood in the school playground and compensated for her difficulties by being a social extrovert. The following sentences give an idea of the stage she had reached:

Target	Response
THE HAMBURGER IS TASTY	The hamburger is ['seɪtsɪ]
THE KITCHEN IS TIDY	The [ṣɪʔ.kɪsn̩] is tidy
THE HELICOPTER IS RESCUING THE CLOWN	The ['hɛlɪklɒkə] is ['ɹɛṣɪn] the clown

Further intervention was obviously required, but in addition to the remaining articulatory errors there was a further cause for concern. It was apparent that Anna's difficult behaviour was not purely a response to her speech impairment. In the classroom, she was experiencing increasing difficulties with language-based activities and the development of literacy skills; spelling was a particular problem. Clearly, a fresh perspective on Anna's problem was necessary – a psycholinguistic perspective that would identify the underlying pattern of processing strengths and weaknesses.

Anna completed a battery of psycholinguistic speech processing tasks. Table 4.1 summarizes results from the speech and language assessments that were administered when Anna was CA 7;7. It is presented here as background information and to indicate the widespread nature of her spoken language difficulties. Anna's performance on the *Wechsler Intelligence Scale for Children* (Wechsler, 1992) revealed that her cognitive abilities fell within the lower average range. Although there was no significant overall difference in her verbal and performance results, there was significant subtest variation, suggestive of specific learning deficits.

From Profile to Programme

The Profile to Programme (P→P) process is directly derived from the psycholinguistic framework for children's speech and literacy difficulties presented in Book 1 (Stackhouse and Wells, 1997), summarized in Chapter 1 of this volume. One of the key concepts behind the P→P process is that the speech processing profile is central not just to your assessment of a child, but also to the child's intervention programme. It forms the hub of the clinical process, as Figure 4.1 illustrates.

Table 4.1: Results of Anna's speech and language test battery at CA 7;7 years, showing raw score and age equivalence results, and standard scores where these are relevant

Name of test	Raw score	Standard score	Age equivalent
Verbal comprehension: *Test for Reception of Grammar* (Bishop, 1989)	12		5;7
Receptive vocabulary: *British Picture Vocabulary Scales* (Dunn, Dunn, Whetton, et al., 1982)	39	66	3;11–4;9
Expressive Language: *Renfrew Action Picture Test, Information*	35		7;0–7;5
Renfrew Action Picture Test, Grammar (Renfrew, 1989)	18		3;6–3;11
Renfrew Bus Story, Information	25		5;5
Renfrew Bus Story, Mean Length of Utterance (Renfrew, 1991)	8		4;1–5;0
Speech Discrimination: *Auditory Discrimination and Attention Test* (MorganBarry, 1988)	12	–2.2	
Speech production: *The Edinburgh Articulation Test* (Anthony, Bogle, Ingram, et al., 1971)	29	< 53	<3;3
Literacy: *Carver Word Recognition Test* (Carver, 1970)	25		5;6
Auditory memory: *Illinois Test of Psycholinguistic Abilities, Auditory Sequential Memory* (Kirk, McCarthy and Kirk, 1968)	21	30	5;8

The psycholinguistic framework is here taken to include both the speech processing profile (Appendix 1, this volume) and the model (Appendix 2, this volume) from Book 1. It is shown as the centre of a figure of eight. The top sphere represents assessment and the bottom sphere intervention. The sequence of arrows indicates that assessment and intervention are linked clinical processes, both of which originate from and refer back to the psycholinguistic framework. The P→P process offers six practical steps towards an intervention programme. Step One and Step Two focus on analysis of assessment results, first at a macro level of detail and then at a micro level of detail. Step Three and Step Four focus on intervention planning. Step Five sees the intervention plan put into action. Finally, Step Six analyses the outcome of intervention, and brings the process full cycle.

In this chapter we take up the story when Anna has completed a battery of speech processing tasks which stemmed from the psycholinguistic framework. We shall consider in turn each step in Figure 4.1, structuring our thinking about Anna's intervention programme by means of a set of questions. Steps One and Two are covered in this chapter, the remaining steps in the next chapter.

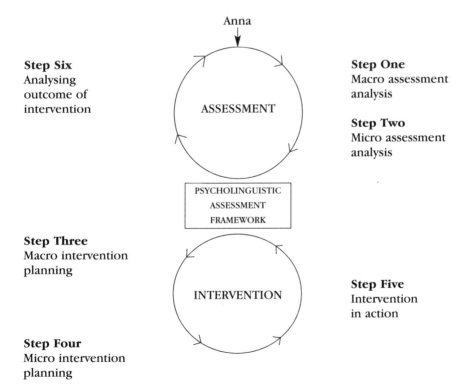

Figure 4.1: The Profile to Programme (P→P) process, showing the psycholinguistic framework as the hub of both assessment and intervention.

Step One: Macro Assessment Analysis

Question 1: Which levels of the psycholinguistic framework have been assessed?

This question invites the therapist/teacher to draw together all the measures that have been administered and pinpoint them on the speech processing profile. You may have set about the assessment with a psycholinguistic approach in mind from the outset, or perhaps be applying it retrospectively. It does not matter: the essence of the psycholinguistic approach is how you think about the tasks you have administered rather than what you administered. The correspondences between tasks and questions on the speech processing profile are discussed extensively in Book 1, Chapters 2 and 3. Figure 4.2 provides a summary of those correspondences, and can be used as a guide for pinpointing the level of processing to which a particular task corresponds.

In order to ascertain which levels of the psycholinguistic framework have been assessed, it is helpful to start with a written list of the tasks that the child has completed. Here the term 'task' is used to cover any test measure, whether informal or formal (see Chapter 3, this volume). Alongside the task name, it is useful to write down key features that characterize the task design. These would include consideration of processing channel (e.g. input or output); modality of stimulus presentation (e.g. visual, auditory) and of response (e.g. silent, spoken); type

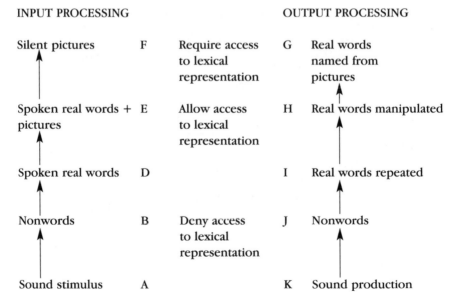

Figure 4.2: Quick search guide for pinpointing the levels of processing to which tasks correspond on the speech processing profile (Book 1).

of linguistic stimulus (e.g. word, nonword, sentence); instructions given, and so forth. This helps to identify the level on the speech processing profile to which the task corresponds. Table 4.2 illustrates this format by presenting the battery of speech processing tasks administered to Anna.

ACTIVITY 4.1

Aim: To identify which levels of the psycholinguistic assessment framework have been tapped by the tasks administered in Anna's speech processing battery.

For this exercise you will need to refer to Anna's task battery provided in Table 4.2 and to the blank speech processing profile from Book 1, reproduced as Figure 4.3.

(a) Identify the level on the profile to which each of the listed tasks corresponds, by referring to Figure 4.2. Write the letter of the corresponding question in the blank column provided in Table 4.2. Those readers not familiar with the speech processing profile are advised to refer to Book 1, which explains its structure and rationale. Examples of tests for each question are given in Book 1 Appendix 2.

(b) Transfer this information by circling the letter at the appropriate level on the speech processing profile (Figure 4.3).

Check your responses with Key to Activity 4.1 at the end of this chapter, then read the following.

The rationale for assigning speech processing tasks to particular levels of the speech processing profile is covered in detail in Book 1, and will not be repeated here. At this point we shall simply check through the list and highlight a quick method for doing this activity, using Figure 4.2. We shall start with the input channel. The first search is for any task that has used a nonlinguistic stimulus. Here, you will have noted Anna's pure tone hearing test under level A. The second search is for any task using nonword stimuli; these are automatically grouped under level B, regardless of other task design features. Here, you will have noted tasks of rhyme judgement, rhyme detection and auditory discrimination. The third search is for any task using spoken real word stimuli without pictures. These will be under level D and here you will have noted further tasks of rhyme judgement, rhyme

Table 4.2: Anna's battery of speech processing assessment tasks at CA 7;7

Task name	Stimulus modality	Stimulus type	Channel tested	Processing level
Naming	Picture	1 word	Output	
Rhyme production	Spoken target	1 word	Output	
Rhyme judgement (AB)	Silent pictures	2 words	Input	
Rhyme judgement (AB)	Spoken	2 words	Input	
Rhyme judgement (AB)	Spoken	2 nonwords	Input	
Rhyme detection (ABX: match X to A or B)	Silent pictures	3 words	Input	
Rhyme detection (ABX: match X to A or B)	Spoken	3 words	Input	
Rhyme detection	Spoken	3 nonwords	Input	
Auditory discrimination (AB: same – different)	Spoken	2 words	Input	
Auditory discrimination (AB: same – different)	Spoken	2 nonwords	Input	
Auditory discrimination (ABX: match X to A or B)	Spoken	3 nonwords	Input	
Auditory lexical decision (yes/no word-to-picture match)	Spoken + picture	1 word	Input	
Speech repetition	Spoken + picture	1 sentence	Output	
Speech repetition	Spoken	1 word	Output	
Speech repetition	Spoken	1 nonword	Output	
Single sound repetition	Spoken	1 consonant or vowel	Output	
Hearing test	Electronic signal	Pure tone	Input	
Correction of own spontaneous speech	—	—	Feedback + self-monitoring	

SPEECH PROCESSING PROFILE

Name   Comments:

Age

Date

Profiler

INPUT	OUTPUT

F

Is the child aware of the internal structure of phonological representations?

G

Can the child access accurate motor programs?

E

Are the child's phonological representations accurate?

H

Can the child manipulate phonological units?

D

Can the child discriminate between real words?

I

Can the child articulate real words accurately?

C

Does the child have language-specific representations of word structures?

J

Can the child articulate speech without reference to lexical representations?

B

Can the child discriminate speech sounds without reference to lexical representations?

A

Does the child have adequate auditory perception?

K

Does the child have adequate sound production skills?

L

Does the child reject his/her own erroneous forms?

Figure 4.3: Blank speech processing profile for Activity 4.1.

detection and auditory discrimination. The fourth search is for any task using spoken word stimuli plus pictures. These will be grouped under level E since they allow the child to access lexical representations. This corresponds to the detection of speech errors, in the auditory lexical decision task in Anna's battery (Table 4.2). Lastly, search for any task using silent picture stimuli (no speech). These are automatically assigned to level F on the framework.

Now we shall do the same for the output channel. The first search is for any task involving oral movement or sound production (but not word production), at level K. Here, you will have single sound repetition. The second search is for any task requiring nonword production. These are always grouped under level J and in Anna's case there is one nonword repetition task to be noted. Above this processing level, all stimuli use real words. The focus of the third search, then, is for production by repetition. Under level I, you should have noted both word and sentence repetition. The focus of the fourth search leapfrogs up to level G: any task involving production by picture naming is always at level G. Anna did one task at this level. Now, by default, you should be left with output tasks at level H: those involving production by manipulation of phonological units. Here, you will have noted Anna's rhyme production task.

What you have now achieved is a visual summary of Anna's task battery portrayed on the speech processing profile, i.e. you have grouped the tasks in terms of the processing demands they made on her. This visual display invites you to check on the completeness of your assessment profile to date. In Anna's case, you can now see that all levels except C have been assessed, and that more than one task has been administered at some levels. Completeness is a privilege rarely afforded to us in clinical life; in reality, a profile like this will be built up gradually over time; but it is an aim worth striving for, because a reasonably complete profile generates clear hypotheses which can lead to effective intervention.

Question 2: In comparison to other children, which levels show processing breakdown and to what extent?

This question addresses the external comparison between a child's performance and that of their peer group. We need to know which of Anna's task results were clinically significant, indicating the need for intervention. Tables 4.3 (input) and 4.4 (output) present her z-scores based on a chronological age–peer comparison. For the moment, we can ignore the detailed breakdown of scores at each level in Tables 4.3 and 4.4; the aim at this point is a macro view of her overall performance. In the tables this is represented by the bold average scores, where a minus score indicates the extent to which her performance is out of alignment with her peer group.

Table 4.3: Anna's speech processing performance at CA 7;7 years compared to normally developing 7-year-olds. Scores of < –1.5 are significant. Scores of <–3.0 are highly significant. Scores in bold print show averaged percentages or averaged z-scores.

Input tasks	Controls mean score	Anna's raw score	Raw score percentage	z-score
Level F:				
Rhyme detection – silent/picture				
AB	11.7	12/12	100	0.64
ABX	11.9	9/12	75	–9.35
			87.5	**–4.9**
Level E:				
Detection of speech 'errors'/lexical decision				
One-syllable words	38.2	37/40	92	–0.74
Two-syllable words	38.8	31/40	77	–6.96
Three-syllable words	37.6	31/40	77	–4.35
			82	**–4.0**
Level D:				
Rhyme detection (ABX)	11.9	9/12	75	–1.63
Rhyme judgement (AB)	11.9	9/12	75	–9.35
Discrimination of real words				
Consonant sequence contrast	8.8	4/9	44	–12.0
Consonant feature contrast	8.8	8/9	88	–1.77
			70	**–6.2**
Level B:				
Discrimination complex nonwords				
Consonant sequence contrast	8.6	3/9	33	–11.43
Consonant feature contrast	9	2/9	22	(off-scale)
Discrimination nonwords ABX				
One-syllable	17.5	16/20	80	–0.81
Two-syllable	17.95	15/20	75	–1.69
Three-syllables	16.85	10/20	50	–3.7
Rhyme judgement nonwords	11.8	8/12	66	–7.31
Rhyme detection nonwords	11.2	10/12	83	–1.2
			58	**–5.3**

This information has been transferred to the speech processing profile shown in Figure 4.4. As suggested in Book 1, a system of ticks and crosses has been used to rank her z-scores. Informal data were available for levels K and L and this has been added in on the basis of my clinical impressions. Her audiometry results are reflected at level A. Overall, the profile shows extensive processing breakdown in relation to her peer

Table 4.4: Anna's speech processing performance at CA 7;7. years compared to normally developing 7-year-olds. Scores of < –1.5 are significant. Scores of < –3.0 are highly significant. Percentages in bold print are averages at each processing level. z-scores in bold print show z-scores derived from raw score totals. The shaded test scores are not included in calculations, being the only sentence-based task within the battery.

Output tasks	Controls mean score	Anna's raw score	Raw score percentage	z-score
Level G:				
Naming pictures				
One-syllable	18.8	10/20	50	–10.38
Two-syllable	18.45	7/20	35	–8.9
Three-syllable	17.1	5/20	25	–5.13
Total	54.35	22/60	**36.6**	**–8.38**
Level H:				
Rhyme production	11.4	0	0	**(off-scale)**
Level I:				
Real word repetition				
One-syllable	18.4	10/20	50	–9.77
Two-syllable	17.85	8/20	40	–8.16
Three-syllable	17.8	9/20	45	–3.41
Total	54.05	27/60	**45**	**–9.17**
Sentence repetition:				
One-syllable target words	18.8	9/20	45	–9.51
Two-syllable target words	18.3	6/20	30	–10.34
Three-syllable target words	17.6	4/20	20	–5.89
Total	54.7	19/60	32	–8.21
Level J:				
Nonword repetition				
One-syllable	16.2	10/20	50	–3.39
Two-syllable	17.05	8/20	40	–4.95
Three-syllable	15.95	7/20	35	–4.1
Total	49.2	25/60	**41**	**–5.29**

group; the z-scores clearly indicate the extent of her difficulty and justify Anna as a high priority therapy candidate. It is sobering to reflect that this is the picture of a girl who had achieved broadly intelligible speech after years of therapy. According to her mother, staff at school and family friends questioned her need for further help, saying, 'She seems to talk OK'. Here we see what trouble there was beneath the surface.

SPEECH PROCESSING PROFILE

Name   Anna

Age   7;7

Date

Profiler

Comments:

Key :   • normal range: +1.5 to –1.5 (✓)
        • mild: <–1.5 (×)
        • mild-to-moderate: <–2.5 (××)
        • moderate: <–3.5 (×××)
        • moderate–severe: < –5.5 (××××)
        • severe: < –7.5 (×××××)

INPUT

F

Is the child aware of the internal structure of phonological representations?

| × × × | (–4.9) |

E

Are the child's phonological representations accurate?

| × × × | (–4.0) |

D

Can the child discriminate between real words?

| × × × × | (–6.2) |

C

Does the child have language-specific representations of word structures?

No data

B

Can the child discriminate speech sounds without reference to lexical representations?

| × × × | (–5.3) |

A

Does the child have adequate auditory perception?

| (Medical records) | ✓ |

OUTPUT

G

Can the child access accurate motor programs?

| × × × × × | (–8.38) |

H

Can the child manipulate phonological units?

| × × × × × | (off scale) |

I

Can the child articulate real words accurately?

| × × × × × | (–9.17) |

J

Can the child articulate speech without reference to lexical representations?

| × × × | (–5.29) |

K

Does the child have adequate sound production skills?

| (Clinical impression) | × × |

L

Does the child reject his/her own erroneous forms?

Figure 4.4: Anna's speech processing profile with *z*-scores.

A macro profile such as this allows one to look at the pattern of performance from several points of view. For example, one can make a first scan for balance of performance between input and output channels of processing. This may reveal that, taken overall, input skills are better than output skills, or vice versa. A second scan can be made to look for balance of performance between top-down and bottom-up processing. This may reveal that on either input or output sides of the profile, or both, the boxes higher up reveal a different pattern of perform-ance from those lower down. Ticks higher up indicate intact top-down processing of lexical and other linguistic information; while ticks lower down indicate intact peripheral processing of auditory input or motor output.

ACTIVITY 4.2

Aim: to analyse Anna's macro profile looking for patterns of perform-ance.

For this activity you need refer only to the macro profile of z-scores ranked by crosses in Figure 4.4.

Scan One: look at the balance of Anna's performance between the input and output channels of processing. Is there an obvious overall discrepancy?

Scan Two: look at the balance of Anna's performance between top-down and bottom-up levels of processing. Is there an obvious overall discrepancy in terms of the requirement to access lexical representa-tions (i.e. top levels)?

Check your responses with Key to Activity 4.2 at the end of this chapter, then read the following.

In Scan One, you will have noted that, in relation to her peer group, Anna's performance on the output side of the profile was more conspicu-ously impaired than on the input side of the profile. Three output levels – G, H and I – are ranked with five crosses, indicating a severe deficit, with z-scores of -7.5 or below. However, it was a clinical revelation to find that Anna had such extensive processing weaknesses on the input side of the profile too. Research in the 1970s and 1980s put the clinical emphasis squarely on output difficulties in children with developmental verbal dyspraxia. More recently, however, psycholinguistic research into cases like Anna's has highlighted the hidden input deficits of these children, with clear implications for change to our clinical practice.

In Scan Two, the input side shows no clear evidence of a top-down vs bottom-up split: Anna's performance at level D, real word auditory discrimination, is slightly more conspicuously impaired than other levels, both higher and lower. On the output side, there is some evidence that higher levels are particularly impaired: levels G, H and I show more crosses than the lower levels J or K. In relation to her peers, then, Anna was particularly poor at output tasks which required her to produce speech through reference to her stored lexical representations (levels G, H).

Finally, there is level L to consider: the external feedback link which makes the child's output become self-input. Here, Anna has been given a three-cross ranking on the grounds that she very rarely corrected her habitual articulation errors in spontaneous conversation, but had begun to do so at the level of single-word production on task. For example naming COMPUTER: "[kəmpu pətutə] – oh whatever!"

What we have learnt about Anna from normative comparison using z-scores

- In comparison to her peer group, Anna's speech processing skills range from being moderate to severely impaired and justify her as a priority therapy case, even though her speech is intelligible.
- Both input and output channels show pervasive impairment, with output processing being more severely affected.
- Output processing is more impaired on tasks involving her lexical representations.

These performance dissociations between and within input and output processing require further analysis before clinical hypotheses and therapy implications become clear.

Question 3: In an intra-personal comparison, which levels show comparative processing strength or weakness?

This question addresses the *internal* comparison of a child's perform-ance at different levels of processing, irrespective of how the child's performance compares to that of their peer group. Sometimes the technique of peer-group comparison can present a somewhat distorted picture of a child's profile of abilities. For example note how, at level D, Anna's rhyme detection and judgement tasks receive z-scores of -1.63 and -9.35 respectively. However, the raw score for both tasks was 75 per cent. Both are input tasks, tapping into the child's awareness of rhyme, and the response format for each task is a binary choice. In rhyme detection the child has to decide which of two test words the target word rhymes with; and in rhyme judgement, the child has to decide whether or not two words rhyme. A score of 75 per cent is above chance level, indicating that Anna has some understanding of each task. Thus, her raw scores indicate some competence on both tasks, in terms of her knowledge of what rhyme is about, and this information is clearly relevant for intervention planning. The great difference in z-scores reflects the fact that by 7 years of age, children with normally developing speech and language find the rhyme judgement task very easy, while the rhyme detection task still presents some challenges.

For these reasons, both z-scores and raw scores are important and provide complementary information for intervention planning. The importance of raw scores is that, where there is a strength/weakness disparity, we can apply an intervention strategy of working from strengths towards weakness. Anna's raw test scores, which appear in Tables 4.3 and 4.4 in the form of percentages, have been transferred to a further speech processing profile in Figure 4.5.

At this point, a third visual scan of the profile is recommended. Comparing top vs bottom processing is useful, but obviously a gross analysis of the profile. There is overlap in the processing demands of tasks at different levels of the profile and this necessitates a detailed teasing out of comparative performance. To take an extreme example, one could not conclude that poor performance on naming at level G was the result of difficulty with access to motor programs unless performance at lower levels was comparatively normal (cf. Book 1, pp.99–101). The reason for this is that processing demands at level G overlap with those at levels I, J and K. Table 4.5 presents an analysis of overlap between levels, which might be useful as a clinical guide.

The bold letters in the top row of Table 4.5 indicate the level of processing that the task is designed to test. This is marked with an × within the table. The italicized letters in the left column, and their corresponding dots, indicate other levels of processing that might be involved. Let us consider a task of real word repetition as an example. The designated level on the profile is I: *Can the child articulate real words accurately?*. There is major overlap with input levels, since the child has to hear and decode the word if s/he is to repeat it: level A (hearing); levels B and D (discrimination); possibly level E (accuracy of phonological representations). On the output side, there is overlap with lower levels, since in order to repeat the nonword accurately, the child needs to have intact motor skills: level J (motor programming) and level K (sound production).

As Table 4.5 shows, even though a task may be designed to test a discrete level of processing, execution of the task often involves the child in using other supporting levels as the task stimulus and response are routed through the processing system. Examination of the tasks

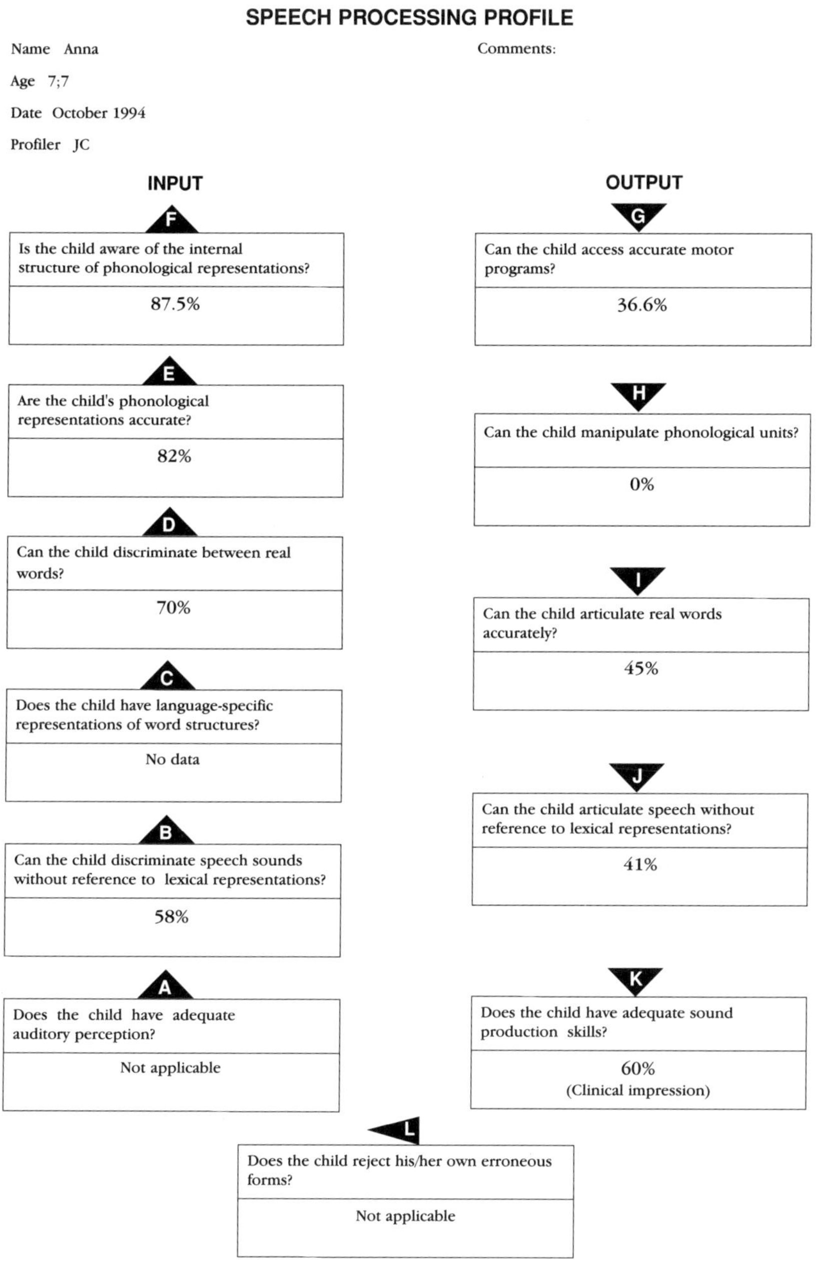

SPEECH PROCESSING PROFILE

Name Anna

Comments:

Age 7;7

Date October 1994

Profiler JC

INPUT

F

Is the child aware of the internal structure of phonological representations?

87.5%

E

Are the child's phonological representations accurate?

82%

D

Can the child discriminate between real words?

70%

C

Does the child have language-specific representations of word structures?

No data

B

Can the child discriminate speech sounds without reference to lexical representations?

58%

A

Does the child have adequate auditory perception?

Not applicable

OUTPUT

G

Can the child access accurate motor programs?

36.6%

H

Can the child manipulate phonological units?

0%

I

Can the child articulate real words accurately?

45%

J

Can the child articulate speech without reference to lexical representations?

41%

K

Does the child have adequate sound production skills?

60%
(Clinical impression)

L

Does the child reject his/her own erroneous forms?

Not applicable

Figure 4.5: Anna's speech processing profile: raw scores (expressed as percentages).

Table 4.5: Clinical guide to potential overlap between levels of processing, for tasks at each level.

	A	B	C	D	E	F	G	H	I	J	K	L
A	×											
B	•	×										
C	•	•	×									
D	•	•		×								
E	•	•		•	×							
F						×						
G							×		•	•	•	
H	•	•		•	•			×	•	•	•	
I	•	•		•	•				×	•	•	
J	•	•		•					•	×	•	
K	•	•							•		×	
L	•	•		•	•							×

Key: bold letters in the top row indicate the level of processing the task is designed to test, marked within the table by ×. The points that appear on the same line to the right and left of the designated ×, indicate other levels of processing that might be involved in performance of the task.

shows that they may have some levels of processing in common. The next analytic step is therefore to compare the child's performance on tasks that systematically include and exclude particular levels of processing. On the face of it, task overlap might seem an unfortunate complication, but in reality it is the very aspect of the speech processing profile that provides the opportunity to generate hypotheses, because it reveals patterns of dissociation in performance. One is working like a detective, solving a processing mystery! In fact, the more overlap there is, the more potentially revealing dissociations there are to tease apart.

We shall now apply this third scan to Anna's data, searching for dissociations between levels of processing. In each paragraph below, the implications arising from the comparative analysis are expressed in terms of the speech processing model from Book 1, reproduced here as Figure 4.6.

We shall take the *output* side of Anna's profile first:

Output: comparing level K with levels J, I and G

In Figure 4.5, the percentage score at level K is 60 per cent, based on clinical records rather than test results. Although Anna's control of nonspeech oral movements was now reasonable, she had a persisting difficulty in producing some single fricatives (e.g. /ʃ/) and affricates

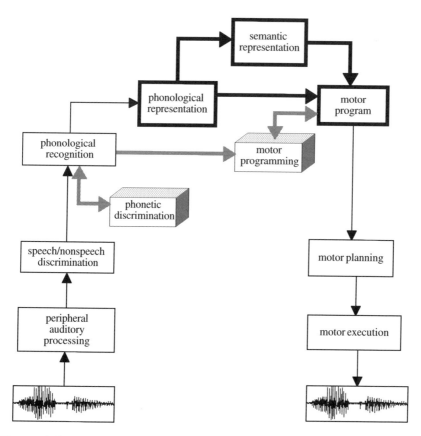

Figure 4.6: Speech processing model from Book 1 presented as a basis for interpreting performance dissociations between levels of processing.

(e.g. /tʃ/), and in co-ordinating contrasting sequences of consonants in diadochokinetic tasks, e.g. /f - s - l/. However, despite these residual difficulties, it appeared that her sound production skills were better than her word level production accuracy suggested. Her performance at higher levels of output, i.e. above level K, was certainly poorer: repetition of nonwords (level J: 41%, $z= -5.29$), repetition of real words (level I: 45%, $z= -9.17$) and naming (level G: 36.6%, $z= -8.38$).

In conclusion, although some difficulty with articulatory skill was evident, motor execution difficulties alone could not account for all of Anna's output difficulties.

Output: comparing level J with level I

In terms of z-scores, real word repetition at level I (45%, $z= -9.17$) was worse than nonword repetition at level J (41%, $z= -5.29$), though marginally better in terms of raw scores. In a normative study of children aged 3 to 7 years by Vance, Stackhouse and Wells (1995), summarized in Book 1 (p.46), the older children scored better on real word repetition than on nonword repetition, whereas the younger children performed similarly on both types of word. Given Anna's age, one might have expected a greater difference between her real word and nonword processing, in favour of real words, but in fact Anna's performance on one- and two-syllable words was virtually identical for both levels I and J. The 41 vs 45 per cent discrepancy came from three-syllable words, a point we shall discuss under Step Two of the P→P process.

In summary, there was little difference between Anna's real word and nonword repetition performance at levels I and J, in terms of raw scores. As the two tests are comparable in terms of procedures and scoring systems, it can be concluded that her performance on both is equally affected by pervasive output processing problems. This suggests two alternative hypotheses:

(a) on-line motor programming (for nonwords) and stored motor programs (potentially accessed for repeated real words) were equally impaired;
(b) Anna routed repetition of both real and nonwords through her motor programming system, which was impaired.

The lack of discrepancy between real and nonword processing that Anna showed is unusual in children aged 7 years. Taken together with her low scores for her age, on both tasks, this suggests that Anna was processing words like a younger child of 3 or 4 years of age.

Output: comparing level G with level I

Anna's performance on naming (level G, 36.6%) was worse than her performance on real word repetition (45%). For example, she named HOSPITAL as ['hɒspɪlt], but repeated it as ['hɒspəwɪlt], and named KANGAROO as [kæn'dʒ'ʷu], but repeated it as [kæŋgə'ɹu]. As discussed in Book 1, this dissociation can have a variety of different sources. The poorer result when Anna was forced to access the word from lexical representation (level G) could be a result of inaccurately stored phonological representations, incomplete stored motor programs, or poor links between either of these and her semantic representations.

To summarize, the pattern of associations and dissociations on output tasks suggests that in Anna's case incomplete stored motor programs were the predominant source of error, with inaccurate phonological representations being contributory. Her motor programming skills were comparatively stronger, i.e. under the real word repetition condition she was able to use the auditory information available from the adult model to override and update her pronunciation of words.

Now we shall consider the input side of Anna's profile through Activity 4.3 below.

ACTIVITY 4.3

Aim: to search for dissociations in performance between levels of input processing and consider the implications in terms of the speech processing model.

To complete this activity you will need to refer to Figure 4.4 (z-scores) and Figure 4.5 (raw scores). Have a blank sheet of paper at hand for making notes.

Compare level B with level D.
Compare levels B and D, with level E.

In each case, address the following questions:

1. Is there a difference in Anna's performance on the levels in question, as measured by raw score percentages ?
2. What does the difference or lack of difference imply about Anna's underlying processing strengths and weaknesses?
3. Are these differences reflected in Anna's performance as measured by z-scores? If not, what might this indicate?
4. Relate these implications to the speech processing model in Figure 4.6.

Check your responses with Key to Activity 4.3 at the end of this chapter, then read the following.

Comparing level B with level D

You will have noted that, according to the raw scores, Anna's ability to perform discrimination tasks involving nonwords (level B: 58%) was weaker than for real words (level D: 70%). Two implications arose. The first was that Anna was processing these two types of word differently. The second was that Anna found it more difficult to discriminate phonological contrasts when forced to rely on the transitory acoustic presentation of a word, i.e. the process of 'phonological recognition' on its own. She found it easier when she was able to refer to her stored form of the word, i.e. when phonological recognition is supported by access to the phonological representations. The fact that the z-scores show the opposite pattern – Anna has overall a better z-score for the nonword tests – shows that the same observations can be made about normally developing children: they generally perform worse on nonwords compared to real words, as they get older – presumably because in nonword discrimination, support is not available from already established phonological representations, whereas knowledge of real words increases with age. This being the case, Anna's slightly superior performance on real words is predictable.

Comparing levels B and D with level E

Here, you will have noted that Anna's discrimination was better when pictures and speech were combined (level E: 82%, $z = -4$) in comparison to pure spoken presentations (level D: 70%, $z = -6.2$; level B: 58%, $z = -5.3$). This implied that, although some of Anna's underlying phonological representations were inaccurate, her discrimination skills were more reliable when processing was routed via semantics to access those phonological representations tested at level E, than when processing was allowed to bypass them (level D) or denied access altogether (level B). In this case, the raw scores and z-scores are in line. This supports the view that level E is relatively strong for Anna, compared to D and B.

I noted that the picture material gave her time to rehearse her decisions, as if she was repeatedly accessing her own representation to check for a match between the phonology of the word stored mentally and the phonology of the word I had spoken. The only risk of her rehearsal strategy was that her own production errors sometimes confounded her decisions : for instance, she thought /gəˈsɑ/ was correct because she pronounced GUITAR as [gəˈsɑ].

Finally, we can compare specific levels of input and output.

Comparing level F with level H

Whereas Anna scored an average 87.5 per cent on silent picture rhyme tasks (level F), she was unable to produce any rhyming words (level H). I remember her saying to me, 'Cat hat — that's all I know'. There is thus a marked dissociation at these levels, both of which involve metaphonological skills. This dissociation suggests that Anna's rhyme production difficulty had a motor programming basis: she was aware of rhyme and could detect it with moderate success, but had no idea of how to build motor programs around a rhyme pattern. An alternative for her on the rhyme production task (level H) could have been to search for rhyming material among the motor programs she already had (i.e. for words already in her lexicon). One reason why she was unable to do this may well be because Anna's stored motor programs were inaccurate, as identifed above in the comparison of output levels.

Comparing level B with level J

Anna's nonword discrimination at level B (58%, $z = -5.3$) was better than her nonword production at level J (41%, $z = -5.29$), as measured by her raw scores; however, both levels showed severe difficulty, as is reflected in the similar low z-scores. Vance (1998) suggests that one reason children might perform poorly on nonword production is that they do not discriminate the words accurately. This could certainly be part of the explanation for poor nonword production in Anna's case. She lexicalized many of the nonwords presented for repetition, for example she pronounced target /snaɪk/ as "snake" and target /glɛv/ as "glove". This suggests that she was not perceiving the words accurately at the phonological recognition stage, in a bottom-up fashion; instead she was using a top-down approach, influenced by phonological representations already stored in her lexicon.

The following points summarize what we have learnt about Anna in Question 3.

What we have learnt about Anna through intra-personal comparisons

- Input processing is stronger than output processing.

Within input processing:

- discrimination without access to phonological representations was a relative weakness;
- discrimination involving access to phonological representation was a relative strength;
- metaphonological discrimination routed silently via semantics into phonological representation was her greatest strength.

Within output processing:

- weaknesses were pervasive across processing levels;
- motor execution was a relative strength;
- repeated real words appeared to be routed through motor programming (like nonwords), which was a relative weakness;
- stored motor programs were an even greater weakness.

Step Two : Micro Assessment Analysis

Step Two of the P→P process moves on to a micro level of analysis. In Tables 4.3 and 4.4, you will have noticed the variation in task performance within levels, some of which was discussed in the previous section. To take just one example, note how within level B Anna's *z*-scores range from off the scale to –0.81 and her raw score percentages range from 22 to 83 per cent. What accounts for this variation? Clearly we would miss a great deal of information by looking only at her overall performance at different levels. As the next two questions reveal, this information is important when planning intervention.

Question 4: Which task design variables influence performance?

Each question on the profile can be addressed by a range of different tasks, and a child's performance may differ according to the task. In other words, for a particular profile question, the child may find one task easier than another. As in Step One, we can distinguish between factors that make one task harder than another for normally developing children in general, as opposed to factors that make the task harder for the individual child. For example, normally developing children tend to find tasks with nonwords harder than tasks with real words – a tendency that increases with age as their knowledge of real words expands and becomes more secure. Similarly, in many tasks children find stimuli consisting of long words harder than tasks using short words. This observation has two implications for assessment and for intervention.

(a) In order to decide whether a child is specifically helped or hindered by a particular task design feature, three steps of analysis are required: first, we should inspect the variability in their performance on that task factor in comparison to the variability of normally developing children (e.g. by using *z*-scores); second, we should inspect the variability in their personal performance on the task factor (e.g. by using raw score percentages) and third, we should compare the direction of variability between these two forms of comparison

(b) When selecting a task to assess a particular level (by addressing a particular question on the profile) we need to avoid a task that is likely to prove too easy for the child – particularly if normally developing children of the same age are likely to be at ceiling on the task. On the other hand, when selecting material for intervention at a particular level, it may be desirable to start off with material that is deliberately easy.

Tasks addressing a single level of processing can be analysed in terms of the variables of task design. These might include stimulus modality, format of task presentation, syllable number and stimulus word design (for further detail, see Chapter 3, this volume). As an example, we can consider the various tasks used to assess Anna's input skills at level D, as presented in Table 4.3. In level D, there are the following variables:

(a) Discrimination involving phonological awareness (i.e. in rhyme tasks), vs discrimination not involving phonological awareness.

(b) Detection vs judgement.

(c) Contrast of consonant sequence vs feature contrast at one place in the word.

We can then note whether any of these variables affects Anna's performance, in the first instance looking separately at her z-scores and raw score percentages and then comparing the direction of variability between the two.

(a) There is no clear evidence of the effect of phonological awareness demands, since Anna had widely diverging scores on tasks involving phonological awareness ($z = -1.63$, z = -9.35) and also on tasks which do not require phonological awareness, ($z = -1.77, z = -12$).

(b) For the detection task and the judgement task, the raw score percentages are equal at 75 per cent. Anna's personal performance shows no variability when task format is changed from detection (ABX format) to judgement (AB format). However, the z-scores show a strong effect of task format. When compared with normally developing children, Anna's performance is barely significant on the detection task (–1.63), but strongly significant on the judgement task (–9.35). This means that, while Anna found both task formats to be of equal difficulty, normally developing children in fact find judgement (AB) easier than detection (ABX). The implication for Anna's intervention plan was to improve auditory judgement skills at this level of input processing. She needed help to listen attentively to the detailed acoustic similarities and differences between two stimulus words, as is required in an AB judgement task, as opposed to finding a guaranteed and overall match between two stimulus words, as is possible in the ABX detection task.

(c) On the basis of raw score percentages, Anna has more problems with items where the consonant sequence is contrasted (44%), than with contrasts at a single place in the word (88%). The z-scores show an equally significant difference, and in the same direction. Not only does Anna personally find consonant sequences more difficult (44%), but this performance is in addition strongly significant when compared to normally developing children (–12.0). The clinical implication in this case is that intervention should aim to improve Anna's consonant sequence contrasts, but do so in a carefully graded manner in view of the difficulty she experiences with the task.

The following activity provides an opportunity to practise task design analysis, using the remaining input tasks undertaken by Anna.

ACTIVITY 4.4

Aim: to perform a task analysis on Anna's input performance.

To complete this activity you will need to refer to Table 4.3 and to Key to Activity 4.1(b) (Figure 4.7). Consider each question on the speech processing profile in turn.

(a) Note which variables of task design are manipulated, in the way that has been illustrated for level D.
(b) Note which variables appear to affect Anna's performance at each level.

Check your answers with Key to Activity 4.4 at the end of this chapter, and then read the following.

Certain trends appear across the input profile. The main design variables affecting Anna's performance are related to the nature of the stimulus word. The first of these is the complexity of the word at level B. Note how the direction of variability is matched for raw score percentages and for z-scores. Anna found complex words difficult (33% and 22%), and in addition this performance was strongly significant in comparison to normally developing children (–11.43 and 'off-scale'). By comparison, Anna found simple words relatively easy (80% and 75%) and this performance was less conspicuous in comparison to normally developing children (–0.81 and –1.69), with the exception of three-syllable words which are discussed below. The clinical implication arising from this pattern of performance is that intervention should aim to improve Anna's performance on complex words, but do so in a carefully graded manner, beginning with simple word stimuli. The second factor that shows variability is word length (in terms of syllables), as illustrated at levels E and B. At level E, the direction of variability of percentages and z-scores is not matched. Note how Anna appears to find two- and three-syllable words of equal difficulty, scoring 77 per cent, yet her z-score for two-syllable words is of greater significance (–6.96 as opposed to –4.35). This gives clear direction for intervention planning: word length should be carefully controlled and work can begin at the two-syllable level. At level B, the direction of variability is matched. While Anna's performance is not markedly different for one and two syllables (80% and 75%), nor highly conspicuous in comparison to normally developing children (–0.81 and –1.69), it is both personally poor (50%) and comparatively conspicuous (–3.7) for three syllables. While intervention should aim to address her difficulty at the three-syllable level, work should initially be graded at the two-syllable level to build confidence.

Broadening out the scope of comparison to look at tasks across levels of processing, it is noticeable that Anna's performance was helped by tasks involving multi-modal stimuli. Note how her rhyme judgement improves in terms of percentage and z-scores when both speech and pictures are presented (level F), in comparison to speech alone (level D).

Finally, there are the output tasks to consider. The number of variables is fewer in the output tasks that Anna undertook compared to the input tasks.

ACTIVITY 4.5

Aim: to perform a task analysis on Anna's output performance. To complete this activity you will need to refer to Table 4.4. Consider each question on the speech processing profile in turn.

(a) Note which variables of task design are manipulated, as you did in Activity 4.4.

(b) Note which variables appear to affect Anna's performance at each level.

Check your answers with Key to Activity 4.5 at the end of this chapter, and then read the following.

On the output tasks Anna's performance, as measured by her raw scores, shows effects of sentential context and of word length. The longer the word, the more incorrect responses she gave. However, her z-scores do not show the same pattern. For example, for level G (Naming), she scored 50 per cent on one-syllable words, and 25 per cent on three-syllable words, but in fact her z-score was worse for the one-syllable words ($z = -10.38$) than for the two- ($z = -8.9$) and three-syllable words ($z = -5.13$). This indicates that the normal controls also performed worse on the longer words. A similar observation can be made about the effect of sentence context on repetition: even though there is a substantial difference in raw scores (45% for words in isolation, as opposed to 32% for words in a sentence) there is not a great difference in the z-scores. This indicates that the controls were rather worse at repeating a real word accurately when the word was in the context of a sentence.

This set of results highlights two important factors for intervention planning. The first was the influence of syllable number on Anna's output performance. Her four top percentage (raw) scores were for tests that use one-syllable words. This suggests a motor programming basis to her production difficulties: whether they were real words or nonwords, named or repeated, what seemed to matter to Anna was the articulatory load of the target word. The second revelation was the influence of linguistic presentation, i.e. sentence vs word. Like younger normally developing children, Anna's articulation was influenced by the syntactic, semantic and memory factors the sentence context embodies.

It was noted earlier that Anna was not able to produce rhyme strings. This was the only task at level H, so no further analysis is possible. However, we can also note that the stimuli for this task, and thus the anticipated responses, were one-syllable words. This means that Anna's poor performance here cannot be attributed to articulatory load in quite the same way as for the repetition and naming tasks.

Question 5: Which sound system factors influence performance?

This is a truly micro stage of the P→P process. In Book 1, the point is made that patterns of processing breakdown are sometimes restricted to specific parts of the phonological system. For instance, Zoe (Book 1, Chapter 9) displayed auditory processing difficulties specifically with the voice–voiceless contrast, and these were reflected in her speech; whereas her output problems with postalveolar consonants could not be linked to auditory processing deficits. It follows, therefore, that speech sound errors within one word may have different underlying sources of processing deficit. Before we draw up an intervention plan for Anna, we need to know more about the specifics of her phonetic capabilities and her phonological system. For instance, are her discrimination difficulties general or perhaps specific to a few consonant contrasts? Equally, what specific targets for production would be appropriate at this stage of intervention?

Examples of Anna's word- and sentence-level production errors, and of her word discrimination errors, are presented below.

Input processing

Nonword discrimination – Anna failed on the following contrasts:

/kɛs/	~	/kɛt/
/vɪn/	~	/zɪn/
/rɔf/	~	/rɔs/
/wʊtʃ/	~	/rʊtʃ/
/tʃi/	~	/tsi /
/glɛb/	~	/glɛv/
/ˈslɔpə/	~	/ˈlɔpə/
/ˈæfɪlɒnt/	~	/ˈælɪfɒnt/
/ˈjælɒɪ/	~	/ˈlæjɒɪ/

Auditory discrimination of real words – Anna failed on the following contrasts:

s~t	PLACE – PLATE
st~ts	GUESSED – GETS
dz~dʒ	/spʌndz/ accepted for SPONGE
p~pl	/peɪt / accepted for PLATE
f~s	/'famwidʒ/ accepted for SANDWICH
st~sk	/'stukə/ accepted for SCOOTER
sl~l	/'lɪpə/ accepted for SLIPPER
s~ʃ	/'pærəsut/ accepted for PARACHUTE
t...k ~ k...t	/'hɛlɪtopkə / accepted for HELICOPTER
k~g	/gəm'pjutə / accepted for COMPUTER

These lists of discrimination errors provide a focus for intervention planning. Anna was particularly susceptible to processing breakdown on feature contrasts within the fricative and affricate consonant classes, and between these and the plosive class. She also failed to detect some consonant cluster contrasts involving /l/. Phoneme sequence errors were common across consonant classes. My margin notes record her saying, 'Too hard – sounds all the same' when I presented her with /'jælɒɪ/ ~ /'læjɒɪ/. It is also interesting to note a plosive voicing error.

Output processing:

Naming:

BRUSH	→	[bwʌs]
SPONGE	→	[spʌndz]
TORCH	→	[tɔts]
WATCH	→	[wɒts]
FISH	→	[fɪs]
FEATHER	→	['fɛvə]
YELLOW	→	['lɛləʊ]
KITCHEN	→	['kɪʔsn̩]
FLOWER	→	['faʊwə]
BISCUIT	→	['bɪsik]
GUITAR	→	[gə'sɑ]
SPAGHETTI	→	['spɛgɪ]
CARAVAN	→	['kævəræn]
PYJAMAS	→	[jə'wɑməs]
HOSPITAL	→	['hɒpl̩]

Sentence repetition:

THE PARROT IS SITTING ON A TREE   → the [ˈpæwə] is [ˈtɪsɪŋ] on a [swi]
THE COMPUTER IS ON   → the [kəmˈpu] on
HIS PLATE IS EMPTY   → his [pleɪʔ] is [ˈempəlɪ]

Broadly speaking, Anna's errors at word level involved consonants
rather than vowels, and were centred within the fricative and affricate
consonant classes. Consonant clusters involving /l/ were susceptible
to error. The /l/ – /j/ contrast was subject to consonant harmony
process. In addition, she had residual difficulties in plosive consonant
sequences involving a change in place of articulation, particularly in
words of two and three syllables, e.g. GUITAR, HOSPITAL, SPAGHETTI.
Beyond the one-syllable level, metathetic errors were common e.g.
[ˈkævəræn] for CARAVAN, as was syllable reduction e.g. [kəmˈpu] for
COMPUTER. At sentence level, these errors were magnified, with
evidence of phonological processes operating across word boundaries e.g. PLATE influencing the production of EMPTY in 'his [pleɪʔ] is
[ˈempəlɪ]'.

An interesting comparison can be made between the types of sound
error for input and output processing. You may have noticed some
commonalities already, e.g. the difficulties with fricatives and affricates.
This could mean that Anna's output difficulties with these consonants
are to be accounted for in terms of her corresponding input difficulties:
she was not producing the contrasts because she was not perceiving
them. This is a likely causative factor, given Anna's history of input difficulties. However, her current profile suggests that she also has
significant output difficulties with these consonant contrasts, over and
above her input difficulties. To take just one example of output
breakdown, consonants such as /ʃ/ and /tʃ/ were among those that she
could not yet produce, even at the single-sound level.

We can now summarize the results of the two parts of the micro
analysis, in the form of a list of implications for intervention planning
for Anna.

Input

1. Begin with one-syllable words and progressively increase syllable
   number.
2. Work from feature contrasts at a single place in the syllable towards
   sequence contrasts at onset and rime, and sequence contrasts across
   syllables.

Output

1. Work from one-syllable words towards two-, and then three- and four-syllable words.
2. Work on the major areas of speech error: fricatives and affricates; consonant sequences; /l/ clusters.
3. Work on words in isolation, before words in a sentence context.
4. Combine output work with work on input and representation.

What We Have Learnt About Anna from Steps One and Two

Steps One and Two of the P→P process have uncovered many different facets of Anna's speech processing difficulties. These have implications for the plannng of intervention, which will be pursued in the next chapter. The main findings, and their implications, are summarized below.

Input processing

1. Discrimination without access to phonological representations is a relative weakness; conversely, discrimination involving access to phonological representation is a relative strength.
2. Metaphonological discrimination, routed silently via semantics into phonological representation, is her greatest strength.
3. Discrimination at single place in syllable is easier than discrimination of sequences within the syllable or across syllables.

Implications for input intervention

1. Begin with one-syllable words and progressively increase syllable number.
2. Work from feature contrasts at a single place in the syllable towards sequence contrasts at onset and rime, and sequence contrasts across syllables.
3. Use stored phonological representations (i.e. higher-level knowledge) to support work on speech sound discrimination.

Output processing

1. Weaknesses are pervasive across processing levels.
2. Output processing is more impaired on tasks involving lexical representations.
3. Motor execution is a relative strength.

4. Repeated real words appeared to be routed through motor programming (like nonwords), which is a relative weakness.
5. Stored motor programs are an even greater weakness.
6. Longer words are harder than monosyllabic words
7. Specific areas of difficulty for speech output are: fricatives and affricates; consonant sequences; /l/ clusters.
8. Pronunciation in connected speech is more difficult than for single words.

Implications for output intervention

1. Work on words in isolation, before words in a sentence context.
2 Work from one-syllable words towards two-, and then three- and four-syllable words.
3. Work on preword articulatory skills, e.g. single sound sequencing/ blending, as a basis for working on motor programs.
4. Target major areas of speech error: fricatives and affricates; consonant sequences; /l/ clusters.

General

1. In comparison to her peer group, Anna's speech processing skills range from being mild/moderate to severely impaired and justify her as a priority therapy case, even though her speech is largely intelligible.
2. Both input and output channels show pervasive impairment
3. Input processing is relatively stronger than output processing.

General implications for intervention

1. Work from input to output.
2. Phonological awareness: overtly teach a strategy to produce rhyme using visual materials.
3. Combine output work with work on input and representation.

In view of Anna's pervasive deficits, and as her representations, input and motor execution are all relative strengths compared to her spoken output, the presentation of multimodal stimuli is indicated. This would include pictures (which access representations); speech (which uses her input channel) and articulation picture symbols (which access motor execution).

Summary

This chapter has described Steps One and Two of a systematic process, called Profile to Programme, which provides a question-driven method of analysing speech assessment data in order to generate a detailed psycholinguistic profile. Key points are as follows:

Step One Involves Macro Assessment Analysis

Question 1: Which levels of the psycholinguistic framework have been assessed?

- Take stock of the breadth and depth of your assessment.
- Survey it visually on a profile sheet.

Question 2: In comparison with other children, which levels show processing breakdown and to what extent?

- Consider which results are clinically significant and require intervention.

Question 3: In an intra-personal comparison, which levels show comparative processing strengths or weaknesses?

- Consider which tasks the child found easy and which difficult.
- Consider the implications for therapy planning.

Step Two Involves Micro Assessment Analysis

Question 1: Which task design variables influence performance?

- Consider which task variables increase or decrease the processing load for the child.

Question 2: Which sound system factors influence performance?

- Consider how the child's different sound errors may stem from different underlying sources of processing deficit.

Table 4.6: Key to Activity 4.1(a) Anna's task battery showing the processing level for each task. The letters correspond to questions on the speech processing profile

Task name	Stimulus modality	Stimulus type	Channel tested	Processing level
Naming	Picture	1 word	Output	G
Rhyme production	Spoken target	1 word	Output	H
Rhyme judgement (AB)	Silent pictures	2 words	Input	F
Rhyme judgement (AB)	Spoken	2 words	Input	D
Rhyme judgement (AB)	Spoken	2 nonwords	Input	B
Rhyme detection (ABX: match X to A or B)	Silent pictures	3 words	Input	F
Rhyme detection (ABX: match X to A or B)	Spoken	3 words	Input	D
Rhyme detection	Spoken	3 nonwords	Input	B
Auditory discrimination (AB: same – different)	Spoken	2 words	Input	D
Auditory discrimination (AB: same – different)	Spoken	2 nonwords	Input	B
Auditory discrimination (ABX: match X to A or B)	Spoken	3 nonwords	Input	B
Auditory lexical decision (yes/no word-to-picture match)	Spoken + picture	1 word	Input	E
Speech repetition	Spoken + picture	1 sentence	Output	I
Speech repetition	Spoken	1 word	Output	I
Speech repetition	Spoken	1 nonword	Output	J
Single sound repetition	Spoken	1 consonant or vowel	Output	K
Hearing test	Electronic signal	Pure tone	Input	A
Correction of own spontaneous speech	—	—	Feedback + self-monitoring	L

KEY TO ACTIVITY 4.1(b)

SPEECH PROCESSING PROFILE

Name   Anna   Comments:

Age   7yrs 7mo

Date

Profiler

INPUT	**OUTPUT**

F

Is the child aware of the internal structure of phonological representations?
Rhyme detection and (silent) judgement

G

Can the child access accurate motor programs?
Naming

E

Are the child's phonological representations accurate?
Auditory lexical decision

H

Can the child manipulate phonological units?
Rhyme production

D

Can the child discriminate between real words?
Rhyme detection and judgement; and discrimmination

I

Can the child articulate real words accurately?
Real word repetition Sentence repetition

C

Does the child have language-specific representations of word structures?

J

Can the child articulate speech without reference to lexical representations?
Nonword repetition

B

Can the child discriminate speech sounds without reference to lexical representations?
Nonword and discrimmination; rhyme detection and judgement

A

Does the child have adequate auditory perception?
Pure tone hearing test

K

Does the child have adequate sound production skills?
Single sound repetition

L

Does the child reject his/her own erroneous forms?
Self-monitoring

Key to Activity 4.1(b) Anna's speech processing profile showing the levels assessed by her task battery, with component tasks written below.

Figure 4.7: Anna's task battery, showing processing level for each task.

KEY TO ACTIVITY 4.2

Scans of Anna's macro profile

Scan One

The output side of the profile is more conspicuously impaired than the input side.

Scan Two: Input

There is no clear evidence of a top–bottom split.

Scan Two: Output

A slight top–bottom split is evident: levels G,H and I are more conspicuously impaired than levels J or K.

KEY TO ACTIVITY 4.3

Compare level B with level D

- Is there a difference in Anna's performance on the levels in question, as measured by raw score percentages?

  Yes: level B (nonwords) is weaker than level D (real words).

- What does the difference or lack of difference imply about Anna's underlying processing strengths and weaknesses?

  Suggests that Anna is using different input processing routes for real and nonwords.

- Are these differences reflected in Anna's performance as measured by z-scores?
  If not, what might this indicate?

  No: the pattern is reversed. This indicates that for normally developing children, nonword discrimination is harder than real word discrimination.

- Relate these implications to the speech processing model in Figure 4.6.

Anna's raw scores suggest that her phonological representations, which can be used for real word discrimination, are stronger than her phonological recognition, which is needed for nonword discrimination.

Compare levels B and D with level E

1. Is there a difference in Anna's performance on the levels in question, as measured by raw score percentages?

   Level E (pictures + speech) is better than levels B and D (speech only).

2. What does the difference or lack of difference imply about Anna's underlying processing strengths and weaknesses?

   It suggests that her auditory processing is improved when she has access to the word's phonological representation via its semantic representation (from the picture).

3. Are these differences reflected in Anna's performance as measured by z-scores? If not, what might this indicate?

   Yes.

4. Relate these implications to the speech processing model in Figure 4.6.

   The relative strength of Anna's phonological representations is more than a mere reflection of the pattern of normal development.

KEY TO ACTIVITY 4.4

(a) Which task design features are varied?
   (i) involvement vs non-involvement of rhyme (i.e. phonological awareness) in discrimination task (levels B, D);
   (ii) judgement vs detection (levels B, D);
   (iii) AB vs ABX task (levels B, F);
   (iv) complex (with clusters) vs simple (without clusters) – here, for nonwords (level B);
   (v) sequence contrast vs feature contrast (levels B, D);
   (vi) word length: one vs two vs three syllables (levels B, E).

(b)Which factors appear to affect Anna's performance at each level?
  (i)   judgement vs detection (levels B, D);
  (ii)   AB vs ABX task (levels B, F);
  (iii)   complex vs simple words (level B);
  (iv)   sequence contrast vs feature contrast (level D);
  (v)   word length (levels B, E).

KEY TO ACTIVITY 4.5

(a)Which task design features are varied?
  (i)   word length (levels G, I, J);
  (ii)   context, i.e. word in isolation vs word in sentence (level I);

(b)Which factors appear to affect Anna's performance at each level?
  (i)   word length (on the basis of raw scores);
  (ii)   context.

Chapter 5
From Profile to
Programme: Steps 3–6

JULIETTE CORRIN

In this chapter, our study of Anna moves on from 'what was wrong' to 'what we did about it'. One of the hallmarks of psycholinguistic work is detailed analysis, of the kind exemplified in Chapter 4. The assumption is that time spent on analysis saves time in therapy intervention because one is 'hitting the right targets' from the start. This being the case, much of the hard work in planning an intervention programme has already been covered in the previous chapter. If Steps One and Two felt like motoring uphill, Steps Three and Four which now follow are the downhill run! To refresh your memory, the Profile to Programme (P→P) cycle is presented again as Figure 5.1. This illustrates how Steps Three and Four are generated from the psycholinguistic framework.

Step Three: Macro Intervention Planning

In Step Three, we focus on macro intervention planning. This involves drawing together the information you have already gathered and formulating a hypothesis-based intervention plan. Two questions are addressed: What *general* intervention plans are indicated? and: What *specific* intervention plans are indicated?

Question 1: What general intervention plans are indicated?

The general intervention plan summarizes the information gathered in Step One of the P→P process. The three questions asked in this first step were:

(1) Which levels of the framework have been assessed?
(2) In comparison to other children, which levels show processing breakdown and to what extent?

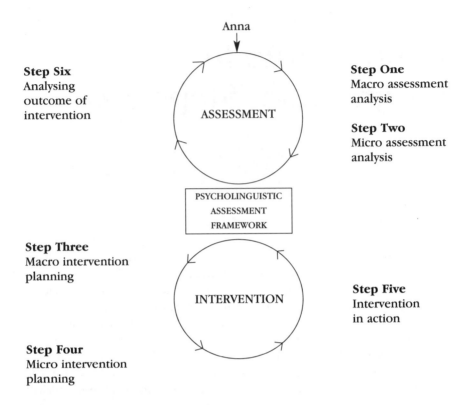

Figure 5.1: The Profile to Programme (P→P) cycle.

(3) In an intra-personal comparison, which levels show comparative strength or weakness?

Before reading further, take an opportunity to refer back to the section at the end of Chapter 4, 'What we have learnt about Anna from Steps One and Two'. We can now convert these findings into a set of clinical hypotheses. The statements are expressed in the present tense, reflecting their origin in my clinical notes.

(a) Anna's input processing skills are a relative strength and, if improved further, will act as a resource to improve her output processing skills. Work on input processing will therefore support output processing. In particular, Anna's inaccurate stored motor programs and relatively poor on-line motor programming skills may be helped by her awareness and knowledge of the internal sound structure of the words she has to pronounce.

(b) Anna's profile shows that her phonological representations are stronger than her lower-level input processing skills. Intervention will be effective if her strengths are reinforced and used to improve her weaknesses, thus working with a top-down approach, i.e. from tasks that require access to lexical representation, to those where lexical representation may be accessed but are not essential, and finally to tasks where there is no possibility of accessing lexical representations.

(c) On the output side Anna's top-down processing is relatively weak. Intervention will be effective if her strengths are reinforced and used to support her weaknesses. This will involve a bottom-up approach, i.e. from tasks which do not access lexical representations, to those that allow or require lexical access. In particular, Anna's motor programming skills will be facilitated by improved control at the motor execution level of single sound production and sequencing.

We can map Anna's general intervention plan on to the speech processing model, as in Figure 5.2.

The numbered arrows in Figure 5.2 refer to the correspondingly numbered points from the general intervention plan. The overarching arrow (1) directed from input processing towards output processing indicates that, as a general principle, you would strengthen input skills first and then use these to scaffold Anna's weaker output skills. On the input side, the model shows a series of arrows 'bunny hopping' from stage to stage in a top-down fashion (2). Finally, on the output side, the model shows a series of arrows 'bunny hopping' from stage to stage in a bottom-up fashion (3).

The illustration highlights the two-pronged approach planned to address Anna's inaccurate stored motor programs. As the arrows show, this would be addressed by working from input towards output, and within output, by working from bottom to top. To make this more tangible: the plan was ultimately to induce a change in Anna's stored motor programs by helping her to think and know about the internal structure of the target word (phonological representations), and have control of the individual sounds involved in the word (bottom-up on the output side, from motor execution) – and then try to pronounce it with supporting visual cues.

Question 2: What specific intervention plans are indicated?

The specific intervention plan makes use of information gathered in Step Two of the P→P process. As a reminder, the questions covered in that second step were:

SPEECH PROCESSING MODEL

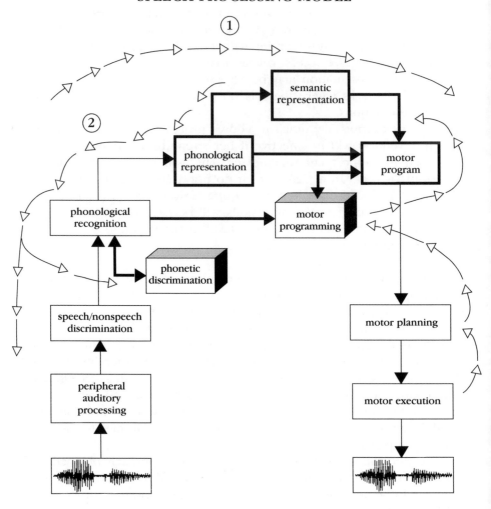

Figure 5.2: Anna's general intervention plan mapped on to the speech processing model.

1. Which task design factors influence the child's performance?
2. Which sound system factors influence the child's performance?

In Anna's case, my intervention plans fell into two broad groups:

(a) With her literacy difficulties so evident in the classroom, it was prudent to work on Anna's phonological awareness skills, through rhyme. Since rhyme taps into a key aspect of the structure of phonological representations (Book 1, Stackhouse and Wells, 1997, pp.158–162), improved awareness of rhyme should lead to (i) more precise phonological representations as a basis for accurate input processing; (ii) more accurate motor programs as a basis for speech output; and, as a result, (iii) a firmer basis for the development of literacy skills through establishing more accurate phonological–graphemic correspondences.

(b) The need to work on Anna's sound system was obvious from the difficulties identified with certain classes of speech sound, including fricatives and affricates, and also consonant clusters. These led to reduced intelligibility.

I viewed these as separate, but overlapping objectives each requiring a specific plan for intervention, as set out below. Before reading further, it may be helpful to refer back to the summary in Chapter 4 of what was learnt about Anna from micro-analysis, to get an idea of how findings from the micro assessment analysis in Step Two of the P→P process are woven into an intervention plan.

Phonological awareness work

1. Anna's rhyme input skills are a marked strength relative to her almost non-existent output skills. Normative data suggest that children first develop some rudimentary rhyme output skills before learning to discriminate and reflect upon rhyme input (Vance, Stackhouse and Wells, 1994). Anna's understanding of the rhyme concept will be facilitated if she first experiences rhyme production, albeit in an artificial manner, e.g. by repeating a rhyme string spoken by the therapist, who will give appropriate cues for articulation. In this way she can develop familiarity, at the level of motor execution, with the articulatory setting that is shared by words that have the same rime. For instance, FEET, SEAT, SHEET, HEAT, MEAT, NEAT, etc. all have the same front, raised tongue position and spread lips, which also affects the pronunciation of the onset consonant through co-articulation. Practice at the level of motor execution can lead to the establishment of a rime element /-it/ in motor programming, which Anna can then draw on in tasks such as rhyme production. Once she has achieved some competence with the mechanics of rhyme production, the focus can return to rhyme input work.

2. Anna's rhyme discrimination skills will be facilitated by working with a top-down approach, drawing on her semantic and phonological representations of picture words and her ability to reflect on their internal sound structure e.g. segmentation of words into onset and rime. Visual support of sound picture symbols and/or

letters will help her to see the rhyme pattern she hears, particularly for nonword stimuli. This visual support will be withdrawn gradually so that Anna learns to discriminate rhyme on an auditory basis alone. Detection tasks would precede judgement tasks.

3. Anna's rhyme output skills will require further work following the introduction described in (1) above. The support of colour-coded sound picture symbols and/or letters should help her to produce rhyme patterns visually as a basis for production practice. Visual support would be gradually withdrawn with the ultimate aim of Anna producing rhyme strings spontaneously from auditory presentation of a target word.

ACTIVITY 5.1

Aim: to map Anna's specific rhyme intervention plan on to the speech processing profile.

For this activity, refer to the blank speech processing profile reproduced as Figure 5.3. Take each of the three statements above and map it on to the profile using arrows to indicate how intervention moves between levels. Label these plans 1, 2 and 3 accordingly. You will need to consider which levels of processing are implicated in each plan, and the relationship between levels.

Check your response with Key to Activity 5.1, then read the following.

---

1. Your profile should show linked arrows from level K to J and I, representing Anna's preliminary introduction to rhyme production in a mechanical 'bottom-up' fashion (label 1).
2. Next, your profile should show linked arrows from level F down to E, then to D and B, representing Anna's 'top-down' work on rhyme discrimination (label 2). You might have noted that the top arrow between levels E and F is bi-directional. This reflects a combined intervention strategy when rhyme input work began. Anna was invited to look at pictures, listen to words and jointly reflect with me upon their internal onset-rime structure, using sound picture symbols. I was not testing her, but teaching her. Both sets of arrows for plans 1 and 2 show dots at the point where one arrow leads to another. The concept conveyed is that it is the relationship between two levels that is carried forward, providing a bridge to the next weakest level of processing.
3. Lastly, your profile should show how input skills at levels F, E and D were brought to bear upon further rhyme production work at

SPEECH PROCESSING PROFILE

Name   Comments:

Age

Date

Profiler

INPUT   **OUTPUT**

F

Is the child aware of the internal
structure of phonological representations?

G

Can the child access accurate motor
programs?

E

Are the child's phonological
representations accurate?

H

Can the child manipulate phonological units?

D

Can the child discriminate between real
words?

I

Can the child articulate real words
accurately?

C

Does the child have language-specific
representations of word structures?

J

Can the child articulate speech without
reference to lexical representations?

B

Can the child discriminate speech sounds
without reference to lexical representations?

A

Does the child have adequate
auditory perception?

K

Does the child have adequate sound
production skills?

L

Does the child reject his/her own erroneous
forms?

Figure 5. 3: Blank speech processing profile for Activity 5.1.

level H (label 3). Picture symbols and letters visually supported Anna's knowledge of the internal sound structure of the target word from which she was to generate a rhyme string (level F), while she also had a chance of determining the phonological representation of the target word by hearing me say it (level D or E).

Sound system work

In what order should we tackle the different sound system objectives that have been identified for Anna? This decision is informed by (a) knowledge of the sequence of normal phonological development; (b) the aim to improve Anna's intelligibility; and (c) a knowledge of the speech sounds that Anna was already able to produce accurately. The order will be as follows:

> fricative contrasts;
> plosive (and other) sequence contrasts;
> cluster contrasts;
> affricate contrasts.

In each case, the intervention plan will be broadly as follows:

(1) It is hypothesized that Anna's input skills will be facilitated by working with a top-down approach. Word targets will therefore be supported by pictures and sound symbols that assist her in visually predicting (pre-stimulus) or checking (post-stimulus) the sound contrast she hears, and reflecting upon the structural position within the word where the sound contrast occurs. The picture material should ensure that Anna processes words lexically, thus providing an impetus for change to inaccurate stored phonological representations. Real word stimuli will precede work on nonword stimuli, which she finds considerably more difficult. Work on nonword stimuli will be supported visually by sound picture symbols and presented first in detection/ABX tasks, which she generally finds easier than judgement/AB tasks. Number of syllables in all real word and nonword contrasts will be controlled for.

(2) Work on Anna's output skills at level K (motor execution/sound production) will overlap input work described in (1) above. The use of sound picture symbols to visually support her discrimination skills will provide natural opportunities for single-sound production practice. For example, when Anna has completed the discrimination task of pointing to the sound picture symbol for /s/ or /ʃ/, corresponding to the word-initial sound she hears me say in a target, e.g. SHEET or SEAT, she will then be invited to practise production of the problem target /ʃ/ at an appropriate level of

difficulty e.g. a repeated sequence /ʃ ʃ ʃ/ or a contrastive sequence /p ʃ p ʃ/.

(3) Once performance on input processing (levels F, E, D and B) and output processing (level K) has been improved as described above, these two relative strengths will be brought to bear on her most intractable problems, namely, inaccurate stored motor programs and deficits in on-line motor programming and motor planning. It is these aspects of processing that primarily account for task failure at levels G, H, I and J. A detailed example of how this can be done will be given in Step Four.

Step Four: Micro Intervention Planning

The P→P process has now reached the final stage of session planning. Step Four is a mental exercise that takes place prior to each session. While it is impossible to reproduce here all Anna's intervention records, there are certain guiding principles for psycholinguistic session planning which can be illustrated from a typical session. Two questions are addressed:

(1) What overall design of session would be effective?
(2) How should each task be designed?

My approach to intervention reflects our department's work at the Nuffield Hearing and Speech Centre and specifically our use of the *Nuffield Dyspraxia Programme* (Connery, 1992). As the tasks in this section will show, consonant and vowel picture symbols are a key to the *NDP*. The use of pictorial symbols teaches the child an association between a speech sound and a picture of an object, as illustrated in Figure 5.4 below. In psycholinguistic terms, this association provides a

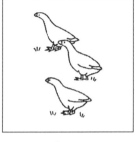

/ g / for 'geese'

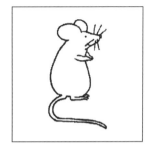

/ i / for 'mouse'

Figure 5.4: An example of the pictorial symbols used in the *NDP*. The object picture cards become elicitation cues for speech production tasks.

link between phonological and semantic representations, in effect creating a visual phonology for the child which underpins their spoken phonology. Once established, the picture symbols become elicitation cues within a therapy programme. In this way, the child is therapeutically supported to:

(a) hear what they see;
(b) think about what they see;
(c) say what they see.

Question 1: What overall design of session would be effective?

The concept of overall session design is particularly important when working with a psycholinguistic approach. The reason for this is that the task sequence is critical to the therapeutic process. Whereas in assessment it is desirable for tasks to have minimal overlap in order to separate out the levels of processing (B, D, E, etc.), in intervention it is desirable for tasks to have maximal overlap in order to bridge between levels of processing. The method of therapy is one in which we scaffold the child's emergent ability by presenting them with a sequence of overlapping tasks that bridges their transition from a stronger to a weaker level of processing. At the Nuffield Centre we have used the speech processing profile as a visual framework for session design and this is illustrated in Anna's example session below. The profile acts to remind us when we are working within a level and when we are moving the child between levels. In fact, once the framework of levels (A–L) becomes part of one's mental architecture, it can provides a clinical shorthand for team communication (cf. Popple and Wellington, this volume). We hear ourselves saying things of this sort: 'I'm moving Tom up to level E today!'.

The following two points summarize considerations in answer to Question 1:

• plan systematic moves between levels of processing;
• plan an overlapping sequence of tasks that scaffolds the child's move from a stronger to weaker level of processing.

Question 2: How should each task be designed?

Chapter 3 of this book provides detailed coverage of task design considerations. Apart from the design factors that we have focused on in analysis of Anna's data (e.g. modality of stimulus/response; word type; syllable number; phoneme class), there are related factors such as task commands and procedure to consider. How the task is presented and explained to the child can be as critical as the task itself. One point to stress is the importance of designing an overlapping sequence of tasks: the aim is to increase the child's processing load by manipulating one task variable at a time, keeping all else constant if possible. For this reason, it is particularly helpful to work with a constant word set. This makes it possible systematically to compare task performance between tasks and levels of processing. Furthermore, it ensures semantic familiarity with the stimuli.

Step Five: Putting Intervention into Action

This section illustrates excerpts from Anna's therapy programme. Although work on rhyme and sound production skills were combined within actual sessions, here they have been separated out so that they can be followed more easily. The presentation of Anna's rhyme skills programme focuses on change over time, showing examples of early, intermediate and late stages of intervention. By contrast, the presentation of her sound skills programme focuses on session planning at a single point in time. In both programmes the tasks may look quite familiar. In intervention based on the psycholinguistic framework, the tasks themselves do not have to be novel. The emphasis is on the rationale for selecting particular tasks and for presenting them in a particular order.

Anna's rhyme skills programme

The three stages of therapy directly mirror the three-step intervention plan presented at the beginning of the chapter and illustrated in Key to Activity 5.1.

An early therapy stage

According to the hypothesis set out within the specific intervention plan, Anna's understanding of the rhyme concept would be facilitated if she first experienced rhyme production (level H). Since she had no functional skills in rhyme production, she had to be explicitly taught. It was necessary to scaffold her abilities in a bottom-up processing fashion, combining aspects of processing at levels K, J and I, to eventually induce success at level H. This intervention plan has already been illustrated in the Key to Activity 5.1: label 1. The task illustrated below in Figure 5.5 shows how Anna was taught a visual and mechanical strategy for rhyme production.

In this task, Anna began by producing a single sound onset, e.g. [d] followed by the nonword rime [ɒg] (levels K and J). She then repeated the whole word DOG, at level I. Anna and I discussed the fact that it

Rhyme wheel

Processing levels: K, J and I.

Task type: blending of segments to produce a word or nonword; judgement of word type; spoken word-to-picture matching.

Materials: A spinning wheel in which the inner circle remains stationary and the outer circle can be spun around. Picture cards for the constant rime segment are edged in red and stuck to the inner circle (marked with bold borders). Picture sounds for the changing onset sound are edged in blue and stuck to the outer circle (marked with dotted borders).

Target words: rhyming words – JOG, DOG, LOG and nonword /wɒg/

NDP key: /w/ – worm; /d/ – drum; /l/ – lolly; /j/ – yo-yo; /g/ – geese; /ɒ/ – hop

Presentation:

Step 1: "Spin the wheel and choose a blue sound. Add the red sounds and say the word. Spin the wheel again to change the blue sound and make another word. Listen – the two words rhyme. Now let's spin the wheel again. Listen, that word also rhymes."

Step 2: "Spin the wheel and choose a blue sound. Add the red sounds and say the word. Does that make a real word? If so, find the corresponding picture for the word and paste it in the blank box underneath which the word is written." (An example for target word DOG is shown below).

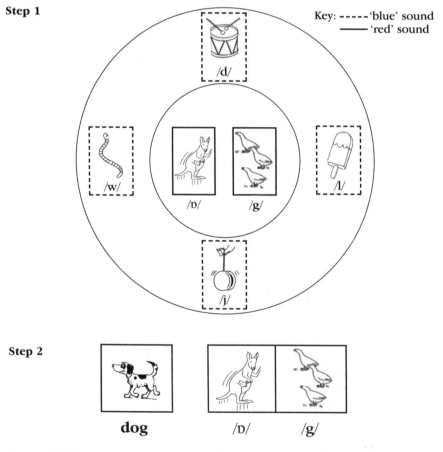

Figure 5.5: Task from an early stage of Anna's rhyme programme focusing on rudimentary skills in rhyme production: rhyme wheel.

made a real word. She identified the corresponding picture symbol sequence below and pasted the real picture of a dog next to it. After three trials, Anna could see the colour-coded pattern for rhyme production she had created and hear herself saying: 'dog, wog, log, jog'. Her memory about the rhyme concept was aided by the cue: 'red for rhyme: the red sounds stay the same; change the blue'. At subsequent sessions, letters were included to assist her recognition of rhyme patterns as a spelling strategy.

An intermediate therapy stage

The early stage heightened Anna's awareness and interest in rhyme as an output activity. The next stage in the intervention plan was to switch focus to her input skills, strengthening her input rhyme processing by drawing on her semantic and phonological representations of pictured words, and on her ability to reflect on their internal sound structure.

ACTIVITY 5.2

Aim: to practise designing specific tasks that derive from a given psycholinguistic rationale.

Design any two therapy tasks which would support the intermediate stage in Anna's intervention plan for rhyme. In each case, consider the following design features:

    (a) processing level(s) involved in the task;
    (b) task type;
    (c) target stimuli and distractor stimuli;
    (d) materials required;
    (e) presentation and instructions to the child.

For further discussion of task design, you may wish to refer to Chapter 3 in this volume. While there is no single correct answer to this Activity, read the Key to Activity 5.2 at the end of this chapter for a description of tasks that were implemented in Anna's programme. Then read the following.

The 'Rhyming Picture Windows' task targeted level F on the psycholinguistic framework: awareness of the internal structure of phonological representations. Using a top-down approach, the aim was to scaffold Anna's phonological processing by drawing on her semantic strengths at story level. The task required her to:

look at the picture of Mr Mog (accessing phonological representations via semantics);
listen to the stimulus sentence e.g. 'Mr Mog went for a ...' (phonological discrimination/recognition);
search for the missing rhyme word by opening the picture
windows;
in each case segment the pictured word into onset and rime e.g. D
+ OG;
judge whether it matched with the target M + OG;
and judge whether it made sense semantically e.g. 'Mr *Mog* went
for a: log, pig, *jog*'.

The search was done in silence, thus focusing the task at level F. We had
done a picture vocabulary check at the start to ensure these words were
accessible from Anna's stored phonological representations. The choice
of word targets reflected the fact that Anna had discrimination difficulties amongst short vowels. She responded best to tasks working on one
short vowel at a time, in an 'auditory bombardment' fashion (see
Chapter 2). In this task, Anna had only to listen out for the vowel [ɒ],
rejecting all others. The distractor vowels [ɛ] and [ɪ] were chosen as a
stark contrast. The choice of a closed syllable CVC stimulus, e.g. DOG,
as opposed to an open CV syllable, e.g. TOE, reflected the fact that she
found a VC rhyme segment e.g. [ɒg], more acoustically salient than only
a VV (long vowel or diphthong) e.g. [əʊ]. As a homework output
processing activity she was asked to memorize the nonsense rhyming
story.

The 'Rhyming Postman' task targeted levels E and D on the
psycholinguistic framework. Compared to the previous task, there was
reduced semantic support because stimuli were single words not story
sentences. As a rhyme judgement task, it required Anna to:

(a) look at the picture (access phonological representations via
    semantics);
(b) listen to the stimulus word spoken (phonological
    discrimination/recognition);
(c) judge whether the rime segment [ɒg] matched with the sound
    symbol pictures on the posting box (accessing phonological
    representations via her stored visual inventory of *NDP*
    symbols).

Once the activity was complete, she enjoyed doing a visual rhyme
check, seeing whether the *NDP* symbols and graphemes on the reverse
side of the pictures matched with those on the post box. In our work at
the Nuffield Centre, we have found that school-aged children like Anna

take well to a combined presentation of *NDP* symbols and letters. Initially, we give visual dominance to the *NDP* symbol with a small letter inscription on a corner of the picture card. Later the dominance can be reversed. The presence of *NDP* symbols serves as a useful phonic basis for building letter–sound links.

An advanced therapy stage

By the advanced stage, Anna was ready to tackle her weakest input processing skill, namely nonword rhyme discrimination. To do this, a 'Rhyming Teddies' activity was devised to target level B on the psycholinguistic framework, relying only on the novel incoming acoustic stimulus: see Figure 5.6.

Rhyming Teddies Task
Processing level: B.
Task type: nonword rhyme detection.
Skills: phonological discrimination; 3 stimuli held in working memory; rhyme knowledge; matching.
Targets: /ˈsɒɡɪtɪ – ˈnɒɡɪtɪ – ˈpɒɡɪtɪ – ˈʃɒɡɪtɪ/.
Materials: a key teddy named /ˈsɒɡɪtɪ/ and 7 other teddies.
Presentation: Story: "/ˈsɒɡɪtɪ/ is looking for lost members of his family – the /ˈɒɡɪtɪ/ rhyme family; listen and look as each toy is touched and named; which one rhymes with /ˈsɒɡɪtɪ/? Listen to the pair you have chosen, do they rhyme e.g. /ˈsɒɡɪtɪ/ – /ˈpʌɡɪtɪ/?".

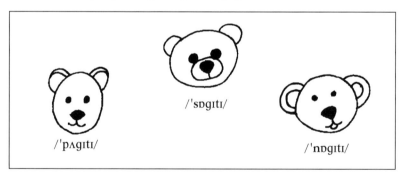

Figure 5.6: Illustration of an activity used in Anna's rhyme programme at an advanced stage of intervention: rhyming teddies task.

To compensate for the reliance on auditory processing, three soft teddies were used to create a visual anchor for the nonword stimuli, thus helping Anna to store them in working memory. Using an ABX design task presentation (see Book 1, p.93 for details), she was required to look and listen as I touched and named each teddy with a nonword, to hold all three stimuli in memory and detect which of the two teddies, A or B, rhymed with the target teddy X, in this case named /'sɒgɪtɪ/. The choice of key word was based on the acoustic salience of the rhyme portion /'ɒgɪtɪ/ and its inherent prosodic rhythm when produced in a rhyming string e.g. /'sɒgɪtɪ – 'nɒgɪtɪ – 'pɒgɪtɪ/. Once she had made her choice between A or B, I repeated the names of the nonword pair she had chosen as a rhyme check e.g. 'Listen Anna, do these rhyme: /'sɒgɪtɪ – 'pɛgɪtɪ /?'. At times, Anna would use whispered rehearsal of the nonword names to help her task decision, but I discouraged this because her pronunciations tended to drift from the target and thus confound her choice.

The final thrust of the therapy programme focused on rhyme production skills, bringing what she had learnt about rhyme as a procedure and her improved rhyme discrimination skills to bear on the task of producing rhyme skills at level H. To visualize this third stage of the programme, refer back to Key to Activity 5.1, label 3. The 'Rhyming Flip-Up' activity shown in Figure 5.7 required Anna to access the phonic representation of the written letter that formed the rhyme onset, e.g. <d> and blend it with the written rhyming portion <oggity> to produce a spoken nonword i.e. /'dɒgɪtɪ/.

Task two: 'Rhyming Flip-up'
Processing level: I, leading to H.
Task type: rhyme blending and production.
Skills: letter–sound links; phonic blending; phonic search; motor planning for articulation.
Targets: any nonwords that rhyme with /'sɒgɪtɪ/.
Materials: flip-up book split between onset and rhyming portion: flip over the onset to make a new rhyme.
Presentation: 'Say this rhyming portion /'ɒgɪtɪ/. Flip over to choose an onset letter sound e.g. <l>. Blend onset and rhyming portion: /'lɒgɪtɪ/. Now here is a blank page: think up your own onset sound, write it down, and make a new rhyme.'

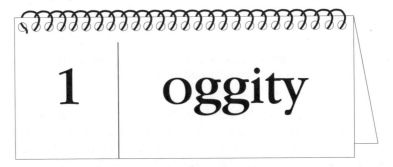

Figure 5.7: The 'Rhyming Flip-up' task. Illustration of an activity used in Anna's rhyme programme at an advanced stage of intervention: 'Rhyming Flip-up' task.

Letters were now the dominant type of symbol, with *NDP* pictures serving as a background phonic check. In this task, Anna had to assemble a new motor program from an onset and a rhyming portion that were supplied. The visual presentation of the onset and the rhyme gave Anna something to refer back to, thus facilitating the motor programming aspects of the task. Once skilled at the activity, the flip-up book was loaded with some blank onsets to encourage spontaneous production. The choice of nonwords forced Anna to use a phonic (as opposed to semantic) strategy in generating the string, and reduced the chance of alliteration errors such as /'pɛgɪtɪ 'pɒgɪtɪ/; it was simpler for her to change the onset of the nonword than reconfigure the rhyming portion /'ɒgɪtɪ/ into a new nonword such as /'ɛgɪtɪ/. As a final step, the flip-up book was removed and Anna was asked to repeat the nonword string from memory. This was tape-recorded as a self-evaluation rhyme check, thus turning the product of her output task into the stimulus for an input task, and bringing the cycle of processing back to level D of the psycholinguistic framework (see Key to Activity 5.1).

Anna's sound system programme

In this presentation, the focus changes. Whereas the rhyme programme was used to illustrate stages of intervention, the sound system programme will illustrate stages within just one session.

Anna had difficulty with the phonological contrast /s/ and /ʃ/, treating them both as /s/. As a general principle, she responded well to sessions which focused on one contrast such as this, taking it 'on tour' around the levels of the speech processing profile, as illustrated in Figure 5.8. The session presented here shows an intermediate stage of intervention when certain strengths of input and output were brought to bear upon her resistant deficit in motor programming.

Sample session: Part one

The first part of the session consisted of three tasks corresponding to numbers 1, 2 and 3 in Figure 5.8. A constant CV word set was used that contrasted the onset target /ʃ/ with the error /s/, using either real word or nonword minimal pairs as the task required. The tasks are illustrated in Figure 5.9.

Task 1 is an auditory lexical decision task (see Book 1, p.37). Anna was familiarized with the target picture set of /ʃ/ initial CV and CVC words e.g. SHOW, SHOE, SHORE, SHIRT, SHEEP. She was required to detect my errors in pronouncing the words, distinguishing between an increasingly fine set of phonological contrasts as I homed in on her /s/ – /ʃ/ error pair. For example, Anna was shown a picture of a SHOE and was asked: 'Is this a /mu/? Is this a /bu/? Is this a /fu/? Is this a /su/? Is this a /ʃu/?'

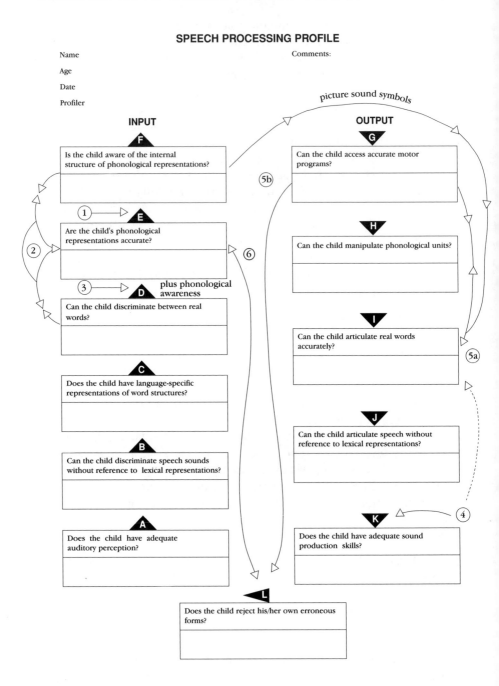

Figure 5.8: A session design for work on Anna's sound system. The /ʃ/ – /s/ contrast taken on tour around the profile. Numbers 1–5 relate to tasks illustrated in Figures 5.9, 5.10 and 5.11 that follow. Number 6 is not illustrated in a separate figure but described in the text.

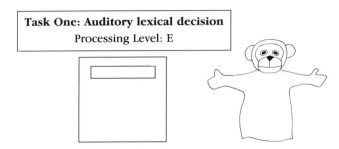

Task One: Auditory lexical decision
Processing Level: E

Targets: SHOW, SHOE, SHORE, SHIRT, SHEEP.
Distractors: rhyming words or nonwords e.g. for target SHOE: /mu/ /bu/ /fu/ /su/.
Presentation: "Put a token in the posting box if you hear Monkey Muppet say the word correctly".

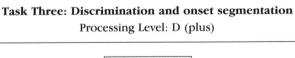

Task Two: discrimination and onset segmentation
Processing Levels: Level E (F+D)

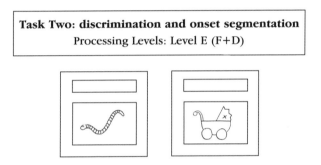

Targets and distractors as in Task One.
Presentation: "Look at this picture e.g. SHEEP. Listen for the sound at the beginning of the word. Does it begin with /ʃ/ or /s/? Post the picture into the right box."
NDP Key: /ʃ/ – hush baby in pram; /s/ – sound of snake.

Task Three: Discrimination and onset segmentation
Processing Level: D (plus)

Targets and distractors as in Tasks One and Two above.
Presentation: "If you hear me say /ʃ/ at the beginning of the word then post a token in to the posting box. Listen: SHEEP."

Figure 5.9: Three tasks for input processing work. In Task Three, the reference to D 'plus' takes in to account the phonological awareness element that the task requires, over and above real word discrimination that characterises Level D.

Task 2 is a sorting and posting activity, designed as a bridge from Task 1 to Task 3. *NDP* symbol cards were used: a snake to represent /s/ and a baby asleep in a pram to represent /ʃ/. The arrows in Figure 5.8 show how Task 2 stems from level E: Anna was shown a picture, but also heard the stimulus word spoken. It also draws on elements of level F: she was required to reflect upon the internal sound structure of words and segment the onset sound. Finally, it scaffolds down to level D, since auditory presentation potentially allowed her to bypass lexical representation. Tasks such as this facilitate learning by scaffolding processing across several levels. One is effectively teaching, not simply testing. For instance, the spoken stimulus can be manipulated to prolong the onset sound e.g.[ʃ:::u], with the addition of obvious lip rounding, or indeed with the addition of a cued articulation visual gesture (Passy, 1993a). The processing demand can be increased gradually by removing these parts of the scaffold one by one, e.g. normalizing the spoken stimulus, removing visual cues of articulation, and so on. Anna was able to evaluate her own performance on this task by checking that the pictures posted through the /s/ slot had the *NPD* symbol for /s/ – the snake – on the reverse, and that the pictures posted through the /ʃ/ slot had the symbol of the pram on the reverse.

Task 3 was Anna's greatest input challenge of the session. The presentation was auditory only, with no pictures and no visual articulation cues. Anna was asked to listen to a target word e.g. SHEEP, to reflect upon its internal sound structure and post a token if the onset sound of the word matched the *NDP* picture symbol depicted on the front of the box. The presentation was auditory only, with no pictures and no visual articulation cues. She also had to reflect upon the internal sound structure of the word. The /ʃ/ word set was increased to include some CVC words e.g. SHIRT, SHEEP, in order to counteract learning effects from the previous task. I have come to think of these segmentation 'posting box' tasks as being 'level D-plus' because of the phonological awareness element they require.

Sample session: Part two

With input primed, the session turned to output processing. In Task 4, Anna was given sound production practice for /ʃ/ in a contrasting sequence with another consonant, using *NDP* picture symbol playing cards. Three sound contrasts were used. To build confidence, we began with /p/ ~ /ʃ/, then moved on to /f/ ~ /ʃ/, and finally to her error pair /s/ ~ /ʃ/. The 'barrier game' involves one player giving the other sufficient information as to how to arrange their materials, such as cards or building blocks, into a matching design from behind a barrier screen: see Figure 5.10. The child arranges a sequence of five *NPD* cards (involving just two sounds, e.g. /s/ ~ /ʃ/) in a random order, e.g. SNAKE PRAM SNAKE SNAKE PRAM. The child then 'reads' this sequence to the therapist, by producing the sound on each card: [s] [ʃ] [s] [s] [ʃ]. The presence of the barrier means that the therapist has to rely on the child's sound production in order to arrange an identical series of sound symbol cards on the therapist's side of the barrier. If the child has been successful in making articulatory contrasts between the two target sounds, the child's series of cards and the therapist's series of cards will be revealed as the same when the barrier is removed. If there is a mismatch, then this stimulates the child to try harder to make the contrast next time. The roles can then be reversed, so that the therapist produces a sequence of sounds which the child has to reproduce by arranging the picture cards in the correct order. For Anna, it certainly added some meaningful communication and fun to a potentially dull articulation activity.

Task Four: Barrier Game
Processing level: K.
Task type: consonant sequencing.
Skills: single sound production in an alternating sequence.
Targets: /s/ /ʃ/.
Materials: two matching sets of NDP picture sound symbols; a barrier.
Presentation: "Lay out your /s/ and /ʃ/ cards in any order that you like behind the barrier so that I cannot see them. Now slowly point to each card in line and say the sound. I will listen and lay out my cards in the same order that I hear you say the sounds. When we remove the barrier, our cards should be arranged in the same order."
NDP Key: /s/ – snake; /ʃ/ – hush baby in pram.

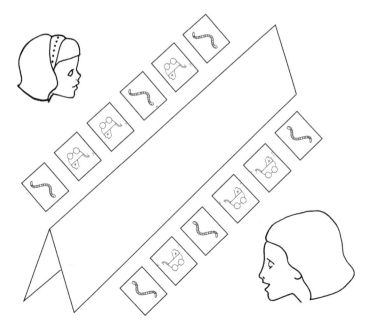

Figure 5.10: Task Four from Anna's sample session for sound system intervention: the barrier game.

As noted in Figure 5.8, Task 5a was the pinnacle of the session. The three-layered spinning wheel (Figure 5.11) gave Anna the opportunity to combine her target consonant /ʃ/ (layer one) with a randomly selected long vowel (layer two) as a single prolonged syllable, e.g. [ʃːːɑːː]. She then had to determine whether the resulting word was a real word or nonword, and choose the appropriate picture (layer three). For example, if she combined /ʃ/ from layer one with /u/ from layer two, she should choose the picture of SHOE from layer three. If the spin of the wheel resulted in /ʃ/ + /ɑ/, resulting in a combination that does not form a real word, then Anna should choose a nonsense character from layer three.

Having nonsense character drawings that she could select and assign to nonwords appealed to Anna's sense of humour. As an articulatory transition task, it involved levels K (single sound production), level J (blending and possible nonword production) and level I (blending and possible real word production). Following this blending activity, Anna's performance was tested at the most demanding level G, by asking her to spontaneously name the composite pictures (see Task 5b in Figure 5.8).

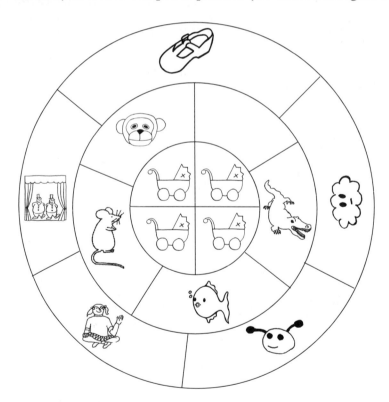

Figure 5.11: Task Five of Anna's sample session for sound system intervention: the spinning wheel task.

Sample session: Part three

The stimuli for Task 6 were Anna's own tape-recorded responses from spontaneous picture naming generated in the second part of Task 5 above. She was asked to judge the correctness of each picture name in turn as it was replayed to her. This task corresponds to level L on the framework, using her own output as input, and taking processing back to level E, which is where the session had started.

Step Six: Analysing the Outcome of Intervention

As illustrated in Figure 5.1, this is the last step in the P→P process, bringing the figure of eight full cycle. Within the psycholinguistic approach, the outcome of each session contributes further data to help solve the processing puzzle. In this way our original hypotheses about the nature of processing breakdown are continually being revised, and change as an outcome of intervention is also monitored. A psycholinguistic framework can be used as a central data bank for recording session outcomes, and as a way of comparing a child's performance across tasks and therefore across levels of processing.

The next activity offers an opportunity to practise this step of the P→P process, by using outcome data from the sample session illustrating Anna's sound system programme, which was described in Step 5. The results of Anna's performance on the six tasks in that session are presented in Figure 5.12.

ACTIVITY 5.3

Aims: to determine the implications of Anna's performance on sound system therapy tasks for a hypothesis about her current processing breakdown, and for planning of the next session.

To complete this activity you will first need to review Figure 5.8 showing the sound system intervention plan set out on the speech processing profile. Then reread the description of the six tasks from Anna's session, referring to the figures. Next, study the results presented in Figure 5.12. Compare Anna's performance across the different tasks and address the following questions below.

(a) Within this specific session, which were Anna's clear strengths and weaknesses ?
(b) Compare her performance across the tasks/levels of processing and write down a revised hypothesis for her processing breakdown on the /s/ ~ /ʃ/ error pair. (For the original hypotheses, refer back to

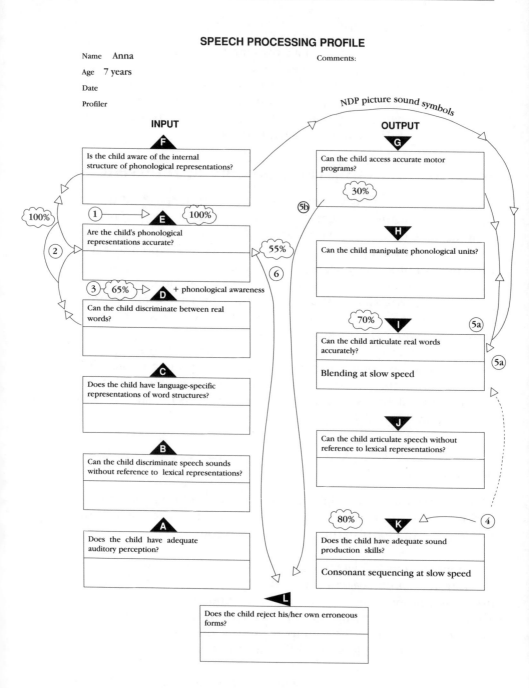

Figure 5.12: Results of Anna's performance on the [ʃ] – [s] error pair during one session. Refer to percentage figures.

the section on sound system work, under 'Question 2: What specific intervention plans are indicated?').

(c) What implications arise for the planning of the next session ?

Check your responses with Key to Activity 5.3 at the end of this chapter and then read the following.

The result of Task 1 shows that Anna's stored phonological representations for the small, working set of CV and CVC target words is now accurate. Equally, in Task 2, she can reliably segment the onset sounds and discriminate between /s/ ~ /ʃ/, when shown pictures of the words and given articulatory cues. However, her performance deteriorates in Task 3 when she is required to perform the same task, but without pictures or articulatory cues, i.e. relying on acoustic information alone. Taking these three input tasks together, the revised hypothesis for Anna's input processing of this word set is that she is not making reliable use of acoustic cues to distinguish between the /s/ ~ /ʃ/ error pair. The implication for future sessions might be to approach level D in a bottom-up fashion, working intensively on discrimination from single sound level upward, intensifying the acoustic contrast by having Anna listen to pre-recorded sound sequences while wearing headphones. The ultimate test will be her discrimination of nonwords.

Task 4 shows an encouraging improvement in control of [ʃ] articulation at single sound level. Likewise, in Task 5a Anna is reasonably able to blend [ʃ] with a following V or VC to make a CV or CVC word, provided that her articulation is slow and careful. The revelation comes in Task 5b when she is asked to spontaneously name the same pictures, scoring only three correct out of 10. Putting the results of Tasks 4 and 5 together, it is apparent that Anna has made considerable gains in her articulatory control of the [ʃ] consonant, from single sound level through to CVC level within the target word set, but has yet to update her stored motor programs to reflect this improved motor programming ability. The good news is that she now has the articulatory ability to produce the words correctly; the bad news is that the old motor programs have not yet been ousted. Whereas Anna had reliably rejected my incorrect pronunciations in Task 1, Task 6 shows that she does not reliably reject her own, even when presented 'off-line' on a tape-recording: she has been too long accustomed to hearing herself say [s] instead of [ʃ] at the beginnings of these words. The implication for future sessions is to continue a combined attack on updating her stored motor programs, by practising production at level I and encouraging her to reflect on the accuracy of her productions at level L.

Conclusion

Figure 5.13 shows a summary of the P→P process. The arrows highlight that assessment analysis at Steps One and Two is the backbone of the process. Once the macro and micro analysis is complete, the specific intervention plans flow forward quite logically. The crux of psycholinguistic intervention is this issue of specificity: intervening at the levels of processing, with the tasks and on the speech sound contrasts where it really matters. This strikes a strong chord with current professional concerns about outcome measurement. We are pressed to demonstrate the efficacy of our intervention and the psycholinguistic approach certainly facilitates this by offering a systematic, theoretically grounded approach to intervention. As a consequence, we have insight not only into what changed, but also into how and why it changed.

Far from being the end of a chapter, Anna's story as presented here led to a new beginning in her clinical management and fostered a significant change to the clinical approach within our department at the Nuffield Centre.

Summary

Step Three involves macro intervention planning.

Question 1: What general intervention plans are indicated?

- Summarize the information gathered in Step One.
- Convert findings into a set of hypotheses.

Question 2: What specific intervention plans are indicated?

- Summarize the information gathered in Step Two.
- Identify areas to be targeted in intervention.

Step Four involves micro intervention planning.

Question 1: What overall design of session would be effective?

- Plan systematic moves between levels of processing.
- Plan an overlapping sequence of tasks that scaffold the child's move from a stronger to weaker level of processing.

Question 2: How should each task be designed?

- It is helpful to work with a constant word set.
- Aim to increase child's processing load by manipulating one task variable at a time.

PROFILE-TO-PROGRAMME PROCESS SUMMARY

STEP ONE ──────────────▶ STEP TWO

Macro Assessment Analysis   **Micro Assessment Analysis**

Which levels of the psycholinguistic   Which task design factors
framework have been assessed?   influence peformance?
In comparison to other children,
which levels show processing   Which sound system factors
breakdown and to what extent?   influence performance?

STEP THREE

Macro Intervention Planning

What general intervention hypotheses   What specific intervention
are indicated?   hypotheses are indicated?

STEP FOUR

Micro Intervention Planning

What overall design of session   How shall each task in the
would be effective?   session be designed?

STEP FIVE

Putting Intervention into Action

Working on a specific processing   Working on a specific processing
skill over time: early, intermediate   skill within one session: a multi-
and advanced stages of intervention.   faceted processing approach.

STEP SIX

Analysing the Outcome of Intervention

Implications for future ◀───────── Comparing strengths and
intervention sessions.   weaknesses
                                          in session performance.

Implications for hypotheses of processing breakdown. ◀────┘

Figure 5.13: Summary of the 'Profile to Programme' process.

Step Five involves putting intervention plans into action.

- The tasks used do not have to be novel.
- Clarify rationale for selecting particular tasks and for presenting them in a particular order.

Step Six involves analysing the outcome of intervention.

- Original hypotheses about the nature of a child's processing breakdown are revised in the light of the outcome of each session.
- This systematic approach to intervention provides a means of measuring outcome in terms of what has changed; why and how.

KEY TO ACTIVITY 5.1

Figure 5.14: Key to Activity 5.1: Anna's rhyme intervention plan mapped on to the speech processing profile

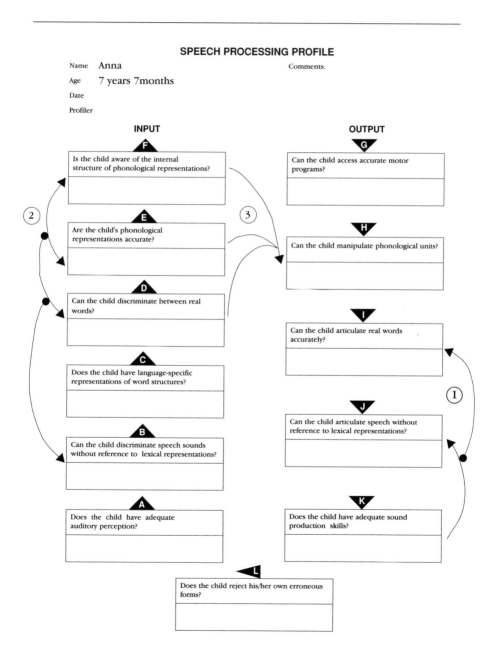

SPEECH PROCESSING PROFILE

Name   Anna

Age   7 years 7months

Date

Profiler

Comments:

INPUT

OUTPUT

F Is the child aware of the internal structure of phonological representations?

G Can the child access accurate motor programs?

E Are the child's phonological representations accurate?

H Can the child manipulate phonological units?

D Can the child discriminate between real words?

I Can the child articulate real words accurately?

C Does the child have language-specific representations of word structures?

J Can the child articulate speech without reference to lexical representations?

B Can the child discriminate speech sounds without reference to lexical representations?

A Does the child have adequate auditory perception?

K Does the child have adequate sound production skills?

L Does the child reject his/her own erroneous forms?

KEY TO ACTIVITY 5.2

Task One: 'Rhyming Picture Windows'
Processing level(s): F, plus story semantics.
Task type: rhyme judgement/gap-fill story.
Skills: sentence level semantics ; rhyme knowledge; segmentation; matching
Targets: DOG, LOG, JOG, FOG. Distractors: DIG, LEG, PIG, LOCK.
Materials: miniature pictures hidden behind opening windows on double sided A4 paper.
Story: Mr Mog went for a jog in the morning fog. He saw a dog and fell over a log. Poor Mr Mog.
Presentation: Look and listen vocabulary check. Listen to this sentence e.g. 'Mr Mog went for a ...' silently search for the missing rhyme picture; does the sentence rhyme and make sense, e.g. 'Mr Mog went for a jog ?'.

Secret Rhyming Windows (Sample)

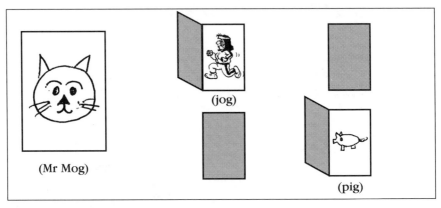

Task two: 'Rhyming Postman'
Processing level(s): E and D.
Task Type: real word rhyme judgement.
Skills: rhyme knowledge, segmentation, matching.
Targets: DOG, LOG, JOG ,FOG Distractors: DIG, LEG, PIG, LOCK.
Materials: 8 picture cards with *NDP* symbols and letters on the reverse side as a visual rime check.
Presentation: Look at the picture and listen to this word e.g. DOG: does DOG sound like OG?: if so, post the picture in the box. When the game is complete check the pictures in the box : do the *NDP* symbols and letters match those on the post box ?

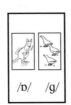

Front of card   Back of card

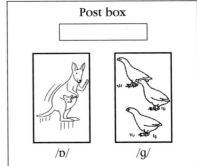

Post box

/ɒ/   /g/

Figure 5.15 Key to Activity 5.2: Ideas for rhyme tasks.

KEY TO ACTIVITY 5.3

(a) Strengths and weaknesses:

Input processing

Anna's clear strengths are auditory lexical decision and real word discrimination with visual cues from pictures and articulation.

Anna's clear weakness is real word discrimination without visual cues from pictures or articulation.

Output processing

Anna's clear strengths are at single sound level and at blended whole word CVC level.

Anna's clear weakness remains spontaneous naming.

(b) Revised hypothesis:

Anna's input processing is weakened by her residual difficulty in detecting acoustic cues.

Anna's output processing shows an improved articulatory ability, but her stored motor programs have yet to be updated to reflect this.

(c) Implications for future sessions:

Target discrimination skills where Anna has to rely increasingly on acoustic cues, withdrawing visual support, taking a bottom-up approach, i.e. working from single sound level upwards.

Target a reconfiguration of Anna's stored motor programs by continuing with input work as described above, by continuing with blending work at word level and encouraging self-monitoring by taped feedback.

Chapter 6
Using Input Processing Strengths to Overcome Speech Output Difficulties

DAPHNE WATERS

This chapter discusses the application of the psycholinguistic framework in assessment and intervention with a 5-year-old boy with a severe developmental speech disorder. It illustrates how a profile of speech processing abilities can integrate with information and data from other sources and perspectives to provide a principled basis for intervention and for evaluating change. This particular child's case illustrates that while phonological analysis and psycholinguistic assessment both made essential contributions to therapy planning, they did not, in themselves, provide sufficient information. Therapists must make a considerable leap from assessment findings to designing therapy appropriate to an individual child's needs as a learner. Chiat (1997) points out that the design of effective therapy has to be seen as a theoretical issue in its own right. Similarly, in relation to adults with acquired disorders of communication, Byng (1995) has argued that we have to recognize that questions about therapy constitute a whole new theoretical domain.

The chapter will illustrate that devising effective therapy for severe developmental speech disorders involves several essential stages. First, it requires an analysis of what needs to change in an individual child's surface spoken language behaviour. Second, it involves investigation of constraints and strengths that underlie current level of functioning. The final, and least often documented, step involves devising a means to facilitate the process of learning and discovery that must take place if speech patterns are to change.

Children with developmental speech disorders form a heterogeneous population that does not lend itself to large group research. Therefore the development of theory and practice in relation to their management depends on clinicians reporting and discussing their experiences with individual children so that a body of knowledge can be built up over time which can encourage a 'theory of practice' to emerge and evolve. It is hoped that the case discussed in this chapter will contribute to that process.

Alan: Background Information

The child (Alan) who is the focus of the chapter was first seen by the speech and language therapy service at CA 3;8. He presented with a severe developmental speech disorder in the absence of any identifiable causative factors and significant family history, except that his father was reported to have 'had a lisp' as a child. He was the second of two children in a loving and supportive family and his older sibling had typical speech and language development. Alan's family were all monolingual speakers of the Edinburgh variety of Scottish English.

From CA 3;11 to 4;3 Alan attended a phonological awareness group designed to prepare young children with phonological delay/disorder for individual therapy. No observable changes in his speech output occurred during that period. He then took part in individual therapy sessions from CA 4;4 to 4;8, in which the Metaphon approach was adopted (Howell and Dean, 1994). The focus of this therapy was mainly on Alan's error pattern of replacing syllable initial fricatives with stops, e.g. SUN → [dʌn]. No identifiable changes occurred in his pronunciation patterns following this period of intervention. Assessments carried out during this time indicated that Alan's severe speech difficulties occurred in the context of otherwise age-appropriate language abilities (Table 6.1).

By now Alan was very aware of not being understood and was increasingly reluctant to take part in assessment or therapy activities that drew attention to his speech, often refusing to co-operate and exhibiting 'difficult' behaviour in the clinic and at home. He entered mainstream school at CA 4;11. Teachers were immediately concerned about him, reporting disruptive and often aggressive behaviour in class and in the playground. All those involved felt that these behaviour patterns were the result of his frequent experience of failure in communicative interactions with adults and with his peers. He did not understand the reason for communicative breakdowns and reacted with a mixture of anger, fear and aggression. His coping strategies included refusing activities where he expected failure, demanding to take control of interactions and taking refuge in elaborate solitary play activities in which other children and adults were, at best, allowed to be spectators.

Around the time of his fifth birthday a further period of therapy was arranged. Initially this consisted of one 45-minute session per week

Table 6.1: Alan's assessment results: C.A. 4;0 – 4;9

Assessment	CA	Result
[1]articulation	4;0	SS 69
	4;4	SS 61
	4;9	SS 57
		Raw score remained almost static over this period: hence the decline in SS with age
[2]receptive vocabulary	4;0	age appropriate
[3]verbal comprehension	4;4	AE 5;0 – 5;2
		SS: + 0.8
[4]expressive language measure	4;4	Scores for Information and Grammar were both judged to be age appropriate. Accuracy of scoring is questionable because of intelligibility difficulties

[1] *The Edinburgh Articulation Test* (Anthony, Bogle, Ingram, et al., 1971);
[2] *British Picture Vocabulary Scales* (Dunn, Dunn, Whetton, et al., 1982);
[3] *Reynell Developmental Language Scales* (Reynell and Huntley, 1985);
[4] *Renfrew Action Picture Test* (Renfrew, 1989);
SS, standard score;
AE, age equivalent.

with the author. Later an additional weekly session was introduced in the same clinic but carried out by Alan's community therapist. There was regular weekly consultation between the two therapists to discuss findings and plan session aims and activities.

At the age of 5 years Alan presented with speech which was unintelligible except for short utterances in context. His mother understood more than anyone else did, but even she was not always able to 'translate'. There had been no identifiable changes in his speech output forms for at least 16 months. In spite of his lack of success in communicating his message he was an eager conversationalist. So long as no attention was drawn to his pronunciation he would converse about topics of his own choice using long, grammatically complex utterances which appeared to include an extensive vocabulary.

Therapy targeting a particular identified systemic simplification pattern in his speech output (stopping of word initial fricatives) had not been effective and, in view of Alan's withdrawal of co-operation in the clinic, a radical rethink was required. Developing a new approach required more extensive evaluation of his speech output patterns and his underlying speech processing strengths and difficulties.

The Search for a Rationale for Therapy

The contribution of phonological analysis

Phonological analysis procedures reveal how a child's speech sound system compares to the adult target system and/or to the speech patterns of typically developing children of similar chronological age (Grunwell, 1992). They give a descriptive, rather than an explanatory account of a child's difficulties and enable us to organize our observations of the changes that need to take place in a child's speech to increase intelligibility, thus assisting in decision-making about treatment goals.

The limitations of perceptually based analysis of speech data must be acknowledged. First, the descriptive account (and hence the indications for therapy) will vary according to the theoretical framework underpinning the particular analysis procedure adopted: for example, segmental error analysis, as in *The Edinburgh Articulation Test* (Anthony, Bogel, Ingram, et al., 1971), phonological process analysis, as in the Metaphon screening and probe assessments (Dean, Howell, Hill, et al., 1990), or non-linear analysis procedures (Bernhardt and Gilbert, 1992). Some phonological analysis had already been carried out on Alan's speech data, mainly within a phonological process framework of description, which had led to therapy targeting a particular error pattern (stopping of word initial fricatives). This therapy had not had a successful outcome. Second, limitations of perceptually based phonological analysis have been revealed by instrumental investigations that demonstrate 'covert contrasts' which are not detectable by a listener (see, for example, Gibbon, 1990; Scobbie, Gibbon, Hardcastle, et al., 1998; Gibbon, 1999; Dent, this volume). These findings suggest that, for some children at least, explanation for some apparent neutralizations of phonological contrasts is more likely to involve difficulties with speech motor processing (programming, timing, and co-ordination of articulatory gestures) rather than with lack of knowledge of phonological contrasts. Potential underlying difficulties such as these are not revealed by linguistic analysis alone, but *can* be explored within a psycholinguistic model of speech processing. First, however, information gained from the phonological analysis itself will be summarized.

Tables 6.2 and 6.3 show samples of Alan's single-word and connected speech data collected when he was approximately 5 years of age. Tables 6.4 and 6.5 show his consonant phonetic inventory and distribution.

Alan's realizations of disyllabic and polysyllabic words preserved the correct number of syllables with appropriate stress (see, for example, items 20, 42, 132 in Table 6.2). Syllable structure types were restricted to CV, VC, CVC, CVCC and CVCCC. That is, Alan did not use syllable

Table 6.2: Transcribed single-word speech data: CA 5;1 – 5;6 years

ITEM	Alans's pronunciation		ITEM	Alan's pronunciation	
1. boat	[bop] 1 1		41. ten	[dɛn]	
2. bus	[bʌpɸ] 1 1 1 1	[bɪf] 1	42. telephone	['dzɛwəboʊm]	
3. ball	1		43. top	[bɒp]	
4. big	[bɔː]		44. tin	[dɪn]	
5. book	[dɪd]		45. tape	[bap]	
6. boot	[dʉt] 1 1 1 1 1		46. tiny	['danɪ]	
7. bit	[bʉp] 1 1		47. toothbrush	['dʉsdɪs]	
8. bat	[bɪp]		48. tree	[dzɛə]	
9. bead	[dat]		49. twelve	[bɛʊɸ]	
10. bin	[bɛːb]		50. train	[dzan]	
11. bear	[dɪn]		51. truck	[gjʌk]	
12. bell	[dɛʌ]	[daʌ]	52. two	[dzu]	[du] 1 1
13. box	[daʊ]		53. garage	['dajadz]	
14. bridge	[dɒts]		54. got	[dɒt]	
15. blue	[dɪdz] 1 1		55. go	[do]	
16. bluetak	[bu]		56. glue	[dju]	
17. brick	['du'da]		57. key	[dɛə]	
18. brush	[dat] [dɪs]	[gak]	58. cat	[dat]	
19. pink			59. car	[gɑː]	
20. pelican	[dzɪnts]		60. comb	[bom] 1 1 1	
21. pine cone	['dɛwədʌn]		61. cup	[bʌp] 1 1 1 1	
22. pan	['g̃aŋ'g̃oŋ]		62. cold	[boːb]	
23. pin	[dan]	[bam]	63. cork	[gɔk]	
24. pear	[bɪm]		64. crossing	['dɒsɪn]	
25. pen	[daə]	[dzaə]	65. clock	[gɒk]	
26. peg	[bam] 1 1 1		66. cloth	[gɒx]	
27. point	[gag]	[gɛg]	67. lorry	['ʒɔwʌ]	['dzɔwʌ]
28. penny	[dɒnt]		68. lights	[dzaːts]	
29. picture	[bɛmʌ]		69. lollypop	['zɔbɒ]	
30. plastic	['dɪtsʌ] ['dasdɪʔ]		70. lamp post	['landost]	
31. doll			71. look	[lut]	
32. duck	[dzɔː] 1 1		72. yes	[dzɛs]	
33. dolly	[gʌk] 1 1		73. round	[jɔnd]	
34. dog	['dzɔwə]		74. ring	[(ʒ)ɪn]	
35. dustbin	[dɒd] ['dɪsdɪn]		75. rubber	['ʊɪpə]	
36. this			76. wellington	['dawəntən]	
37. thirteen	[nus]		77. one	[dʒɔn]	
38. think	['dɛtɪn]	['datsdɪn]	78. man	[nan] 1 1 1	
39. things	[dɪnts]		79. motorbike	['notʌdaːt]	
40. three	[dɪnts]		80. measuring tape	['nɛzəm'bap]	
			81. mummy	['mʌmɪ]	
			82. metal	['nɛtʊ]	

ITEM	Alan's pronunciation	ITEM	Alan's pronunciation
83. fire engine	['daɛndzən]	113. nine	[naən]
84. four	[dɔ]	114. numbers	['mʌmbʌs]
85. five	[baɣ]	115. next	[nɛst]
86. fourteen	['dɔtɪn]	116. knife	[nɛəs]
87. fifteen	['dɪsdɪn]		
88. fit	[dɪt]	117. shops	[bɒpɸ] ı ı ı
89. farmer	['bɑmə]	118. sheep	[bɪːp] ı ı ı
90. farm house	['bɑmʔaʊs]	119. shark	[gaːkx]
91. fish	[bɪɸ]	120. shoe	[dju] [dzu]
92. fan	[dzan]	121. shell	[dzaʊ]
93. fork	[ḡɔk]	122. shells	[daʊs]
94. frying pan	['daəmbam]		
95. flowers	['dɔwʌs]	123. chimney	['bɪmʊɪ]
		124. Jo	[dzjo]
96. six	[ḡɪq]	125. Jim	[bɪm]
97. seven	['dɛsən]	126. jar	[dɛː]
98. centre	['dɛntə]		
99. safety clip	['baʔɪbɪp]	127. hot	[ʔɒt]
100. safety pin	['bɛstɪbɪm]	128. house	[ʔaʊs]
101. sock	[gɒk] ı ı ı	129. hairbrush	[ʔaːdɪs]
102. soap	[bop]		
103. soft	[dɒst]	130. aeroplane	['aːbam]
104. sun	[djʌn]	131. easy peasy	[ɛzə'bɛːɣɛ]
105. sunglasses	['dʌndɛsəs]	132. elephant	['dawədʌnt]
106. sunflower	['djɪndɔə]	133. ambulance	['andzəʔants]
107. scissors	['dɪsɛs]	134. alarm clock	[ʌw'amgɒk]
108. school	[gu]	135. eleven	['dɛsən]
109. straw	[dzɔ]	136. early	['ɜwə]
110. screwdriver	['dubaɸa]	137. egg	[ag] ı ı
111. spoon	[bʉm]	138. animal	['anʌdu]
112. sponge	[bʌmz]		

Items in Table 6.2 are grouped according to target initial phoneme.
Multiple tokens of a realization are indicated by the symbol appearing outside the square brackets.

Table 6.3: Transcribed connected speech data: CA 5;1 – 5;6

Orthographic transcription	Alan's transcribed form	
I do want to do some drawings	[ə 'du nɒnə du nə 'dzɔn̩ts]	1
that reminds me…the drawing paper	[na ə'nandz mɪ…ʌ 'dsɔːn 'bapa]	2
a proper word	[ʌ 'pɒpʌ zjɔd]	3
tiny little book	['danɪ nɪʔ 'dʉt]	4
I do like it	[aɪ 'du 'daɪt ɪt]	5
still too big	['dzaː 'du 'dɪt]	6
hang on a minute	[an ɔn ə 'nɪnɪt]	7
actually, you do get houses like that	['aχədə ə 'du dɛt ʔausəs a nat]	8
the bridge too small?	[ə dɪts du 'nɔ]	9
mustn't cross at the corner	[nʌsʌ dɒs at ə 'gɔːŋʌ]	10
turn that round	[dzɔn na 'dzɔnd]	11
there's something missing	[ʌs dɪnsɪ'mɪfɪm]	12
no, that's not how it goes	['no nats nɒt aʊ ə 'do	13
I know how it/that goes	'naʊ no ʔaʊ nə do	
it goes like that	na dos na 'nat]	

Table 6.4: Alan's phonetic inventory (consonants) based on data collected between the ages of 5;1 and 5;6

	Labial	Dental	Alveolar	Post-alveolar	Palatal	Velar	Glottal	Other
Nasal			n			(ŋ)		
Plosive	p b		t d			k g	ʔ	(q)
Fricative	(ɸ)	f (ɣ̥)	s z z̥	ʒ		(x)		(χ)
Affricate			ts ds dz	(dʒ)				
Approximant	w	(ʋ)	l		j			
Other								

Table 6.5: Phonetic distribution (consonants)

Single consonants

	Word Initial	Within Word	Word Final
Nasal	m n	m n	m n (ŋ)
Plosive	b d g ʔ	b d t ʔ	p b t d k g (q)
Fricative	z̥ ʒ	s ɣ̥ (χ)	ɸ f ɣ̥ s (x)
Affricate	d͡s d͡z (dʒ)	d͡z	t͡s d͡z (p͡ɸ)
Approx.	l	w (ʋ) j	

Consonant clusters

Word Initial	Word Final
gj	nt nts st

initial consonant clusters (for example, Table 6.2, items 15, 17, 65, 108, 111). His consonant inventory was surprisingly complete. Only the following phonemes were absent: velar nasal /ŋ/; voiceless post-alveolar fricative /ʃ/; the interdental fricatives /θ/ and /ð/; voiceless post-alveolar affricate /tʃ/; alveolar approximant /ɹ/ and glottal fricative /h/. However, Table 6.5 shows that the distribution of many consonant phonemes was restricted. Voiceless consonants did not appear word initially. There were no fricatives in word initial contexts. However, affricated alveolar stops (and occasional velar stops with palatal release) appeared in word initial positions. These occurred in the context of word initial fricative, affricate, cluster and glide targets (see items 120, 124, 109, 72 in Table 6.2 respectively), but also occasionally in the context of word initial plosive targets (for example items 19, 31, 52 in Table 6.2), therefore no 'rule' was discernible which might predict their occurrence. There were many vowel errors that could not be easily predicted on the basis of either the target or its consonant environment. In particular, the close-front vowel /i/ did not occur in his system, his realization of /ɛ/ was variable (for example, item 26 in Table 6.2), and there were very few occurrences of diphthongs.

By far the most striking pattern to emerge from analysis of the transcribed data was a strong tendency for all consonants within an utterance to be produced at the same place of articulation (for example, items 5, 6, 26, 62 in Table 6.2). This seemed to be an absolute constraint at the level of the syllable, but the tendency was also apparent, although with less consistency, across syllable boundaries (compare, for example items 15 and 16 in Table 6.2). Sometimes, whole connected utterances involved only one place of consonant articulation (usually alveolar), see, for example utterances 1, 4, 5, 7, 9, 13 in Table 6.3. Pronunciations of the same word in isolation were usually consistent on different occasions but there were a few examples of inconsistency, which nevertheless always conformed to the 'one place of articulation' constraint (see Table 6.2, items 17 and 22 in particular). No 'rule' could be found that could predict what place of consonant articulation would be adopted for a particular target syllable or word. Place of articulation appeared often to be predictable from the target coda (for example, items 10, 26, 60, 61 in Table 6.2), but this was not always the case (see items 1, 4, 5, 6 for example). Vowel realizations seemed to be independent of consonant environment.

Analysis of Alan's pronunciation patterns went some way towards defining a new focus and rationale for intervention. Perhaps the most valuable insight concerned what *not* to do: it was apparent from the analysis that a 'minimal contrast' approach to therapy would be of little help since his pronunciation patterns could not be characterized in terms of contrasts (or lack of contrasts) at a segmental level. For example, his realization of word initial velars could not be described in terms of lack of velar/alveolar contrast (see items 57–66 in Table 6.2). The domain of contrast seemed to be the syllable, or possibly the word, and place of articulation seemed to be specified for onset + coda rather than for each separately. The focus of therapy should, therefore, be chiefly at the level of the syllable or larger unit, rather than at segmental level. Among other things, and perhaps most urgently, Alan needed to learn to monitor and manipulate place of consonant articulation at the level of the syllable in order to improve intelligibility, but it was not at all clear what could be done to help him to achieve this. These insights were a first step on the way to knowing how to proceed in therapy. However, the information gained from phonological analysis, while valuable, was not enough.

The contribution of psycholinguistic profiling

For several reasons we needed to know more about the speech processing strengths and weaknesses that Alan brought to the task of achieving intelligible speech. First, this would provide us with possible explanations for his current unintelligibility. Second, it could tell us what constraints we (and Alan) were up against in working towards positive change, and what strengths we could count on to assist him in that process.

The psycholinguistic framework allows systematic exploration, via a series of assessments or 'tapping' tasks, of a child's input and output processing, the status of internal phonological representations and the child's awareness of their structure. However, it is rarely appropriate in a clinical context to spend long periods of time exclusively on assessment tasks. In Alan's case there was a high level of anxiety and sense of urgency on the part of parents and teachers that precluded postponing intervention pending an extended period of investigation. Fortunately, one of the advantages of working within the psycholinguistic framework is that pieces of information that are gleaned by design or good fortune during investigative therapy can be slotted into a child's profile. This approach was adopted in profiling Alan's speech processing abilities.

In the interests of clarity of presentation, the evidence used to compile the profile is presented separately from the discussion of therapy. This is, in fact, an artificial separation since much of the evidence was acquired gradually in the course of therapy 'probe' activities that had been planned on the basis of hunches and hypotheses about his difficulties and abilities. In fact, one of the consequences of working within the psycholinguistic framework seems to be a blurring of the distinction between tasks designed for assessment and those designed for therapy (cf. Corrin, this volume; Rees, this volume). The resulting profile is shown in Figure 6.1. Examples of the evidence used

SPEECH PROCESSING PROFILE

Name   Alan

Age   5;0

Date

Profiler

Comments:

INPUT	OUTPUT

F

Is the child aware of the internal structure of phonological representations?

✓   (emerging)

G

Can the child access accurate motor programs?

× × ×

E

Are the child's phonological representations accurate?

✓ ✓

H

Can the child manipulate phonological units?

× × ×

D

Can the child discriminate between real words?

✓ ✓ ✓

I

Can the child articulate real words accurately?

× × ×

C

Does the child have language-specific representations of word structures?

No data

J

Can the child articulate speech without reference to lexical representations?

× × ×

B

Can the child discriminate speech sounds without reference to lexical representations?

✓ ✓ ✓

A

Does the child have adequate auditory perception?

✓ ✓ ✓

K

Does the child have adequate sound production skills?

×

L

Does the child reject his/her own erroneous forms?

×

Figure 6.1 Alan's speech processing profile at CA 5;0.

to answer each question in the profile are discussed in the following sections.

Input processing: auditory perception and auditory discrimination for speech

Alan had passed all routine screening tests of hearing, he had no history of ear infections and his parents had never suspected any hearing difficulty. We could therefore confidently answer "Yes" to question A, "Does he have adequate auditory perception?". To answer question B, "Can the child discriminate speech sounds without reference to lexical representations?" and question D, "Can the child discriminate between real words?" we investigated Alan's 'same/different discrimination' performance with pairs of real words, e.g. BUS/BUT; PLACE/PLATE and nonwords, e.g.VOST/VOTS; BLAYST/BLAYTS, taken from Bridgeman and Snowling (1988) following the procedure described in that paper. He performed without error on both real word and nonword items. If further evidence were needed it came from his enthusiasm for this activity. We had by now deduced that when Alan was co-operative and enthusiastic in a task it was a strong indication that he was confident of success. Conversely, when he refused a task, or employed elaborate diversion tactics, it was a strong indication that he felt he was going to fail. His verdict on the same/different discrimination tasks was that they were 'easy peasy'.

Alan's response to rhyme judgment tasks provided further evidence relevant to questions B and D. He was very wary of such activities at first because initially we had not made it clear enough that he was only expected to listen and comment (rather than generate rhymes which he was unable/unwilling to attempt). However, once his co-operation was gained it became clear that Alan understood the concept of rhyme and was able to make judgements about nonwords and real words (spoken by an adult) that 'belonged together' on the basis of rhyme match. The game format used was the 'Ed Game' (see Read, 1978). This involved a puppet named Ed who likes only things that sound like his own name (that this, things that rhyme with 'Ed'). A number of pictures, objects and toy characters were presented and named by an adult (for example, BED, FRED, MOUSE, TED, RED, ICECREAM). Alan's task was to decide whether Ed would like each item. Again he was wary at first but soon showed that he was able to match auditorily presented word on the basis of rhyme match. We were confident in answering "Yes" to questions B and D. (No evidence was sought to answer question C "Does the child have language-specific representations of word structures?".)

Accuracy of phonological representations

There was no indication that input processing deficits were contributing to Alan's severe speech difficulties. However, there was still the possibility that, in spite of adequate auditory processing abilities, he may not have extracted and/or stored phonological information from auditory input in a typical way. Perhaps phonological representations were less robust (weaker or 'fuzzier') than in most children of his age and, while adequate for receptive (recognition) purposes, they were insufficient to provide a basis for successful output processing. What kind of evidence would support that possibility? Weak/'fuzzy' phonological representations might be expected to lead to a tendency to confuse words with phonological similarities such as RADIO/RADIATOR, perhaps slow acquisition of new vocabulary and word-finding difficulties (see Constable, this volume). Alan did not exhibit any of these difficulties. Furthermore, he had no difficulty with auditory lexical tasks (see Book 1, Stackhouse and Wells, 1997, Chapter 2). For example, when asked to select a picture, named by an adult, from a minimal pair or minimal set of items, such as TREE/THREE or COAT/BOAT/GOAT, he had no difficulties. Success in this task requires robust and accurate internal phonological representations of the items since, to succeed, a child must rely solely on comparing the spoken stimulus with internal phonological representations of each of the pictured items. The task removes any possibility of using contextual clues. 'Fuzzy' phonological representations would be expected to lead to difficulty with such tasks. Alan made consistently accurate responses, whether the contrast involved onset, vowel or coda. He was also consistently successful in a judgement task where he was asked to say whether a puppet's pronunciation of a picture name was "good" or "silly". The "silly" pronunciations were either minimally contrasting real words, e.g. CAP pronounced [tap] or nonwords, e.g. TREE pronounced [dɹi]. Again, Alan's lack of anxiety and evident enjoyment of the task were noted.

The above evidence suggested strongly that Alan's severe speech difficulties could not be accounted for on the basis of inaccurate or 'weak' internal phonological representations. The answer to question E, "Are the child's phonological representations accurate?" was "Yes". Although we could not be sure that his phonological representations were fully adult-like, it seemed unlikely that they could be sufficiently atypical to account for his extremely deviant output forms.

Awareness of the structure of phonological representations

Alan was now introduced to *silent* rhyme and alliteration tasks in order to address question F, "Is the child aware of the internal structure of phonological representations?". He was asked to make judgements about whether words rhyme and/or about whether words begin with the same sound. The items were presented as pictures and not named by the therapist. (Examples of such activities are described and analysed later in the chapter.) Success in these tasks required (a) that Alan's phonological representations for the items concerned were accurate and (b) that he was able to access those representations, and reflect on their subsyllabic structure. We used these tasks to probe the current extent of Alan's awareness of phonological structure and to decide whether such tasks would be likely to play a useful role in therapy aimed to develop this awareness.

These were unfamiliar activities for Alan and it took a little while before he understood what was required. However, it soon became apparent that he did have an emerging ability to reflect on and silently manipulate the (subsyllabic) structure of internal phonological representations. He was, with encouragement, able to decide on onset and rhyme matches between pictured items without auditory input. Ability to reflect explicitly on the structure of stored, internal phonological representations seemed to be an emerging strength. Question F was therefore given one tick.

Alan had to be reassured that these were 'thinking and listening games' and *not* 'speaking games'. However, on one occasion, he spontaneously suggested an addition to the rhyming set we were working with: SNAKE, RAKE, LAKE, etc. He said, "I know another one that goes with 'Mr Snake' ($\rightarrow$ [net]); it's [gak]". None of the adults around the table were able to interpret this. Alan was frustrated when we did not respond appropriately to his suggestion and after repeating it several times, in exasperation, he rummaged through our pile of pictures and eventually held up a picture of a cake. "See [gak]" he said, "[gak] rhymes with [net]".

ACTIVITY 6.1

Aim: to demonstrate that informal observations can provide important evidence when compiling a child's speech processing profile.

Reflect on the incident described in the previous paragraph. For which of the questions on the speech processing profile does it provide evidence?

See Key to Activity 6.1 at the end of this chapter, then read on.

In spite of knowing, on the basis of his own phonological representations, that SNAKE and CAKE share a common rhyme (which confirmed the answers to questions E and F), Alan was unable to generate output forms that reflected that knowledge. Therefore the answer to question H,

"Can the child manipulate phonological units?" (for output purposes) was "No". The fact that he was unable to 'repair' the communication breakdown which ensued suggests that he had no access to accurate stored motor programs for these words (question G, "Can the child access accurate motor programs?"). Furthermore, Alan's puzzlement and frustration at our inability to appreciate the rhyme match he had discovered strongly suggested that he regarded his pronunciations of these words as adequate realizations of the phonological representations in his lexicon. In other words, he had failed to reject his erroneous output forms and remained unaware of the mismatch between his stored phonological information and the audible end product of his output processing (question L).

Speech output processing

Alan's extremely deviant speech patterns could not be accounted for by either input processing difficulties or by weak or inaccurate phonological representations. The evidence pointed to an explanation in terms of speech output processing limitations. Could we be more precise about which particular aspects of output processing were the principal source of Alan's difficulties? Evidence addressing question K, "Does the child have adequate sound production skills?" was provided by an oro-facial examination, a diadochokinetic (DDK) task and an investigation of ability to imitate single phonemes. No structural abnormalities were found. Alan was able to imitate a range of lip and tongue movements successfully, but side-to-side alternating movement of the tongue was effortful and involved whole head movement, and he had difficulty with tongue elevation. It is worth considering the latter observation in the light of recent findings that seven out of a group of 10 normally developing 5-year-old children had difficulty in achieving tongue elevation (Williams and Stackhouse, 2000).

In a DDK task his repetitions of single syllables /pə/, /tə/ or /kə/ were slow and when the polysyllabic sequence /pətəkə/ was required he found it very difficult to maintain the order of syllables, and sequencing broke down after four slow repetitions. Alan was able to imitate most consonant phonemes in isolation with the exceptions of /ɹ/ and /l/, both realized as [z], and /ð/ which was realized as [n̪]. The velar plosive /g/ was realized variably as [g] or [d]. His imitated realizations of the vowels /i/, /ɛ/ and /ə/ were all [a]. Diphthongs were not attempted. He was very reluctant to imitate CV nonsense syllables, attempting only syllables with /m/, /b/, /p/ and /v/ in onset, which he achieved accurately, except that the bilabial voiceless plosive target was realized as voiced.

These findings indicated some degree of difficulty with speech sound production and with the planning and co-ordination of articulatory gestures. It seemed likely that some aspects of Alan's pronunciation patterns could be related to difficulties in executing articulatory gestures for certain speech sounds, especially absence of /ð/, /ɹ/ and /i/ from the phonetic inventory and the variable realization of /ɛ/. However, it seemed unlikely that limitations in relation to question K could be sufficient to account for all Alan's current speech patterns.

Another possible explanation was that accurate phonological representations, linked to semantic information in the lexicon, were not linked to motor programs that allowed the acoustic correlates of those representations to be reproduced in output: either the motor programs themselves or the mapping between them and phonological and semantic information were 'faulty'. Inadequate motor programs, in turn, might be the result of difficulty with motor programming. If motor programming for speech *was* the major area of difficulty for Alan it would be evident in tasks that required him to imitate auditorily presented speech material as well as in his spontaneous naming responses. The three tasks – spontaneous naming, imitation of real, familiar words and imitation of nonwords – require and allow progressively less involvement of existing, stored motor programs. These three tasks address, respectively, question G, "Can the child access accurate motor programs?", question I, "Can the child articulate real words accurately?" and question J "Can the child articulate speech without reference to lexical representations?". If a child's imitated forms for nonwords are significantly more accurate than spontaneous naming and more accurate than imitations of real words, the implication is that motor programming ability is adequate. That is, the child *is* able to devise accurate motor programs (and plan and execute the required articulatory gestures) when called upon to do so 'from scratch' without drawing on existing motor programs stored as components of lexical representations. In fact, Alan did not seem to be any more accurate when imitating nonwords than he was in other kinds of speech data. We had already found that he was extremely reluctant to attempt imitation of nonsense syllables (even CV syllables), which was almost certainly indicative of inability. He refused to attempt CVC syllables which required two places of consonant articulation, e.g./gɪm/, therefore no further systematic assessment of this ability was undertaken. However, the small amount of evidence we had indicated that his imitated realizations were similar to those found in spontaneous speech. For example, he imitated voiceless plosive targets in CV nonwords as voiced cognates, e.g. /ka/ → [ga], consistent with his spontaneous speech in which all prevocalic consonants were voiced.

This exploration of Alan's speech output processing indicated difficulties at all stages including, and perhaps predominantly, limitations in relation to motor programming. The errors evident in his spontaneous real word output (where output was derived from stored motor programs) seemed, as far as we could judge, to reflect the same limitations evident when he was required to devise new motor programs to reproduce the articulatory and acoustic characteristics of auditorily presented nonwords.

It is interesting to compare Alan's performance on these tasks with Bryan and Howard's (1992) report of the child D.F., whose nonword repetitions were more accurate than either his spontaneous naming responses or his imitations of real words. Bryan and Howard concluded that D.F. had failed to update stored motor programs for words in his lexicon as his motor programming abilities for speech had matured. They describe this as a case of 'frozen phonology' in which stored motor programs (and consequently habitual output forms) were not making full use of the child's current programming ability. In Alan's case it seemed more likely that stored motor programs were inadequate because of *current* limitation on speech motor programming ability.

Summary of the results of psycholinguistic investigation

ACTIVITY 6.2

Aim: to summarize the above evidence using the speech processing model.

Refer to the speech processing model from Book 1, reproduced below as Figure 6.2. Using ticks and crosses, indicated Alan's areas of strength and weakness.

Check your answer with the Key to Activity 6.2 at the end of this chapter, then read on.

Alan had no apparent difficulties with input processing and his internal representations were accurate. He had difficulties at all levels of speech output processing. In particular, we concluded that he had an on-going inability to devise motor programs to reproduce either stored phonological representations or auditorily presented familiar or novel combinations of phonemes.

Considering the child as a learner

Considerable insight had been gained into Alan's speech processing abilities. Were we now in a position, as Chiat (1994) puts it, to know how to help Alan to find ways through his speech processing limitations?

SPEECH PROCESSING MODEL

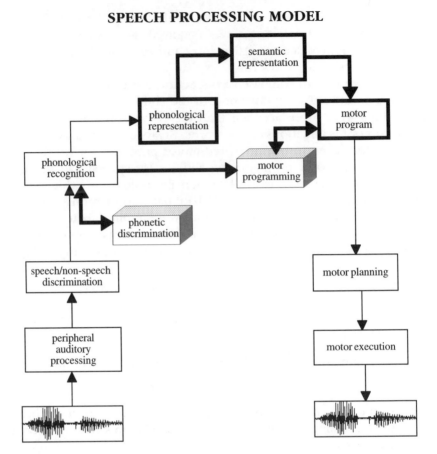

Figure 6.2 Speech processing model for use in Activity 6.2.

The achievement of positive changes in intelligibility would require Alan to use and extend his limited motor programming abilities to attempt modification of the existing inadequate motor programs stored in his lexicon in association with semantic, grammatical and perceptually based phonological representations. However, we still had little idea of how that might be achieved. Marshall (1997) points out that psycholinguistic theories themselves do not grapple with issues of therapy, such as which treatments work for which deficits. This echoes Chiat (1994) who stresses that while psycholinguistic profiling throws light on where problems occur in processing, this does not, in itself, tell us how that problem can be overcome. A successful solution to this question for one child will not necessarily be successful with another. We needed to consider this child as an individual learner.

The most basic step in planning therapy was to decide whether to target Alan's identified output processing deficits directly or, instead, to design therapy activities around his identified strengths. Intuitively it seems logical that therapy should focus on areas of weakness, which are assumed to be causative and maintaining factors in a child's surface difficulties. In Alan's case, this would suggest intervention targeting speech output processing skills. For example, learning to produce the full range of single phonemes accurately, then learning to devise and execute motor programs for various CV syllables and words, then CVC syllables and words, and so on in a systematic way by providing him with models, feedback and opportunities for practice. Such a deficit-based approach would involve the therapist taking the lead in therapy while Alan's role would be to strive for increased accuracy through imitation and practice. Therapy tasks would, of necessity, draw attention to his speech output difficulties. However, it was clear from Alan's history of refusal of just such activities that this was not likely to be a successful strategy. He had clearly indicated his unwillingness to follow instructions passively, his determination to avoid tasks in which he expected to fail, and his need to remain in control of interactions. On the other hand, we had been impressed by his inventiveness, and his pleasure in discovering a new skill or piece of information for himself, while an adult played a supporting and facilitating role. These problem-solving skills and the evidence of emerging reflective awareness of spoken language (Grieve, 1990) in his response to assessment tasks led us to conclude that he would respond best in situations that allowed him to be an active discoverer and user of information rather than a passive learner.

The Rationale for Therapy

On the basis of all the above evidence we hypothesized that Alan could best be helped to overcome his identified output processing difficulties by capitalizing on his speech processing strengths and on his cognitive strengths, rather than by focusing directly on output processing.

ACTIVITY 6.3

Aim: to identify speech processing and cognitive strengths that could be utilized in intervention.

Reflect on the evidence presented so far about Alan's strengths and weaknesses. List aspects of speech processing and cognitive abilities that could be enlisted to assist him to make changes in his speech output.

See Key to Activity 6.3 at the end of this chapter, then read on.

Alan's good auditory (input) processing ability, his accurate phonological representations, and his emerging awareness of their structure were all strengths that could be used to good effect in therapy. Furthermore it would be possible to take advantage of his enthusiasm for activities that require active reflection, deduction and discovery. He would, we believed, be able and willing to attempt the difficult task of devising new motor programs when he felt he had sufficient resources to ensure a reasonable chance of success. It was the role of therapy to provide him with learning opportunities to acquire those resources of knowledge and skill, which were analysed as follows:

(1) He needed greater awareness of acoustic and articulatory charac-teristics of various categories of speech sounds, especially awareness of relationship between place of consonant articulation and auditory and visual cues.
(2) He needed to build on his emerging ability to analyse the structure of adult pronunciations.
(3) He would need to further develop the ability to reflect on the structure of his own (accurate) internal phonological representa-tions.
(4) He would have to learn to apply those same analysis skills to moni-toring his own output forms.

It was hypothesized that his accumulation of knowledge and skills would provide the impetus for attempts to devise new and more successful motor programs. Such a rationale for intervention recalls Piagetian notions of development as a process of "connecting new knowledge with already existing knowledge structures, or changing knowledge structures in the light of new knowledge" (Blachowicz, 1994). It also incorporates the view expressed by Chiat, that therapy should be designed to "unsettle" habitual processing and to "trigger new processing" by engaging the child "in conscious manipulation of aspects of language to which they have access" (Chiat, 1994, p.78). In this view, the child is expected to be an active solver of his/her linguistic problems rather than a passive learner who practises new skills imposed by the therapist.

Therapy

The challenge now was to find therapy tasks to implement this strategy. The psycholinguistic framework and model were particularly helpful at this stage because they allowed us to analyse the speech processing demands made by therapy tasks before introducing them to Alan (see Rees, this volume). Thus tasks could be chosen and designed to meet precise speech processing goals and, we were enabled to introduce tasks that would involve 'difficult' aspects of speech processing in a controlled way.

Examples of each kind of therapy task will now be considered in turn, in the order in which they were introduced to Alan between CA 5;2 and 5;9. The tasks are grouped under six broad goals of intervention:

Goal A: To establish and strengthen links between acoustic information (auditory input) and awareness of articulatory placement.

Goal B: To extend awareness of articulatory placement to phonemes in word onsets in adult pronunciations.

Goal C: To encourage reflection on the phonological structure (onset and rhyme) of words spoken by an adult and on the place of articulation used in onsets and codas.

Goal D: To encourage Alan to reflect on the phonological structure (onset and rhyme) of his (accurate) phonological representations and to become aware of different places of articulation associated with onset and coda .

Goal E: To prompt attempts to devise new, and more successful, motor programs to reproduce phonological representations (for CVC words) in output by encouraging Alan to become aware of mismatch between his own, habitual output forms and his accurate phonological representations.

Goal F: To extend his ability to revise motor programs to words with more complex phonological structures (polysyllabic words/ words with clusters at onset).

If Alan was to succeed in revising his output forms he had to acquire explicit awareness of (among other things) target places of articulation for the range of consonant phonemes. Evidence suggested that he perceived the acoustic properties of speech sounds adequately when they occur in words spoken by others and made use of that information to lay down phonological representations. We wanted to raise this tacit awareness of acoustic properties to conscious level and then link that awareness with knowledge and experience of the articulatory characteristics of speech sounds.

Goal A: to establish and strengthen links between acoustic information (auditory input) and awareness of articulatory placement

The therapy tasks used to address Goal A are now described. Readers will then be asked to consider what aspects of speech processing were involved in each task.

Therapy task 1

A variety of game formats were devised which all shared the following characteristics:

(a) An adult selected a colour-coded pictorial referent, indicating either bilabial (e.g. front carriage of a train, coloured red); alveolar (middle/blue) or velar (back/yellow) place of articulation. The referent was *not* shown to Alan at this stage.
(b) Alan listened (and watched) while an adult produced an isolated consonant sound at the place of articulatory closure indicated by the referent. In the early stages manual cues to articulatory placement were given (Passy, 1993a).
(c) Alan was asked to indicate whether the stimulus was an example of a 'front', 'middle' or 'back' sound. Many commonly used referent devices were used to motivate him to respond: sitting on trains and buses with front, middle and back carriages; feeding pelicans and crocodiles with paper fish at the 'front', 'middle' or 'back' of their mouths, etc. These were adapted from Metaphon therapy activities.
(d) Alan checked his response against the pictorial, colour-coded referent held by the adult speaker.

A speaking role was never required of Alan in therapy task 1. However, his natural desire to take a turn in all aspects of a game did lead him on some occasions to adopt the speaker's role out of choice (therapy task 2 below).

Therapy task 2

(a) Alan selected a colour-coded pictorial referent card (as in task 1) and, in response, produced a consonant sound or a non-speech sound involving bilabial or lingual/palatal contact.
(b) The adults present responded according to whether Alan had produced a 'front', 'middle' or 'back' sound.
(c) Alan compared his referent card with the feedback given by the adults' responses (e.g. sitting in the front carriage of a train).

Alan became fairly confident with this task in a few sessions, although his repertoire of speech sounds remained limited to [b] or [f] 'front', [d] or [s] 'middle' and [g] in response to a 'back' referent. Later, *colour-coded graphemes* were introduced (following the *Sunnybank Colour Coding* scheme, Reid, 1987) to supplement the pictorial referents in order to investigate whether written forms would be of interest to Alan and whether they would be likely to be an asset in future therapy. These written referents proved to be very motivating for Alan, who seemed to regard this as 'grown-up work'.

ACTIVITY 6.4

Aim: to understand the rationale for therapy tasks 1 and 2 (in relation to Goal A).

Reflect on the tasks as described above and then answer the following questions:

(a) What aspects of speech processing are involved in task 1?
(b) What aspects of speech processing are involved in task 2?
(c) Did the introduction of colour-coded graphemes change these tasks in any way?
(d) What contribution did the adults' responses make to Goal A in task 2?

See Key to Activity 6.4 at the end of this chapter, then read on.

The Activities and Keys to Activities that are based on therapy tasks are not intended to give the impression that there is only one way of analysing a task or that there is a 'best' way to address an intervention goal. Different children may well approach and benefit from the same task in different ways. The keys reflect the way we thought about these therapy tasks in relation to this child and readers may well have alternative or additional ideas

Task 1 involved aspects of input processing considered to be strengths for Alan. This task required Alan to reflect on the relationship between acoustic features of phonemes and place of articulatory closure used by adults to achieve those acoustic features. Thus task 1 began the process of establishing consistent relationships between acoustic and articulatory features for certain consonant phonemes of English as spoken in isolation by adult speakers.

In task 2 Alan was required first to devise and execute a motor program to achieve a particular place of articulation, on the basis of the pictorial referent he had selected. He then experienced the results of that attempt, via auditory feedback as well as kinaesthetic and proprioceptive feedback. The likelihood that Alan would recognize when he had achieved a sound with the intended characteristics was greatly increased by the external feedback provided by the adults' responses. That is, the response action performed by an adult assisted Alan in evaluating whether his attempt had resulted in a front/middle/back sound to match the pictorial referent he was holding in his hand. Thus, this task provided a first, tentative step towards linking his own articulatory gestures to acoustic outcomes.

The addition of graphemes (colour-coded for place of articulation) in these tasks probably shifted the tasks from *phonetic* recognition and production of place of articulation towards *phonological* input and output processing and prepared the way for focusing on place of articulation of phonemes in word onsets. Alan had acquired some experience of, and ability to think about, the relationship between articulatory and acoustic characteristics of single consonant sounds spoken by an adult (and, to a lesser extent, sounds spoken by himself). He now needed to develop awareness of articulatory placement associated with word onsets in adult pronunciations of real words.

Goal B: to extend Alan's awareness of articulatory placement to phonemes in onset position

---

ACTIVITY 6.5

Aim: to design therapy tasks to meet precise speech processing goals.

(a) Design a task that builds on the previous tasks and which requires the child to identify the place of consonant articulation (front, middle, back) in word onsets spoken by an adult.

(b) Now suggest a modification of your task that will increase the involvement of the child's own phonological representations of the words spoken by the adult.

You may wish to refer to Chapter 3 of this volume for background on task design.

The Key to Activity 6.5 at the end of this chapter gives the principles on which the design of such tasks is based.

Now read the description of task 3 that we used with Alan to address Goal B.

Therapy task 3

In task 3, an adult chose a picture illustrating a CV word from a selection made up of two or three minimal sets (e.g. PEA, BEE, TEA, KEY, SEA; TIE, GUY; BOW, GO, DOUGH). Place of articulation of word onset was indicated by a colour-coded pictorial and colour-coded grapheme on the reverse of each picture. These were not yet shown to Alan. He was required to identify the articulatory placement the adult speaker had employed to produce the word onset, and to indicate his decision by performing some 'front', 'middle' or 'back' related action, like putting a flag on a carriage of a train. In order to carry out this task he first had to segment the onset from the rhyme of the spoken word. Allowing Alan to check the referents on the reverse of the picture then provided feedback. We then discussed the correctness or otherwise of his decision. Manual cues to articulatory placement were incorporated into the discussion as necessary.

The task, in the form just described, could have been carried out purely on the basis of auditory analysis and recognition (as in task 1), without any involvement of internal phonological representations. To increase the likelihood that Alan's phonological representations of the words would be involved in the task, he was shown the picture prior to hearing the word pronounced by the adult, thus activating semantic and associated phonological information in the lexicon before carrying out the task. This made it likely that, in performing the segmentation and articulatory placement identification, Alan would draw on both immediate acoustic information and on stored phonological represen-tations of the word. This modified task has the potential to establish or strengthen associations among acoustic characteristics, articulatory targets and phonological representations.

The next step was to encourage further reflection on the phono-logical structure of spoken words and to extend awareness of articulatory placement to consonants occurring in codas as well as in onsets.

Goal C: to encourage Alan to reflect on the onset/rhyme structure of words spoken by an adult, and on the place of articulation used in onsets and codas

Therapy tasks 4(a) and 4(b) described below were designed to address this goal. Task 4(a) did not make demands significantly different from the previous task but it served to strengthen links between acoustic cues, articulatory placement and phonological representations of real words while simultaneously continuing to establish links between all of these and written representations of word onsets. It also introduced Alan to the idea of sorting illustrated words according to an aspect of their phonological structure.

Therapy task 4(a)

The same CV real words were used as in the previous task. Alan was asked to look at each picture, listen to each word spoken by an adult, then place the picture beside the appropriate letter (colour coded for place of articulation) which corresponded to its onset. He then checked his decision against the colour-coded pictorial referent and colour-coded letter on the reverse of each picture.

If Alan was to develop new motor programs that would signal syllable onsets and rhymes independently of one other (i.e. with different places of consonant articulation) he needed to acquire competence in reflecting on the rhyme of words as well as on onsets. Therapy task 4(b) was designed to achieve this.

Therapy task 4(b)

The focus of the sorting task now switched to the rhyme of words. Alan listened to picture names spoken by an adult. His task was to post the pictures into the doors of cardboard box 'houses' belonging to various characters such as Mr. Rat, Mr Snake, a King, Mrs Hen, etc. (up to a choice of six). The basis of the game was to match for rhyme, so that pictures of RING and WING and SWING were to be posted into the King's house, and so on. Adults as necessary assisted Alan's decision-making. For example, an adult might turn up a picture of MEN and say, 'Men. Men. Does men rhyme with king? No. Does men rhyme with rat? No. Does men rhyme with hen?' and so on until Alan was sure where to post the picture.

Tasks 4(a) and 4(b) could be performed purely on the basis of an auditory match with no involvement of internal phonological representations. However, since Alan was exposed to illustrations of each item before and during the presentation of the word spoken by an adult, it is likely that semantic information was activated and that the task prompted some reflection on the structure of associated phonological representations. We now needed to design a task that more explicitly required Alan to reflect on his own internal representations.

Goal D: to encourage Alan to reflect on the onset/rhyme structure of his (accurate) phonological representations and to become aware of different places of articulation associated with onset and coda

---

ACTIVITY 6.6

Aims: to design a therapy task that requires a child to think about the structure of stored phonological representations.

Read the descriptions of tasks 4(a) and 4(b) again and suggest how those tasks could be adapted to meet Goal D.

The Key to Activity 6.6 at the end of this chapter gives the principles involved. Now read how this adaptation was achieved with Alan.

Therapy task 5

Alan was now asked to carry out the same sorting games (focused on either onset or rhyme match), without first hearing an adult pronunciation. He selected a picture and was encouraged to carry out the task silently. Everyone present, including Alan, pretended to zip their lips closed while he considered the problem. He reflected on his own phonological representation associated with the semantic information activated by the picture and made the required onset or rhyme matching decision on the basis of analysis of the structure of that representation. When the focus of the sorting task was word onset, Alan was asked to place each picture beside an appropriate colour-coded letter that matched the word onset, thus drawing his attention to articulatory placements associated with word onsets. We also wanted to draw his attention to place of articulation in word codas. This was achieved by including written words on the reverse of some of the rhyming picture sets. Both onset and coda were colour coded for place in these written words (vowels in black). After a rhyming set had been completed (e.g. RAT, CAT, MAT, FAT, HAT), Alan's attention was directed to the written forms on the reverse of the illustrations. We discussed that the words that make a rhyming set all share the same endings (vowel and coda) while their 'beginnings' are all different and have different places of articulation (some 'front', some 'middle' and some 'back'). Alan quickly acquired facility with these silent rhyme and alliteration tasks. We noted that he was quite capable of switching his attention within a single therapy session from word onset to rhyme. This led us to experiment with more demanding tasks that required him to reflect simultaneously on onset and rhyme.

Therapy task 6

Alan was presented with a large set of pictures of CVC words. The set included up to three different rhymes and a variety of onsets. For example pictures of CAT, RAT, BAT, FAT, MAT; MAN, PAN, TAN, FAN, CAN; PIG, BIG and WIG were placed on the table. Representatives of each rhyming set, e.g. CAT, MAN, BIG, were placed at the top of the table while the remaining pictures were placed randomly. Each picture had the written form of the word on the reverse with onset and coda consonants colour coded for place of articulation and the vowel in black.

The adult selected a picture from a duplicate set and said to Alan 'You have to guess which picture I've got in my hand. I'll give you *two* clues. Don't try to guess until you've heard *both* clues. My picture rhymes with CAT ...... *and* ...... it begins with /b/. Which picture is it?'

ACTIVITY 6.7

Aim: to analyse the speech processing and other cognitive demands of task 6.

Reflect on the description of therapy task 6 and then:

(a) Make an analysis of the speech processing steps that Alan must go through in order to be successful in the task.
(b) Consider what other cognitive demands the task makes on Alan. Consider how the colour-coded written forms on the reverse of the pictures could be used to extend the task.

The Key to Activity 6.7 is at the end of the chapter. Now read on.

Clearly this is a very demanding task and would not be suitable for every child of this chronological age. Alan, however, as we predicted, loved the game and was very motivated to succeed.

By this stage Alan had been attending assessment and therapy sessions for about six months. He was now participating eagerly in therapy and no longer seemed to come with an expectation of failure. We felt confident that therapy tasks to date had provided Alan with useful learning experiences. However, up to this point there had been no observable changes in his speech patterns. It was very important at this time to explain our rationale carefully to his parents and teachers and to have frequent discussions between ourselves to remind us of the long-term strategy.

Alan now needed to be assisted to make the transition from awareness of the structure of internal representations to awareness of the fact that his current output forms did not match those representations. Awareness of that mismatch, together with his newly acquired knowledge of the links between acoustic and articulatory characteristics of speech sounds (supported by colour-coded written forms) would, we believed, prompt attempts to devise and execute new motor programs to amend output forms. For the first time it was necessary to involve aspects of speech processing that had been identified as 'deficits' rather than as strengths in Alan's profile. Clearly this would have to be handled with great care or we would risk losing his co-operation all over again, since he had come to expect that he would not be confronted in therapy with the inadequacy of his speech output. Tasks were required that would move Alan gently in the direction of recognizing this mismatch rather than confronting him in a way that could undermine his confidence.

Goal E: to prompt attempts to devise new motor programs by helping Alan to become aware of mismatch between his own output forms and his (accurate) phonological representations

Therapy task 7(a)

Two named puppets were introduced, Jo and Jim. Alan listened to an adult saying an isolated consonant (onset) followed by an isolated rhyme – in this case, either /o/ or /ɪm/. His thinking was assisted by giving him colour-coded written forms of the presented onsets and rhymes and inviting him to glue them together to form written syllables. His tasks were to decide (a) whether the resulting syllable rhymed with 'Jo' or 'Jim' and (b) whether the resulting syllable formed a real word or a nonsense/'rubbish' word. Obviously he first had to silently blend the presented onset and rhyme.

As expected, Alan could do both parts of this task successfully.

Therapy task 7(b)

Alan was now encouraged to try to 'help the puppets to say' each of the synthesized syllables that rhymed with their names. He was encouraged to make use of the colour-coded written forms and also to consult with any of the adults present (especially his mother) about what the synthesized syllable might sound like in output before attempting production himself (via a puppet).

He was very wary of the request to 'say' the syllable and needed a lot of support. It was noted that he was relatively confident in attempting to say the syllable when the synthesized syllable involved an onset + rhyme combination that already occurred in his spontaneous output, i.e. when the syllable was either a CV syllable with voiced plosive onset, or a CVC syllable with voiced plosive onset where both onset and coda shared the same place of articulation, for example /bɪm/. Presumably he drew on existing stored motor programs in these cases. When the target syllable did not meet these criteria he was extremely reluctant to attempt production. However, on the occasions when he could be persuaded to try, there were some signs that he was attempting to achieve a match for acoustic and articulatory features of the target syllables, resulting in some syllable types that had never been heard in his spontaneous speech. For example, when the target syllable onset was a voiceless plosive. e.g. /pɪm/ or TOE, his realization was devoiced throughout. When the target syllable onset was a fricative he at first made no attempt, but later produced a few examples of nonword syllables with a fricative onset, e.g. [fo] and [fɪm]. We felt that this task had had some limited success in moving Alan towards new motor programming attempts under the influence of heightened awareness of the target characteristics of an onset + rhyme combination. The next therapy task also addressed Goal E and was designed to build on this tentative beginning.

Therapy task 8

A set of cards, each with a written colour-coded CVC syllable on it, was used (only three different vowels were used for the cards). If the syllable was a real word the card included a small illustration of the word concealed under a flap in the corner. If the syllable was a nonword there was a black 'blot' concealed under the flap. An adult selected one of the cards. The adult then presented the three sounds of the selected syllable, orally, separated by a gap of approximately one second. Alan was asked to select colour-coded letter tiles for the three sounds presented and to assemble them, in order of presentation, on a plastic rack taken from a Scrabble game. A second presentation was given if the memory load proved too great.

All the CVC real word items were illustrated on cards spread across the floor, with colour-coded written forms on the reverse. He was told that the 'word' he had built on his Scrabble rack might be one of those pictures, or it might be a rubbish word. The game involved Alan throwing a beanbag on to the appropriate picture (or into a wastepaper basket if he decided it was a 'rubbish' word). He could then check his decision by looking at the hidden illustration on the stimulus card and by comparing the letters on his Scrabble rack with the written word on the back of the picture card. He was gently encouraged to say the target syllable at each stage of the game, but this was never forced.

ACTIVITY 6.8

Aim: to analyse the way that choice of stimulus items can change the demands of a therapy task.

The CVC sequences presented in task 8 resulted in a mixture of:
(a) nonwords;
(b) real words which Alan had not seen in print before;
(c) real words which were part of his sight-reading vocabulary, learned in school. (We could not always predict which these were.)

Consider what different demands were made by the task in each of these three cases.

The Key to Activity 6.8 is at the end of the chapter.

Now read the following account of Alan's response to this therapy task.

Alan enjoyed this task immensely. It seemed that he regarded it as focusing on his knowledge of phoneme/grapheme correspondences and his small sight-reading vocabulary. In spite of much encouragement to say the target words/syllables aloud he did not seem to find the task threatening or to perceive it principally as a 'speech task'. He was usually quick to decide if a syllable was a 'rubbish word', implying that he found it easy to blend the presented segments silently and compare the resulting syllable with phonological representations in his lexicon. He was, as might be expected, particularly quick to decide on the 'real word' status of words that were part of his sight-reading vocabulary. As he became more absorbed in the game he tended to name spontaneously the real words he had 'made'. His realizations were his habitual non-adult-like forms. For example, he placed the letters ‹p› ‹i› ‹g› on the rack, considered them silently and said with glee "I know what that is, it's a [ɡɪɡ]". He repeated "It's a big fat pig" → "it's a [ɡɪɡ daʔ ɡɪːɡ]", as he threw his bean bag on to the picture of the pig. But now the carefully designed materials began to play their part in prompting awareness of the inadequacy of his output form. He turned the picture of the pig over to check the colour-coded written word against the letter tiles on his rack. The therapist drew his attention, in a conversational manner, to the fact that the initial consonant ‹p› was 'red' for 'front'. Alan now seemed to draw on all the learning experiences he had taken part in to date and, for the first time, he consciously rejected his habitual output form and attempted to devise and execute a new motor program to reproduce the phonological structure of the word PIG. He said "a [bɪːɡ]" – very tentatively at first and then again with increased confidence as if he recognized that he had achieved a closer match between output, phonological and orthographic representations. In the same session this sequence of events was repeated for several other words, resulting in revised output forms. The word CAT, habitually realized by Alan as [dat] was revised to [gat]; MAN [nan] changed to [man]; BAG [gag] was revised to [bag] and the word PAN [dan] became [ban].

It was clear that a breakthrough had been achieved in the session described above. He was now CA 5;7 and we had been working with him for seven months. He had now begun to understand that his habitual productions did not match what he 'knew' about the phonological structure of words in his lexicon. Colour-coded written forms clearly assisted his reflection on that structure, particularly when he, himself, first blended phonemes to 'discover' a match with an item in his lexicon.

We now used a variety of therapy activities to capitalize on this new learning and new ability and willingness to attempt new motor programs. Therapy task 9 is an example of one of these.

Therapy task 9

Alan was shown an illustrated written sentence with missing letters in the onsets of rhyming words. Here are some examples, with the missing letters in parentheses:

```
<The  (d)og is on the  (l)og>
<The  (p)ea is in the  (s)ea>
<The  (p)ig has a  (w)ig>
<The  (p)ig can dance a  (j)ig>
```

His task was to supply the missing word onsets by selecting the correct colour-coded letters and sticking them on the cards. He was then encouraged to 'tell the story of the picture' while his attention was drawn to the colour-coded word onsets he had just supplied.

Alan's pronunciations of the target CVC words in task were invariably accurate for place of articulation and he took part with enthusiasm and confidence.

At around this time the family became concerned that Alan was beginning to stammer. Intermittent dysfluent episodes occurred in the clinic, particularly when he wanted to communicate new information, when chatting in the waiting room for example. The dysfluencies involved syllable repetitions (whole monosyllabic words, or initial syllables of polysyllabic words). The repetitions were very variable in number and frequency of occurrence, often affecting only the first word in an utterance, but sometimes up to six repetitions occurred on almost every word of an utterance. The situation was discussed at length with Alan's mother, who was asked to try to ensure that, whenever possible, Alan had an adult's full attention when he wanted to talk so that he didn't feel rushed. We also discussed possible explanations for Alan's dysfluency. In particular, that his growing awareness of his output errors was leading him to attempt pronunciation changes (new motor programming) in the course of a conversation. These attempts demanded additional processing time, which may have been disrupting 'down-line' components of output processing. By now, the school summer holidays were imminent and a break from therapy was indicated to allow Alan to consolidate and make use of his new skills and knowledge without pressure of additional new learning.

Goal F: to extend Alan's ability to revise motor programs to words with more complex phonological structures

In the final session before the summer break (at CA 5;9) Alan was given a large set of pictures of polysyllabic words (e.g. LADYBIRD, CATERPILLAR, ALLIGATOR). He was asked to silently match colour-coded written words to the pictures. These were not words that were part of his sight-reading vocabulary and he sometimes needed some adult help, but on the whole he succeeded independently: he reflected on his internal phonological representation of each pictured item and searched for the written word that gave the best orthographic match. He was then encouraged, in a variety of game formats, to name the pictured items while paying attention to the colour-coded written forms. His pronunciations were not fully adult-like: vowel errors, reductions of clustered onsets, and voicing errors were apparent as well as errors involving target phonemes which Alan was unable to imitate accurately, especially /ð/ and /ɹ/. However, his realizations of these polysyllabic words, none of which had ever been used in therapy, were accurate for place of consonant articulation, e.g. LADYBIRD → [ladɪbɜd], CATERPILLAR → [gadʌbɪlə], BUTTERFLY → [bʌdʌfaː]. The constraint which had 'allowed' only one place of consonant articulation in a syllable had been largely overcome. He was now able to devise and execute motor programs that were able to reflect place characteristics of syllable onset and syllable rhyme independently.

Outcomes and Discussion

It was clear that Alan had developed knowledge and strategies that he could begin to use independently to enable him to devise and execute new and revised motor programs. There were now frequent overt attempts at pronunciation revisions in spontaneous connected speech. Progress from this point was rapid. Alan had begun to recognize the nature of the mismatch between his output forms and adult forms. He had also discovered that colour-coded written forms could help him to focus on the phonological structure of a word he was about to produce and help him to monitor his accuracy. He began, with relatively little help, to apply these skills to other aspects of pronunciation such as the voiced/voiceless distinction for plosives and fricatives in word onsets.

By the time he entered his second year of school, at CA 5;11, his behavioural difficulties had resolved in all contexts. He now transferred to the school-based speech and language therapy 'outreach' service, with a new therapist. He was confident in therapy sessions and willing to take part in activities that focused more directly on production accuracy, including therapy directed at expanding his vowel system and his use of affricates. Therapy strategies continued to be based on developing Alan's awareness of an ever-widening range of phonological and phonetic features of words in his lexicon. He was now able to take part in tasks requiring generation of rhyming and alliterative strings of real and nonwords. The intervention continued to make extensive use of written forms and to develop, in collaboration with his teacher, his decoding skills and awareness of analogous written forms, in conjunction with awareness of phonological structure. At CA 6;2 his speech was largely intelligible to adults and children. Dysfluencies still occurred, particularly when he was eager to convey information quickly, but with less frequency. The family dealt with dysfluent episodes with great sensitivity and Alan did not seem to be disturbed by this aspect of his communication.

ACTIVITY 6.9

Aim: To use the speech processing profile to identify change following intervention.

Consider the above account of Alan's progress at CA 6;0. Reprofile Alan on a blank profile sheet (Appendix 1), using ticks to show adequate performance and crosses to show remaining difficulties. Compare his performance at CA 5;0 years (see Figure 6.1). Use * to identify on the profile where positive changes have occurred in comparison with his profile at CA 5;0.

In the Key to Activity 6.9 at the end of the chapter aspects of speech processing in which positive change had occurred are marked * .

During Alan's sixth year positive changes had occurred in all aspects of output processing, with the possible exception of level K, for which we had no new data. Therapy had been directed mainly towards developing awareness of phonological structure (level F) which had been an emerging strength at 5 years and which was now greatly enhanced. There was a further crucial change in relation to question L. That is, Alan was now applying his reflective skills to his own output forms. The profile does not readily capture Alan's enhanced awareness of the relationship between phonological representations (presumably acoustically based) and articulatory characteristics, which we believed to have been a crucial component of therapy. Here, the speech processing model may be more helpful; the role of this awareness might be thought of as supplying information to the motor programming component to facilitate its role in devising instructions for reproducing in output the (acoustically based) components of phonological representations.

At the age of 6 years, in addition to his progress with speech intelligibility, Alan was making excellent progress with literacy skills. This was, in fact, predicted by his speech processing profile at age 5 years, which showed good input processing abilities, accurate phonological representations and the beginnings of awareness of their structure (see Stackhouse, this volume).

His social interactions with his peers had now improved dramatically and, for the first time and to the delight of his family, he chose to invite classmates to his sixth birthday party, which was the subject of the conversation sampled in Table 6.6.

Table 6.6 Alan's connected speech at CA 6;2.

Orthographic transcription	Alan's transcribed form
I had a birthday party one day after	[ʌ had ə 'bʌfde 'pɑti wɒn de 'aftʌ]
It's got a big slide	[ɪs gɒʔ ʌ bɪg slaːɪd]
It's got a wee haunted house	[ɪs gɒʔ ʌ wi 'hɒntəd haʊs]
Nine, but ten including me	[naːn bʌ tɛn ɪnklʉdiŋ mi]
Cheese sandwiches and	[tʃiz 'samɪdʒɪz an mɒs̬'mawoʊz and
marshmallows and sausage rolls	sɒsɪdʒ ɹoəlz ən klɪsps]
and crisps	

Summary

The intervention strategies described in this chapter, which focused on areas of strength, had a successful outcome in Alan's case. As has been emphasized throughout the chapter, rationale for therapy must take account of the individual learning needs and strengths of each child and it may be that these strategies would be less successful with other children with similar speech processing profiles. It is only as large numbers of cases are accumulated in the literature that it will be possible to evaluate the wider application of particular approaches to intervention. However, Alan's case demonstrates the valuable contribution that the psycholinguistic approach can make to all stages in the management of children with developmental speech disorder.

The following points are highlighted in this chapter:

- A profile of speech processing abilities integrates well with information and data gathered from other sources to provide a principled basis for intervention and for evaluating change.
- A child's speech processing profile can be assembled via therapy activities; a large assessment battery is not necessary.
- The information collated on the speech processing profile needs to be supplemented by knowledge of the child as an individual learner.
- Children with similar speech processing profiles do not necessarily respond in the same way to intervention tasks; what works with one may not work with another.
- The psycholinguistic approach allows identification of a child's underlying strengths and weaknesses, and what needs to be changed in a child's spoken language behaviour.

- An understanding of a child's processing strengths and weaknesses allows intervention goals to be programmed from easy to hard.
- Preparatory work on input skills, a relative strength, facilitated the targeting of speech output skills at a later stage in the intervention programme.
- A psycholinguistic analysis of the therapy tasks enabled a more precise targeting of the intervention programme.
- The tasks incorporated in the intervention programme made explicit links: between the components of lexical representations; and between written and spoken language.
- Colour coding and cued articulation were helpful in making these links.

KEY TO ACTIVITY 6.1

This incident provided evidence relevant to:

question E, "Are his phonological representations accurate?" YES;
question F, "Is he aware of the internal structure of phonological representations?" YES;
question G, "Can he access accurate motor programs?" NO;
question H, "Can he manipulate phonological units (for output purposes)?" NO;
question L, "Does he reject his own erroneous forms?" NO.

KEY TO ACTIVITY 6.2

See Figure 6.3.

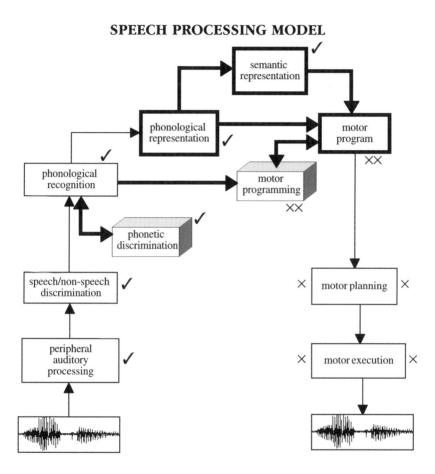

Figure 6.3 Speech processing model indicating Alan's strengths and weaknesses at CA 5;0.

KEY TO ACTIVITY 6.3

The following could be enlisted to help Alan make changes in his speech output:

(a) auditory (input) processing;
(b) accurate phonological representations;
(c) emerging awareness of phonological structure;
(d) quick understanding of instructions and task requirements;
(e) ability to reflect on aspects of spoken language.

KEY TO ACTIVITY 6.4

(a) Task 1 involved auditory input processing including phonetic discrimination.
(b) Task 2 involved both output and input processing:
  (i) Motor programming, planning and execution for single consonant sounds / non-speech sounds;
  (ii) Input processing of auditory feedback;
  (iii) Also processing of proprioceptive and kinaesthetic information resulting from his sound production attempts.
(c) The addition of colour-coded graphemes probably tended to shift the tasks from phonetic to phonological processing.
(d) The adult responses prompted Alan to reflect on what acoustic effects his output attempts had achieved.

KEY TO ACTIVITY 6.5

(a) Principles underlying the design of task 3.
  (i) Stimulus items confined to CV words so that there is no confusion about which part of the word is the focus of the judgement task.
  (ii) Pictorial referents and response games representing each place of articulation carried over from previous tasks to reduce extraneous processing load.
  (iii) All materials designed to allow the child to self-check his/her decisions, rather than having to rely on right/wrong feedback from an adult.
(b) The phonological representation for a stimulus item (linked to semantic information) can be activated by presenting a picture/ object of the item prior to auditory presentation.

KEY TO ACTIVITY 6.6

The main principle in designing such a task is that the child should be given no auditory input. That is, the therapist does not say the items aloud and the child is discouraged from saying the items aloud too. The task is carried out in silence, with items presented as pictures or objects. These visual stimuli activate phonological representations linked to semantic information in the lexicon. (Of course, it can never be certain that a child is carrying out a task without reference to his/her own output forms since s/he may be 'rehearsing' the item names subvocally as a strategy for reflecting on phonological structure.)

KEY TO ACTIVITY 6.7

(a) To be successful in this task Alan had to:
   (i) segment the word CAT as presented by the adult and identify the rhyme
   (ii) reflect on internal representations of all the picture choices, segment the rhyme of each in order to eliminate those which did not match the rhyme in the word CAT;
   (iii) recall that he was searching for a word beginning with /b/;
   (iv) reflect on his phonological representations of the remaining set of items, segmenting each until he arrived at a word with a /b/ onset.
(b) This task makes demands on the child's attention control and concentration as well as on memory.
(c) After each response Alan was encouraged to turn the picture over and look at the colour-coded written word on the reverse of the identified picture, while listening to the adult pronunciation of the word. This focused his attention on links between adult forms, internal representations, and knowledge of place of articulation of onset and coda.

KEY TO ACTIVITY 6.8

The demands made by task 8 were as follows (depending on the type of word).

(a) Nonwords:
  (i) Blend the CVC to form a syllable (silently or orally)
  (ii) Scan the lexicon for a phonological match linked to semantic representation.
  (iii) Recognize lack of such a match and conclude that the syllable is a nonword.
(b) Real words not previous seen in print:
  (i) As above, but this time a match is found in the lexicon.
  (ii) Identify appropriate picture.
(c) Real words in sight vocabulary;
  (i) Look at the CVC letter string.
  (ii) Scan the orthographic component of the lexicon (visual input lexicon) for a visual match.
  (iii) Recognize match and identify picture.

KEY TO ACTIVITY 6.9

Alan's speech processing profile at CA 6;0 is presented in Figure 6.4. Levels where there has been positive change since CA 5;0 are marked with a *.

SPEECH PROCESSING PROFILE

Name Alan   Comments:

Age 6;0

Date

Profiler

INPUT

F

Is the child aware of the internal structure of phonological representations?

✓ ✓ ✓   *

E

Are the child's phonological representations accurate?

✓ ✓ (✓)   (*)

D

Can the child discriminate between real words?

✓ ✓ ✓

C

Does the child have language-specific representations of word structures?

No data

B

Can the child discriminate speech sounds without reference to lexical representations?

✓ ✓ ✓

A

Does the child have adequate auditory perception?

✓ ✓ ✓

OUTPUT

G

Can the child access accurate motor programs?

(✓)   *

H

Can the child manipulate phonological units?

(✓)   *

I

Can the child articulate real words accurately?

(✓)   *

J

Can the child articulate speech without reference to lexical representations?

(✓)   *

K

Does the child have adequate sound production skills?

×   (no new data)

L

Does the child reject his/her own erroneous forms?

✓ ✓   *

Figure 6.4 Alan's speech processing profile CA 6;0.

Chapter 7
Electropalatography:
A Tool for Psycholinguistic Therapy

Hilary Dent

Traditionally, speech deficits have been analysed on the basis of an auditory, or perceptual, assessment: the speech and language therapist records and/or listens to a sample of speech, transcribes phonetically what s/he hears and analyses the transcribed data, examining, for example, types and patterns of error. Such an assessment reflects communication, inasmuch as the therapist analyses what is heard or perceived, but it is also therefore subjective, since two therapists may perceive and analyse the same speech output differently. It is now possible to investigate speech deficits using a range of computer-based instrumental techniques, which isolate one feature of speech production and measure this. While such methods do not mirror the communicative process, they do provide data which are objective and quantifiable.

Electropalatography (EPG) is one such computer-based system, which provides a visual display of tongue contact with the roof of the mouth (hard palate) during speech. Within the clinical context, use of this technique can make available information which may be crucial to an accurate description, and successful treatment of some speech impairments. When applied to assessment, EPG can reveal aspects of articulation (motor execution) which may be important features of the presenting speech deficit, but which may not be accessible during a traditional perceptually based speech analysis. During therapy, the system can allow both therapist and child to examine the detail of atypical (incorrect) articulatory patterns compared with typical model (correct) patterns. It also permits detailed observation of the child's attempts to modify errors and to match model pronunciations.

This chapter provides a brief description of the EPG system and outlines the application of EPG as a clinical tool within the psycholinguistic framework. The discussion focuses on the role of EPG in both the assessment and the therapy processes. Two case studies are presented, to illustrate employment of the technique in the management not only of an articulatory difficulty, but also of auditory discrimination, representational and motor programming deficits.

What is EPG?

The technique of EPG has been applied clinically in assessment and treatment over a number of years and has been reported widely in the literature (Hardcastle, Gibbon and Jones, 1991; Hardcastle, Gibbon and Dent, 1993; Dent, Gibbon and Hardcastle, 1995). Most of the clients have been described within the medical perspective (see Book 1, Stackhouse and Wells, 1997, pp.4–5) as having speech articulation difficulties associated with, for example, cleft palate (Dent, Gibbon and Hardcastle, 1992), dysarthria (MorganBarry, 1995a), dyspraxia (MorganBarry, 1995b), hearing loss (Crawford, 1995) and dysfluency (Wood, 1995).

A central feature of the EPG system is an artificial acrylic palate, similar to a dental brace, which is made individually for each user, and on the surface of which are embedded 62 electrodes (see Figure 7.l).

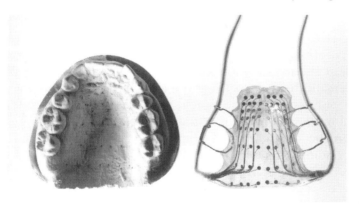

Figure 7.1 Photograph of the artifical palate used in the EPG system: the wires from the electrodes on each half of the palate are fed at the back corners into plastic tubing which connects at its other end with the multiplexer, (see text). Also illustrated is a plaster impression of the upper palate and teeth, from which the palate is contructed. The subject is a child aged 13 years.

The wires from the artificial palate are connected to the EPG unit via a small box (multiplexer unit) which the child wears around the neck. The EPG unit interfaces directly with the computer (see Figure 7.2).

When the palate is worn, tongue contact with the electrodes is recorded. The information can be saved on the computer for later analysis, or can be displayed in real-time on the computer screen. Contact between the tongue and the hard palate is sampled during

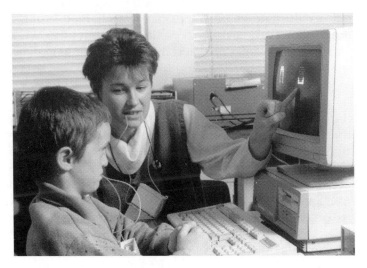

Figure 7.2 Photograph of EPG system in use, illustrating the connections between the artificial palate, multiplexer unit, EPG unit (bottom right corner of picture) and computer. See later for discussion regarding the display on the computer screen.

speech every 10 milliseconds, so that a contact pattern at one point in time and contact patterns over time can be recorded, analysed and displayed. Thus, the system provides information regarding tongue placement and tongue movement during speech. Figure 7.3 illustrates the schematic diagram (palatogram) employed on the computer screen and on printouts from the system to represent the electrodes on the artificial palate and patterns of tongue contact.

When the tongue makes contact with a particular electrode, the corresponding circle in the palatogram is either blocked out, or changes from a small to a larger circle. The top three rows of the palatogram represent electrodes in the region of the alveolar ridge, (the ridge just behind the upper front teeth, which can be felt by running

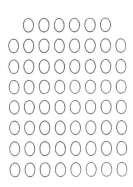

Figure 7.3 Schematic EPG palatogram.

the tip of the tongue backwards along the hard palate from the back of the teeth). The last two rows represent electrodes in the velar region, (at the back of the hard palate, where it meets the soft palate which hangs down centrally at the back of the mouth).

ACTIVITY 7.1

Aim: to identify the pattern of tongue contact with the hard palate which occurs during production of each of the following speech sounds: [t d k p s i].

Say each of these sounds on its own, as many times as you need to, to decide which of the palatograms in Figure 7.4 it corresponds to. Think carefully about what your tongue is doing in your mouth:

   Does it touch the front or the back of your hard palate?
   How the sound is produced?
   Is there a sudden or a continuous flow of air from your mouth?

Write the phonetic symbol for the sound underneath the palatogram which you decide it corresponds to.

Check your answers with Key to Activity 7.1 at the end of this chapter, then read the following.

The sounds [t] and [d] are identical in terms of tongue contact with the hard palate, (they differ only in terms of activity within the larynx or voice box), and therefore have identical palatograms. (This is the case for other pairs of sounds which differ only in terms of activity within the larynx, e.g. [k] and [g]; [s] and [z].) They involve contact between the tip of the tongue and the alveolar ridge and electrodes are therefore activated in the first three rows at the top of the palatogram. The sound [k] involves contact between the back of the tongue and the velar region and electrodes are therefore activated in the last two rows at the bottom of the palatogram. Each of these sounds is a plosive, created by a sudden flow of air from the mouth following the release of a blockage, which is formed by complete contact between the tongue and the palate. Electrodes are therefore activated across at least one complete row during production of these sounds. The sound [p] is also a plosive but the blockage in this case is formed by both lips, rather than the tongue and the hard palate, so no electrodes are activated during production of this sound. Like [t] and [d], [s] involves contact between the tip of the tongue and the alveolar ridge, but this sound is a fricative, created by a continuous flow from the mouth of air which is

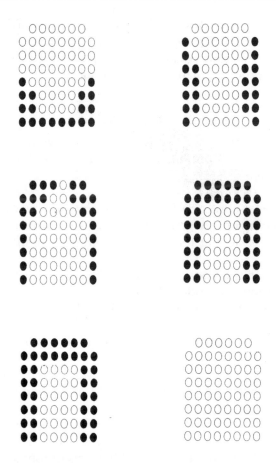

Figure 7.4 Palatograms for Activity 7.1.

turbulent in quality, because it is forced through a narrow pathway (groove) made in the centre of the tongue. This groove is reflected in the palatogram by a triangle of electrodes which are not activated in the centre of the first three rows. During production of [i] there is some contact between the sides of the tongue and the sides of the palate, so that electrodes are activated down both edges of the palatogram, but there is a wide central area involving no contact, so that a continuous flow of non-constricted air from the mouth is possible. This characterizes all vowel sounds.

Having considered single sound production in Activity 7.1, we can now examine word production. Figure 7.5 illustrates a printout from the EPG system of a normal adult speaker's production of the word GOOSE. The printout should be read just as print is, from left to right along each line, following the numbering of the palatograms.

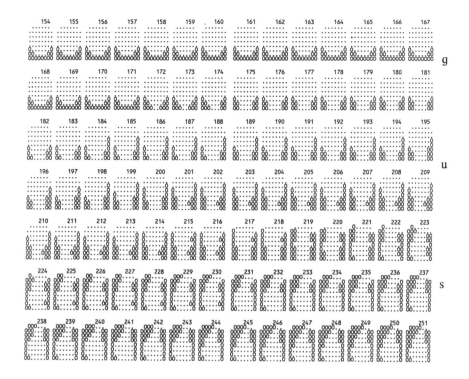

Figure 7.5 EPG printout of GOOSE.

Because the electrodes are sampled every 10 milliseconds, production of a single sound continues across several palatograms. Complete contact across the palate in the velar region is evident during articulation of the initial velar plosive [g], (palatograms 154 to 171). Some tongue contact with the back of the palate is recorded (palatograms 172 to 197), during production of the vowel segment [u], which involves positioning the tongue high up at the back of the mouth. A contact pattern in the region of the alveolar ridge, involving a central groove, can be seen during production of the final fricative [s], (palatograms 225 to 251).

ACTIVITY 7.2

Aim: to interpret a printout from the EPG system of a single word produced by a normal adult speaker.

Examine the printout in Figure 7.6. Mark on the printout which sequences of palatograms you think represent a sound, then, for each sequence, consider which sounds the pattern you are looking at might represent. Write the phonetic symbols for these sounds by the palatograms concerned. Focus on those sections that involve most tongue contact with the palate, as these are easier to interpret. Refer to the points made in and following Activity 7.1. On the basis of the phonetic symbols that you have written down, see if you can guess the word being produced. Some clues: in a phonetic transcription, the word has seven (segmental) symbols; all the consonants are voiceless; and there are two syllables.

Check your answers with Key to Activity 7.2 at the end of this chapter, then read the following.

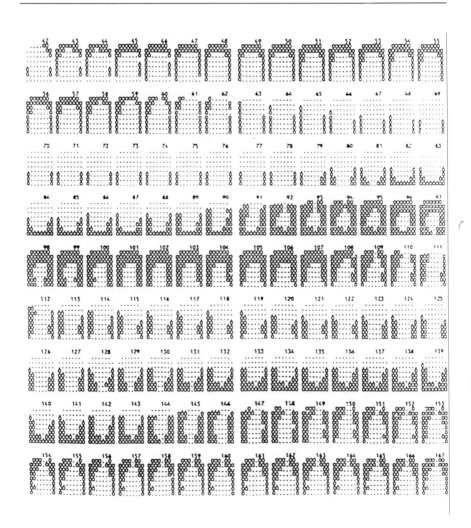

Figure 7.6 EPG printout for Activity 7.2.

The contact pattern in palatograms 43 to 59 and 98 to 108 could represent [t] or [d], as discussed following Activity 7.1. Similarly, the pattern in palatograms 82 to 91 and 132 to 143 might represent either [k] or [g]. The vowel segments, (palatograms 60 to 81 and 109 to 131), are difficult to interpret, but the presence of contact down each side of the palatograms during the second vowel segment suggests that this involves positioning the tongue relatively high in the mouth, closer to the hard palate than the first vowel segment. During the first vowel segment there is much less contact, reflecting a lower tongue position. Palatograms 92 to 97 reveal a 'double articulation', which is not heard in a perceptual analysis of this production: complete contact with both the velar region and also the alveolar ridge is made simultaneously during production of the consonant cluster /kt/ in the middle of the target TACTICS. The fact that EPG analysis can, as here, reveal features of speech production that are not perceptible, will be discussed in more detail below. However, Activities 7.1 and 7.2 have illustrated that the EPG system does not distinguish between sounds that differ only because of the activity of the larynx. The discussion that follows will consequently employ only voiceless sounds as the basis for illustrations.

Use of EPG in Assessment

EPG has two main advantages when compared with traditional methods of speech assessment, which rely on a perceptually based transcription.

1. It can provide much more detail regarding the exact articulatory patterns of speech that is perceived to be atypical.
2. It can reveal patterns of inaudible tongue activity that are not accessible to a perceptually based analysis.

In this section, these two advantages are illustrated with reference to children with developmental speech disorders.

What does EPG provide?

EPG can provide much more detail regarding the exact articulatory patterns of speech that is perceived to be atypical. In Figure 7.7 are typical palatograms for production of [s] and [ʃ]. Also illustrated are palatograms from the speech of three children who were referred for speech and language therapy employing EPG because they had not responded to more traditional therapy techniques.

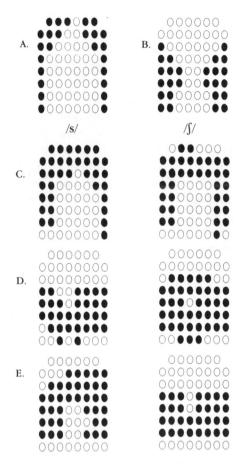

Figure 7.7 Palatograms for target /s/ and /ʃ/.

Each of these children was perceived to be realizing both targets /s/ and /ʃ/ as [ɬ] , e.g. SUN →[ɬʌn], CRASH →[kɹæɬ], POSTER →[pəʊɬtə]. The consonant [ɬ] is the lateral fricative also found in the Welsh language (e.g. in LLANDUDNO). It is clear from the contact patterns, that although the speech errors of these children were perceived to be the same, they had different articulatory patterns (see Gibbon, Hardcastle, Dent, et al., 1996 for more details). Thus, each child had a slightly different 'diagnosis' and, consequently, different needs in terms of therapeutic goals. For example, for production of target /s/, treatment for child C was required to focus only on establishing a central groove, while for child D place of articulation had first to be moved forward in the mouth to the alveolar ridge.

The fact that such articulatory detail is not available to a perceptually based analysis is doubtless one reason why these children could not modify their production patterns successfully prior to EPG assessment:

neither the child nor the therapist would have been able to identify accurately what the child is actually doing when making these erroneous realizations of /s/ and /ʃ/. However, EPG data are not the only prerequisite of an accurate description of such a speech impairment. This point will now be illustrated through a comparison of two of the children whose speech was illustrated in Figure 7.7.

Here is some information about the speech processing skills of the two children: Sophie (Child D in Figure 7.7) and Sam (Child C in Figure 7.7).

Sophie, CA 8;6

Sophie has a mild sensorineural hearing loss in her right ear. Her auditory discrimination of nonwords and real words involving high frequency fricatives such as /s/ and /ʃ/ is below chance level. Her performance on an auditory lexical decision task employing the same real words is also below chance level (e.g. when presented with a picture of a PARACHUTE and asked "Is this a [pæɹəʃut]?"; "Is this a [pæɹəɬut]?", she accepts some error stimuli (see Book 1, Chapter 2, p.37). She is perceived to make the substitutions described above , e.g. SUN → [ɬʌn], CRASH → [kɹæɬ], POSTER → [pəʊɬtə], during naming, real word and nonword repetition tasks. She is not able to imitate [s] and [ʃ] in isolation.

Sam, CA 10;5

Sam has no history of any hearing difficulties. His performance during all types of auditory discrimination and auditory lexical decision task is accurate and consistent. He is perceived to make the substitutions described above, i.e. /s/ and /ʃ/ → [ɬ], during naming, real word and nonword repetition tasks. He is not able to imitate [s] and [ʃ] in isolation.

ACTIVITY 7.3

Aim: to contrast two perceptually identical speech impairments by compiling profiles of the underlying speech processing skills.

Using the two sets of data presented above, complete the profiling sheet presented in Figure 7.8 for both Sophie and Sam. Put a cross if an area is problematic and a tick if it is not. Mark Sophie's performance on the left of each box and Sam's on the right.

Check your answers with Key to Activity 7.3 at the end of this chapter, then read the following.

SPEECH PROCESSING PROFILE

Name   Comments:

Age

Date

Profiler

INPUT

F

Is the child aware of the internal structure of phonological representations?

E

Are the child's phonological representations accurate?

D

Can the child discriminate between real words?

C

Does the child have language-specific representations of word structures?

B

Can the child discriminate speech sounds without reference to lexical representations?

A

Does the child have adequate auditory perception?

OUTPUT

G

Can the child access accurate motor programs?

H

Can the child manipulate phonological units?

I

Can the child articulate real words accurately?

J

Can the child articulate speech without reference to lexical representations?

K

Does the child have adequate sound production skills?

L

Does the child reject his/her own erroneous forms?

Figure 7.8 Blank profile sheet for Activity 7.3.

It is now clear that Sophie and Sam differ not only in articulatory terms, as revealed by EPG assessment, but also in psycholinguistic terms, as revealed by their speech processing profiles. This illustrates a principle discussed in Book 1, Chapter 2: an assessment completed in isolation provides limited information, but completed in conjunction with other tasks it can contribute to a profile of strengths and weaknesses which can be employed as a basis for accurate therapy planning. Therapy for Sophie and Sam must therefore now differ in several ways, rather than in only those suggested above on the basis of the EPG analysis.

Therapy with Sophie

Sophie's discrimination of the /s/ ~ /ʃ/ distinction is poor at all levels assessed. This is likely to be associated with her mild hearing loss, and can therefore be assumed to have been present throughout her development of speech. Her performance on the naming, real word and nonword repetition and single sound imitation tasks suggests a low-level articulatory problem, i.e. an inability to co-ordinate the fine movements of the tongue that are necessary to produce the sounds [s] and [ʃ]. Alternatively, it may well be the case that Sophie has never learned the movements necessary to articulate these sounds simply because she has never accurately perceived them.

The first phase of therapy for Sophie should therefore focus on discrimination (i.e. input) as well as articulation (i.e. output). This should be done simultaneously, using the EPG palatograms for [s] and [ʃ] as visual cues to teach both auditory and articulatory features. For example, the following contrasts could be explored:

[s]
  saying   = front of mouth + narrow gap (on palatogram)
  listening   = louder + hissing noise

vs

[ʃ]
  saying   = further back + wider gap (on palatogram)
  listening   = quieter + slushy noise.

Sophie's performance on the auditory lexical decision tasks suggests that her poor auditory skills have resulted in the laying down of inaccurate phonological representations, faulty stores in memory of phonological information regarding word forms. Furthermore, it is likely that this deficit, perhaps in combination with an articulatory difficulty, has contributed to the laying down of inaccurate motor programs, faulty stores in memory of the sequences of gestures required for the pronunciation of word forms. (For a detailed discussion of phonological representations and motor programs see Book 1, Chapter 6.)

The next phase of therapy should therefore draw on Sophie's newly acquired discrimination and articulation skills in order to help her revise, or update, her inaccurate phonological representations and motor programs. The following therapy programme would be appropriate:

(i)   The therapist pronounces /s/ and non /s/ real words. Sophie has to assign the /s/ real words to the /s/ palatogram. Sophie is encouraged to say each word, using her new articulatory pattern for /s/, before making her decision. Initially, employ simple /CV/ and /VC/ words, such as SEA, ICE, then gradually increase the complexity of the words, moving on to longer items with more syllables, e.g. SATURDAY, OCTOPUS.

(ii) Complete the same stages of therapy for /ʃ/ vs non-/ʃ/ real words.

(iii) Carry out the above stages employing both /s/ and /ʃ/ real words and palatograms in the same activity, so that Sophie has to distinguish carefully between the two sounds in both her production and her discrimination.

(iv) Finally, ensure that Sophie has stored the correct auditory and articulatory features for /s/ and /ʃ/ by completing the same activities without the visual support of the palatograms.

Therapy with Sam

In contrast to Sophie, Sam has no discrimination deficits, and performance on the auditory lexical decision tasks reveals that his phonological representations are accurate. His performance on the naming, real word and nonword repetition, and single sound imitation tasks suggests that he is unable to co-ordinate the fine movements of the tongue necessary to produce [s] and [ʃ]. A hypothesis that this is due to poor discrimination of the distinction concerned, as was formulated for Sophie, is not appropriate. Therapy for Sam should therefore focus on motor execution, although his intact discrimination skills and representational knowledge should be employed to help him achieve differentiation of the target sounds. For example, the auditory features which distinguish /s/ from /ʃ/ could be related to articulatory features of the two sounds, as for Sophie (see above), via the use of minimal pairs such as SEA VS SHE; MESS VS MESH, which Sam is able to perceive. Once he has established new patterns for /s/ and /ʃ/, Sam is still likely to find it hard to modify the motor programs that he has already established for the words in his vocabulary, not least because of his age. One possible therapy strategy would be to practise his new /s/ and /ʃ/ patterns in *nonwords*. This would enable him to practise and consolidate the fine motor skills involved in producing /s/ and /ʃ/ in the context of other sounds, while at the same time avoiding the added pressure of having to modify existing motor programs. The aim would be to increase his chances of successful updating of motor programs and generalization to more complex levels such as spontaneous connected speech.

What does EPG reveal?

EPG can reveal patterns of tongue activity that are not heard in a perceptually based analysis. The case of Emily, who is 9 years old, is a good illustration of this.

Emily, CA 9;0

Emily has no history of any hearing difficulties; her auditory perception skills can therefore be assumed to be intact. Her performance on the *Auditory Discrimination and Attention Test* (MorganBarry, 1989) is appropriate for her age, indicating that her phonological representations for the stimuli tested are accurate. A perceptually based analysis of Emily's speech output has revealed that she sometimes 'backs' alveolar plosive targets e.g. [t] to velar place of articulation, e.g. [k], in her spontaneous speech. Thus, she realized TIME as [kaim], BUTTER as [bʌkə] and PLATE as [pleik]. This suggests that some of her motor programs for words involving these alveolar targets are inaccurate. The pattern also occurred at times in her repetition of nonwords, e.g. [teib] → [keib]; [mɪtə] → [mɪkə]; [bɹaut] → [bɹauk], indicating that she cannot consistently articulate these alveolar targets, even when pre-existing motor programs are not involved. Emily appeared to have difficulty in a single sound imitation task involving these alveolar targets, reflecting some sound production problems, although she is perceived sometimes to produce these sounds accurately. Figure 7.9 presents the speech processing profile compiled for Emily at age 9 years from the assessments summarized above.

On the basis of this information, the following hypotheses can be formulated regarding Emily's processing of speech:

(1) Emily cannot hear the difference between alveolar and velar targets and therefore cannot distinguish between them in her speech.
(2) Emily's phonological representations for some words containing alveolar targets are inaccurate and therefore her production of these words is inaccurate.
(3) Emily has a sound production problem, which affects her articulation of some but not all alveolar targets.

Figure 7.10 illustrates the sequence of tongue movements occurring during Emily's articulation of target velar and alveolar plosives, as revealed by EPG analysis.

SPEECH PROCESSING PROFILE

Name   Emily   Comments:

Age   9;0

Date

Profiler

INPUT	OUTPUT

F

Is the child aware of the internal structure of phonological representations?

G

Can the child access accurate motor programs?

In spontaneous speech the alveolar plosive target in some words is replaced by velar plosive

E

Are the child's phonological representations accurate?

✓ for items in ADAT

H

Can the child manipulate phonological units?

D

Can the child discriminate between real words?

I

Can the child articulate real words accurately?

C

Does the child have language-specific representations of word structures?

J

Can the child articulate speech without reference to lexical representations?

✕ in some nonword stimuli the alveolar plosive target is replaced by a velar plosive

B

Can the child discriminate speech sounds without reference to lexical representations?

A

Does the child have adequate auditory perception?

✓

K

Does the child have adequate sound production skills?

Able to imitate alveolar plosives in isolation, but difficulties apparent

L

Does the child reject his/her own erroneous forms?

Figure 7.9 Emily's profile at CA 9;0.

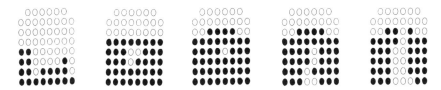

A. target /k/ perceived as [k]

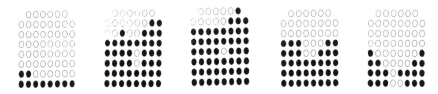

B. target /t/ perceived as [t]

C. target /t/ perceived as [k]

Figure 7.10 Sequences of palatograms taken from a number of points during Emily's productions of targets /t/ and /k/. They illustrate Emily's tongue movements during (A) production of target /k/ perceived by listeners as [k]; (B) production of target /t/ perceived by listeners as [t]; (C) production of target /t/ perceived by listeners as [k].

Her articulation of the target velar /k/ in Figure 7.10 (A) involves complete closure across the back of the hard palate, followed by release of the closure, to allow release of a burst of air. This is the sequence of movement typical of normal articulation of this sound. Emily's production of the target alveolar /t/ is evidently quite different from her articulation of target velar plosives. While perceptual judgements suggested that Emily's productions of alveolar targets were variable, EPG assessment reveals that all of her attempts at these targets in fact involve a consistent but abnormal pattern of tongue movement: complete closure across the back of the hard palate is evident in each of Emily's attempts at alveolar sounds, but there is also contact between the tongue and the hard palate further forward in the mouth, towards the alveolar ridge. The random variability in Emily's articulation occurs when she attempts to release the contact between her tongue and hard palate: sometimes the tongue is lowered from back to front, so that the sound perceived is alveolar, but at other times the tongue is lowered from front to back so that the sound perceived is velar.

ACTIVITY 7.4

Aim: To modify the hypotheses formulated regarding Emily's speech processing, in light of the EPG assessment data.

Consider the EPG data presented in Figure 7.10 and the implications of these, not only for Emily's sound production skills, but also for other levels of her speech processing. Return to the three hypotheses formulated regarding Emily's speech processing and modify these accordingly.

Check your answer with Key to Activity 7.4 at the end of this chapter, then read the following.

The EPG data suggest that Emily has knowledge of the distinction between alveolar and velar plosives and is attempting to mark the contrast in her speech output. However, she has apparently not learned the correct sequence of tongue movements involved in production of alveolar targets such as /t/, with the result that the contrast she is attempting to make is not always perceived by her listeners. Emily's discrimination skills and phonological representations appear, therefore, to be intact. Her motor programs for words involving these alveolar targets, however, may be inaccurate because of the persistence of an isolated motor execution difficulty, which has probably been present throughout speech development. (See Gibbon, Dent and Hardcastle, 1993 for further discussion of this case.)

This description of Emily's speech processing skills demonstrates that the listener's perception of a loss of contrast (such as here between alveolar and velar plosive targets), cannot be assumed to reflect a loss of contrast at the level of the phonological representation. A child may have stored knowledge of a particular phonological contrast, and may indeed be marking this in his/her output, but not in a manner that means that the two distinct articulations produced are perceived as such by the listener.

This section has illustrated how EPG can be employed as an assessment tool to provide information regarding features of speech sound production within the psycholinguistic framework. It has demonstrated also that, as for any procedure, interpretation of EPG data is meaningful only in the context of the results of other investigations. Finally, it has made clear how EPG can provide information that cannot be obtained from any other assessment procedure, and in this way may reveal patterns that are crucial to an accurate description and analysis of the presenting speech difficulty.

Use of EPG in Treatment

EPG is one of a number of computer-based systems that can isolate a feature of speech production, so that it can be analysed during assessment, as discussed above. In addition, the feature can be presented visually during therapy to provide feedback to the client. These systems are being applied increasingly and successfully to the treatment of a range of speech impairments. Figure 7.2 showed the EPG system in use during a therapy session. The 'therapy' mode of the EPG system's software, illustrated on the computer screen, can be manipulated by both therapist and child simultaneously, so that the child can monitor not only his/her own tongue placements and movements, but also, when appropriate, those of the therapist. Visual feedback of tongue placement, contact pattern and movement is available in real time via a single palatogram on the left of the computer screen. A pattern achieved here can be copied to the right of the screen, where it remains in a static display so that it can be discussed, used as a model or compared with subsequent attempts at a target.

Thus, the system has several features that are important in the context of teaching/learning the fine motor skills involved in speech sound production.

(1) It provides a meaningful display that is easily perceived and interpreted.
(2) It allows patterns of tongue contact with the palate to be matched, or compared. For example, a correct vs an incorrect pattern can be illustrated and compared to indicate exactly how the incorrect pattern is erroneous and what modifications are necessary to move towards the correct pattern for the target.
(3) During the early stages of learning, the child can immediately be shown the results of an attempt at sound production; while in later stages this process can be delayed. The latter encourages the child first to monitor his/her production via auditory/kinaesthetic feedback; this is followed by an opportunity to check the articulatory pattern too, by referring to the EPG display.

Two case studies will now be outlined, to highlight the use of EPG as an assessment tool and a therapy technique within the context of the psycholinguistic framework. The first study, of Paul, illustrates the application of EPG to the analysis and modification of atypical fricative productions similar to Sophie's and Sam's errors discussed earlier. The second study, of Jonathan, highlights how EPG can aid in the teaching of auditory discrimination and motor programming skills, and thereby the updating of inaccurate phonological representations and motor programs. Both children were attending a residential school for children with specific speech and language disorders at the time of the investigations and therapy described. They each had long-term, persistent speech disorders as one feature of their complex and severe communication disorders.

Case Study 1: Paul

Paul was CA 9;4 when he entered the school. Assessment at that time revealed that his auditory discrimination of real words (assessed on the *Auditory Discrimination and Attention Test*, Morgan Barry, 1989), was within normal limits for his chronological age. He demonstrated some awareness of the internal structure of phonological representations. For example, he was able to complete onset detection and rhyme tasks such as: "what is the sound at the beginning of PAINT; PILLOW; PANTOMIME?"; and "which of the following words rhyme: BAT; RAT; PIN; CAT?". However, he could not detect codas in tasks such as: "what is the sound at the end of CUP, ROPE, TAP?". He was unable to manipulate phonological strings. For example, he could not blend onsets and rimes accurately, as in: "say [s] then [ʌn] quickly one after the other – what word do they make?", and could not produce rhyming strings, as in: "tell me all the words you can think of which rhyme with HAT". Tongue control and sequencing of sounds were problematic, e.g. Paul repeated the nonword [ˈpʌkətəs] as [ˈpʌtəkəs].

Thus, Paul presented with severely disordered speech output. A perceptually based speech analysis revealed in particular a reduced sound system in word final position, characterized by omission of consonants; a reduced system of fricative contrasts; frequent use of glottal stop; productions of consonant clusters not typical of normal speech development. See Table 7.1 for further details of this analysis.

Intervention focused on highlighting for Paul how phonological representations can be broken down into their component parts, and on teaching him how these can be manipulated. A block of therapy involved segmentation, blending and rhyme production games, using onsets, rimes and codas. All the sounds of the English sound system were employed in these activities, regardless of whether or not they occurred in Paul's system, (see Table 7.1). Consonant clusters were also

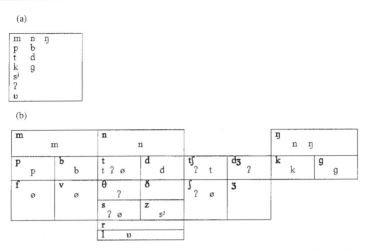

Table 7.1. (a) Paul's system of contrastive phones in word final position and (b) his realisation of target phonemes, at CA 9;4 based on a perceptual analysis (∅ = zero realisation).

included as Paul's skills developed.

Following this therapy, Paul performed accurately and confidently on segmentation, blending and rhyme production tasks involving simple CVC words. He was also attempting the same tasks using more complex words containing consonant clusters and two syllables. A second perceptually based speech analysis at CA 10;2 revealed that Paul's output, although not a focus of treatment, had also developed: he was now signalling word final position and sound contrasts in that position much more consistently, and clusters were realized more accurately. See Table 7.2 for further details of this analysis.

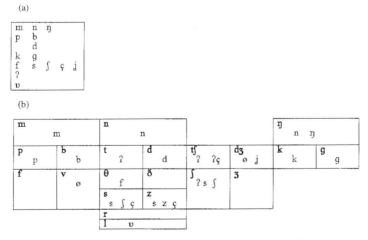

Table 7.2. (a) Paul's system of contrastive phones in word final position and (b) his realisation of target phonemes, at CA 10;2 based, on a perceptual analysis (∅ = zero realisation).

However, Paul encountered persistent difficulties with the fricatives /s/ and /ʃ/ and the affricate /tʃ/, as in SIP; SHIP; and CHIP respectively. In his output, Paul either appeared to fail to distinguish between these sounds, or to select incorrectly from among them. Thus, for example, if attempting to produce the three words SIP; SHIP; and CHIP, Paul might be perceived to say the same for each target, or to say "ship" instead of "sip" or "chip". Furthermore, when completing activities that did not demand a spoken response, such as a rhyme detection task, Paul again appeared to demonstrate confusion between these sounds. For example, when presented with pictures of the following targets: SHOP, CHOP, MOP and CHIP, and asked to point to those that rhyme, Paul would express uncertainty and lack of confidence, pointing to all or none of the pictures. Incorrect selection of the relevant graphemes and digraphs was also seen in Paul's attempts to spell words involving these sounds, for example, SHIP was spelt as ‹sip› and SHRIMP as ‹srimp› (see Stackhouse, 1996, for a discussion of a case in which similar confusions arose in speech production and spelling patterns).

Assessment of Paul prior to EPG therapy

To investigate this persistent deficit further, a number of tasks were designed and administered and the results interpreted within the psycholinguistic framework:

(i) Task 1: Visual Onset/Coda Detection
Two sets of stimulus pictures were used:

> Set S (/s/, /ʃ/, /tʃ/) contained 45 words in which the onset was varied between each of the three sounds, and 45 words in which the coda was varied;
> Set P (/p/, /t/, /k/) similarly contained two subsets of 45 words in which the onset or coda was varied.

See Table 7.3 for examples of words employed in each set.

Table 7.3: Examples of the stimuli employed during the visual onset/coda detection task (task 1)

	SET S				SET P			
	/s/	/ʃ/	/tʃ/	Total	/p/	/t/	/k/	Total
onset	sailor	shelf	chips	45	pencil	tiger	castle	45
coda	tennis	polish	pitch	45	zip	kite	snake	45

For each of the stimulus pictures, Paul was given three cards, on each of which was written one of the three graphemes/digraphs that correspond to the sounds in set S or those in set P. Paul was instructed to look at each picture, and to decide which one of the three sounds was at the beginning of the target word represented by the picture. Figure 7.11 illustrates how the materials for this task were presented.

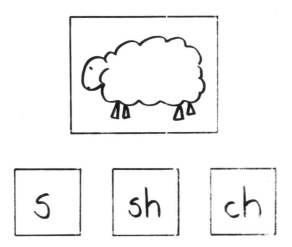

Figure 7.11 Materials for visual onset/coda detection task.

The same procedure was followed for the coda detection task. Paul was instructed to look at each picture presented and to decide which one of the three letter cards represented the sound at the end of the target. He was asked not to say or whisper anything when reaching his decision. Paul's knowledge of phoneme–grapheme links was known to be accurate.

Paul's performance on all the stimuli in set S was inferior in comparison to his scores for the stimuli in set P. He took a long time to make a decision for each of the stimuli involving /s/, /ʃ/, /tʃ/, changing his mind several times. In contrast, he gave a single, rapid response for each of the stimuli involving /p/, /t/ or /k/.

(ii) Task 2: Auditory Lexical Decision (after Locke, 1980)
Each of the stimuli in set S and set P was used as a template to form two additional real word or nonword stimuli: the onset or coda of each item was substituted by one of the other phonemes within the set, so that three possibilities for each stimulus picture, one correct and two incorrect, were available. See Table 7.4 for examples of words and nonwords in each set.

Table 7.4: Examples of the stimuli employed during the auditory lexical decision task (task 2)

		SET S			SET P	
	stimulus	alternative	alternative	stimulus	alternative	alternative
onset	SHOP	/sɒp/	/tʃɒp/	PANDA	/tændə/	/ kændə/
coda	MOUSE	/maʊʃ/	/maʊtʃ/	FORK	/fɔp/	/fɔt/

Each set of stimulus pictures was presented on three different occasions. On each occasion, Paul was shown a picture and asked "Is this a ... ?", using either the correct, or one of the two error alternatives. The order of presentation of each of the three posibilities was randomized. See Book 1, Chapter 2 for more details of this task.

All of Paul's responses during this task were correct. He responded to most of the items in both S and P stimulus sets promptly and with apparent ease, accepting correct and rejecting error alternatives.

(iii) Task 3: Auditory Visual Onset / Coda Detection

The procedurc for task 1 was repeated, but this time Paul heard the target word as the stimulus picture was presented to him. Again, he was instructed not to say or whisper anything while making his decision. He scored between 96 and 100 per cent correct across all conditions. There was no difference in his performance between /s/, /ʃ/, /tʃ/ and /p/, /t/, /k/ items.

(iv) Task 4: EPG Recording and Analysis

Paul was asked to produce a list of items including some /s/, /ʃ/, /tʃ/ minimal pairs, e.g. SUE, SHOE, CHEW; SIP, SHIP, CHIP. This was recorded using the EPG system. Figure 7.12 illustrates the tongue–palate contact patterns seen in typical productions of target /s/, /ʃ/, and /tʃ/, and examples of the patterns seen in Paul's attempts to produce each of these targets.

Paul's contact patterns were clearly atypical: attempts at targets /s/ and /tʃ/ lacked contact in the alveolar region and attempts at target /ʃ/ were characterized by insufficient contact down each side of the palate. Furthermore, Paul's articulation of these sounds was not well differentiated: the pattern for each target involved some contact with the sides of the palate and could not be clearly distinguished from the pattern for each of the other targets.

Table 7.5 summarizes Paul's pattern of performance during each of the four tasks described above.

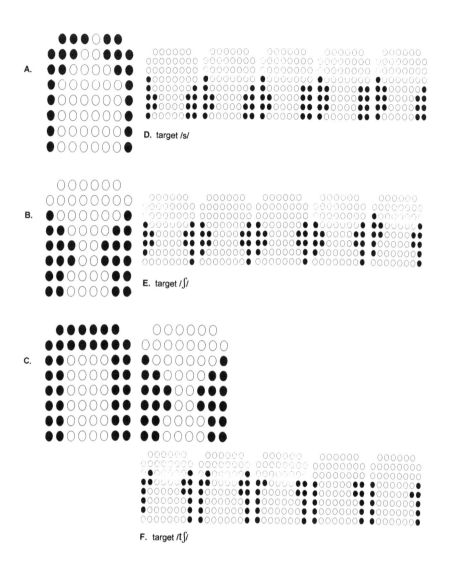

Figure 7.12 Paul's realization of target /s/, /ʃ/ and /tʃ/ before therapy

Table 7.5: Actual and percentage correct responses for each stimulus set during tasks 1 – 3. Percentage figures are given in parentheses. A brief summary of the results of the EPG analysis is presented.

Task		SET S				SET P			
		/s/	/ʃ/	/tʃ/	Total	/p/	/t/	/k/	Total
1: Detection – picture only	Onset	7(47)	10(67)	13(87)	30(67)	15(100)	14(93)	15(100)	44(98)
	Coda	6(40)	7(47)	3(20)	16(36)	15(100)	14(93)	15(100)	44(98)
2: Auditory lexical decision	Onset	15(100)	15(100)	15(100)	45(100)	15(100)	15(100)	15(100)	45(100)
	Coda	15(100)	15(100)	15(100)	45(100)	15(100)	15(100)	15(100)	45(100)
3: As 1, with speech stimuli	Onset	13(87)	15(100)	15(100)	43(96)	15(100)	15(100)	15(100)	45(100)
	Coda	15(100)	13(87)	15(100)	43(96)	15(100)	15(100)	14(93)	44(98)
4: Naming with EPG	Onset	EPG contact patterns /s/, /ʃ/, /tʃ/ atypical and undifferentiated							
	Coda	As above							

ACTIVITY 7.5

Aim: to formulate and test hypotheses regarding speech processing strengths and deficits on the basis of a series of tasks.

For each task presented in Table 7.5, consider what Paul had to do in terms of speech processing, and then examine the results. What are the implications of these for Paul's speech processing skills? Write down your thoughts, then read the following.

During task 1, Paul had to select his phonological representation for the item in the picture, segment the onset or the coda, and match this with one of the graphemes/digraphs in front of him. Paul's difficulty in making decisions regarding the set S stimuli therefore suggested the following hypotheses:
either,

1. Phonological representations for these items were inaccurate,

or,

2. Paul was unable to segment /s/, /ʃ/, /tʃ/ onsets and codas from whole word representations.

    (As Paul's knowledge of phoneme–grapheme links was not impaired, this could not be postulated as a possible cause of his difficulties).

In task 2, Paul again had to select his phonological representation for the item in the picture, and compare this with the word or nonword that he heard. His acceptance of only the correct alternatives across both stimuli sets indicated that his phonological representations for items involving /s/, /ʃ/, /tʃ/ were accurate. Hypothesis 1 was therefore disproved.

During task 3, Paul could segment the onset or the coda of the word that he heard, and match this with one of the graphemes/digraphs in front of him, thus completing the task without reference to his own phonological representations for the stimuli. His accurate pattern of performance across both sets of stimuli suggested that he was able to segment any onset/coda from a whole word. His difficulty with the set S stimuli in task 1 could not therefore be explained by a problem with the segmentation of /s/, /ʃ/, /tʃ/ from whole word representations. Hypothesis 2 was therefore also disproved and Paul's pattern of perform-ance in task 1 was still unexplained.

In task 4, he had to select his motor program for the item in the picture and execute this. The atypical and undifferentiated contact patterns seen in the EPG palatograms may have been laid down in Paul's motor programs for items involving target /s/, /ʃ/, /tʃ/, or may have arisen only at the point of motor execution. Whichever was the case, they represented Paul's articulation of these targets and a third hypothesis could therefore be formulated regarding the cause of his difficulties in task 1:

3.   Paul was silently articulating the items involved when reaching his decisions, using these undifferentiated patterns for stimuli involving /s/, /ʃ/, /tʃ/ and consequently encountering difficulty for these but not for the /p/, /t/ and /k/ stimuli, which he articulated accurately.

This explanation could also account for the confusions seen in his attempts to spell words involving these sounds.

EPG therapy with Paul

The tasks described above indicated that Paul's difficulty articulating /s/, /ʃ/, and /tʃ/ accurately and consistently was affecting not only his speech output, and therefore his intelligibility, but also his ability to segment and blend words involving these sounds, and therefore his literacy development. Furthermore, unlike his other speech output problems, it had not resolved spontaneously as a result of the therapy programme outlined earlier. It was therefore hypothesized that Paul would benefit from a more direct articulatory teaching method, such as EPG: the visual feedback provided by the system could be employed to help Paul to learn correct tongue contact patterns for /s/, /ʃ/ and /tʃ/, thus modifying his motor execution. He might subsequently require support in revising and updating his stored motor programs for words involving these sounds, if these too were incorrect.

   The EPG therapy undertaken involved seven key stages, described below. At each stage the target sounds concerned were discussed in terms of their sound and letter names and the appropriate graphemes and digraphs were employed as visual labels.

(i) Demonstration
The nature of the EPG visual display was demonstrated and explained, focusing in particular on: the relationship between Paul's mouth, tongue, teeth and hard palate and the visual display; the relationship between the contact patterns on the visual display and sounds produced; the differences between Paul's patterns and the correct patterns /s/, /ʃ/, and /tʃ/.

(ii) Gross tongue movement

Paul was made aware, via the visual display, of his ability to achieve and control gross tongue movements, such as raising the back to the velar region and the front to the alveolar ridge.

(iii) Fine tongue movement

Paul was helped to achieve control of the tongue contact pattern for each of the target sounds in turn. He was asked to focus on moving his tongue, without making any sound. The target pattern was displayed on the screen and similar and dissimilar features in this and in each of Paul's attempts to copy it were discussed. Slight modifications were suggested for his next attempt, until a close approximation to the model was achieved. Paul was encouraged to monitor and record his progress for himself and at times he worked with the EPG system independently. He was also asked at this stage to consider how production of the new contact pattern differed from his error pattern, e.g. was his tongue further forward in his mouth; was it touching a different part of his hard palate. Such features were highlighted for Paul to help him become increasingly aware of the tactile and kinaesthetic features of the correct contact pattern. He would then be able to use this awareness in subsequent attempts to achieve the pattern again.

(iv) Alternating tongue movements

Once Paul could achieve and maintain a target contact pattern for five seconds, he was asked to produce it in alternating sequences with other contact patterns for sounds already in his repertoire, such as /t/ and /k/. He then alternated it with his error pattern for the target concerned. Again, all activities were conducted silently. At intervals during this stage, the visual display was blocked from Paul's view, to begin to reduce his dependence on this, and to force him to make use of the tactile and kinaesthetic knowledge he had acquired during this and the previous stage.

By the end of this stage of therapy, Paul was able to achieve and maintain each target contact pattern quickly and accurately without the support of the visual feedback provided by the EPG system. It was hypothesized that he had by now therefore established aspects of new articulatory patterns for use during motor execution. He would also be encouraged to employ the new patterns during motor programming, for new word production and for updating faulty motor programs if necessary.

(v) Coarticulation of target consonants with vowel gestures

Paul was then required to practise motor programming skills using each of his new contact patterns in simple sequences: he was asked to produce silently nonword sequences such as /sɑ/, /eiʃ/, and /tʃai/. This stage helped Paul to learn how the tongue contact pattern has to change slightly to accommodate the different lip, jaw and tongue movements necessary for the production of preceding and subsequent sounds – a phenomenon known as coarticulation. These skills would be necessary for accurate production of words in the future.

(vi) Adding the airstream

Only at this stage was Paul asked to articulate the target sounds audibly, by making the contact pattern then 'blowing' (i.e. adding airstream). Because he had established the patterns firmly during the previous stages, Paul was able to maintain them when he added airstream to produce the target sounds, and thus achieved the correct motor execution for /s/, /ʃ/, and /tʃ/ very quickly at this point. Motor programming was targeted by practising audibly the simple sequences used during the previous stage and also CVC nonwords such as /sip/, /nɔʃ/, and /tʃɑk/.

(vii) Generalizing to real words

Therapy now focused on production of real words: tasks required Paul either to update faulty motor programs, or simply to employ his new contact patterns in the context of real rather than nonwords. He was asked to reflect on a particular picture and written stimulus before attempting production, to encourage him to use his new contact patterns spontaneously. He encountered some difficulty at this stage, particularly as more complex stimuli such as multisyllabic words and words involving consonant clusters were included, e.g. SELLOTAPE, DINOSAUR, TOOTHBRUSH. A range of activities was therefore employed to help Paul to generalize his new articulatory skill to words and then to connected speech.

Assessment of Paul following EPG therapy

As noted above, it was not possible to determine whether Paul's incorrect contact patterns had been laid down in his motor programs or had arisen only at the point of motor execution, (for discussion of different levels of processing see Book 1, Chapter 6). However, the patterns illustrated in Figure 7.13 demonstrate that, whichever was the case, EPG therapy had helped Paul to modify his articulatory patterns for use in words in connected speech.

Figure 7.13 illustrates the tongue–palate contact patterns seen in typical productions of target /s/, /ʃ/ and /tʃ/, and examples of the patterns seen in Paul's productions of each of these targets in connected speech, following therapy using the EPG system. Compare these with the patterns illustrated in Figure 7.12. It is clear that Paul was

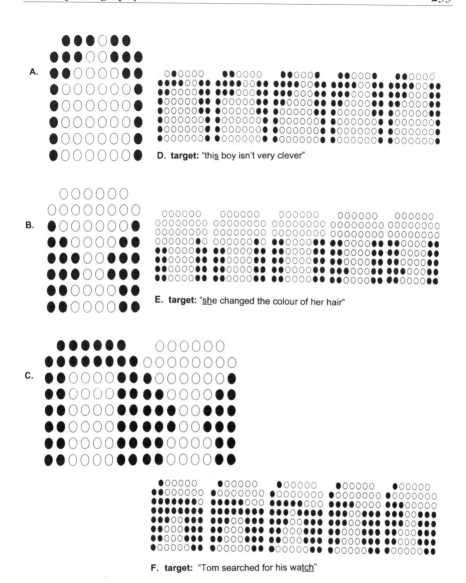

D. target: "this boy isn't very clever"

E. target: "she changed the colour of her hair"

F. target: "Tom searched for his watch"

Figure 7.13 Paul's realization of /S/, /ʃ/ and /tʃ/ after therapy.

now able to differentiate his articulation for these sounds and to produce tongue–palate contact patterns which closely resembled the model patterns.

A perceptual analysis of Paul's speech confirmed these findings: during therapy sessions his production of target /s/, /ʃ/ and /tʃ/ was perceived to be 100 per cent accurate in single words, and accurate 50 per cent of the time in connected speech. He was now able to undertake confidently and successfully segmentation, blending and spelling tasks involving each of these targets. Paul was aware of how both his old and his new articulations felt in his mouth and sounded on production, and he was able to correct errors that he made. He did not, however, do this consistently. For example, when he was tired or excited and had a lot to say Paul continued to use his old articulation pattern and could not monitor himself to revise errors as they occurred. Despite this persistent difficulty, Paul's speech was generally perceived as being more intelligible by people who interacted regularly with him in school.

Case study 2: Jonathan

As with Paul, EPG was employed with Jonathan not to refine specific aspects of particular articulatory patterns, but to assist in the teaching of auditory discrimination and motor programming skills simultaneously, as a foundation for the subsequent modification of phonological representations and motor programs.

Assessment of Jonathan prior to EPG therapy

Jonathan's speech processing skills were assessed when he was CA 11;9. At this age, his speech production skills were the subject of some concern; in particular, his inconsistent and limited use of alveolar (e.g. [t]) and velar (e.g. [k]) plosives, which in spite of considerable intervention were still problematic. Jonathan often omitted these sounds from his speech, or produced an alveolar in place of a velar plosive. This pattern of errors made Jonathan's speech sound immature. Furthermore, as a consequence of these and several other features, his speech was often unintelligible if his listener was unaware of the topic of conversation. A psycholinguistic assessment revealed the following deficits with regard to the alveolar vs velar contrast.

(i) Input
Performance on all types of auditory discrimination task using simple stimuli, nonwords and real words was well below chance level. For example, Jonathan was asked to listen to pairs of real words and nonwords such as those illustrated below and to say whether he thought they were the same or different:

Real words

CAN ~ CAN	PACKING ~ PACKING	BIKE ~ BIKE
CAN ~ TAN	PACKING ~ PATTING	BIKE ~ BITE

Nonwords

/kan/ ~ /kan/	/pukə/ ~ /pukə/	/baʊk/ ~ /baʊk/
/kan/ ~ /tan/	/pukə/ ~ /putə/	/baʊk/ ~ /baʊt/

Jonathan responded inconsistently and was often incorrect; sometimes he said that two identical stimuli were different, sometimes he said that two different stimuli were the same. There was no apparent pattern to his errors, but he said at times that he was unsure of how to respond and it was clear throughout that he found auditory processing of both nonwords and real words very difficult.

(ii) Representations
An auditory lexical decision task, identical in design to the one used with Paul, was constructed for Jonathan based on his alveolar/velar plosive output errors. Each of the stimuli included an alveolar or a velar plosive and was used as a template to form two additional real word or nonword stimuli: alveolar plosives were substituted by either the glottal stop [ʔ], or the bilabial plosive [p]; velar plosives were substituted by either an alveolar plosive, or the bilabial plosive. Thus, three possibilities for each stimulus picture, one correct and two incorrect, were available. See Table 7.6 for examples of some of the real words and nonwords employed.

Table 7.6: Examples of the stimuli employed during the auditory lexical decision task.

Alveolar stimuli			Velar stimuli		
Stimulus	Alternative	Alternative	Stimulus	Alternative	Alternative
TABLE	[ʔeibl̩]	[peibl̩]	CAR	[ta]	[pa]
LETTER	[lɛʔə]	[lɛpə]	ROCKY	[ɹɒtɪ]	[ɹɒpɪ]
BOAT	[bəʊʔ]	[bəʊp]	SMOKE	[sməʊt]	[sməʊp]

As described for Paul, Jonathan was shown a stimulus picture and asked "Is this a...?", using either the correct form, or one of the two error alternatives. Jonathan always rejected as incorrect the alternatives that involved the bilabial plosive [p]. However, he responded inconsistently and was often incorrect when faced with the alternatives involving the glottal stop or alveolar plosives; sometimes he accepted as correct an incorrect version of the target, sometimes he rejected a correct version. Again, there was no apparent pattern to his errors and he expressed his difficulty in processing these stimuli. Jonathan's inability to discriminate correct from incorrect versions of stimuli during this task indicated that his phonological representations for these items were not sufficiently well specified with regard to the alveolar or velar segment.

(iii) Output
The targets used in the auditory lexical decision task were employed in a picture-naming activity and in a real word repetition task, in which Jonathan was asked to repeat exactly each item as it was produced by the therapist. The nonwords used in the auditory discrimination tasks were then employed in a nonword repetition task, in which Jonathan was told by the therapist: "I'm going to say some new English words that you won't have heard before. Say them after me". Table 7.7 illustrates stimuli and responses across these investigations.

Table 7.7: Illustration of the stimuli used and responses given across the series of tasks designed to investigate Jonathan's speech output processing skills

	Alveolar stimuli		Velar stimuli	
Task	Stimulus	Response	Stimulus	Response
Naming	BUTTON	[bʌʔʌ̃n]	COMB	[təʊm]
Real word repetition	BUTTON	[bʌʔʌ̃n]	COMB	[təʊm]
Nonword repetition	/putə/	[pʰuʔʰə]	/kan/	[tʰɑ̃]

Jonathan's output during each of these three tasks was inconsistent:

> Naming: the alveolar plosive /t/ was used appropriately in all word positions, though not consistently: in word medial and word final position it was frequently omitted. The velar plosive /k/ in word initial position was either used appropriately, or replaced by the alveolar plosive; in word medial and word final position, the velar was either again replaced by the alveolar, or omitted.
> Real word repetition: the pattern of errors generally reflected that made during the naming task.
> Nonword repetition: Jonathan found this task particularly difficult and it was not completed; he used no velar segments, replacing them with [t] or omitting them in all word positions.

In isolated sound production, Jonathan managed to repeat the alveolar plosive /t/ and the velar plosive /k/ but his articulation was effortful. Alveolar productions were perceived to involve excessive contact between the tongue and the hard palate, suggesting that the body rather than just the tip of the tongue was employed in the articulation. These productions were consequently indistinct and involved some friction. Attempts at velar plosive production involved excessive lower jaw movement and were perceived to be retracted, i.e. articulated further back in the mouth than the velar region. These sounds, like the alveolar productions, involved some friction. Jonathan thus appeared to find isolated production of the alveolar and velar plosives, in the absence of any context, much more difficult than the use of these sounds within words.

A recording was made, using the EPG system, of Jonathan repeating a list of items which included the real words employed in the tasks described above. Figure 7.14 illustrates the tongue–palate contact patterns seen in typical productions of targets /t/ and /k/, and examples of the patterns seen in Jonathan's attempts to produce these targets.

The EPG data supported the conclusions made above regarding Jonathan's pattern of errors in naming and real word repetition. Figure 7.14 presents data from his realization of two different disyllabic words where target /t/ is in intervocalic position: LITTER and SWEATER. Jonathan's tongue contact pattern for the /t/ in LITTER is very similar to the expected target. In SWEATER, however, there is no tongue contact at the front of the mouth. This illustrates that Jonathan is capable of accurate realization of /t/, but is inconsistent.

Three attempts at target /k/ are illustrated in Figure 7.14. When the target is in onset position, at the beginning of KICK, Jonathan's realization is very similar to the target, with contacts visible across the back of the palate, i.e in the velar region. At the end of KICK, however, there is less evidence of closure: contacts are visible at the sides of the palate in the velar region, but not in the centre of the palate. In the coda of PICK, there is virtually no velar closure. Instead, closure is found in the alveolar region: compare Jonathan's production of the /k/ in PICK with his production of the /t/ in LITTER.

It was thus apparent from the EPG data that on some occasions Jonathan was capable of realizing these target plosive consonants within words, with patterns of tongue–palate contact that closely resembled the model patterns. Thus, his pattern for /t/ involved complete contact across only the first two rows of the palate, and his pattern for /k/ featured complete contact across the last row. When he failed to produce the correct realization, he either omitted the consonant in whole or in part (SWEATER, KICK), or else substituted another: PICK → [pɪt].

Figure 7.15 presents Jonathan's speech processing profile, based on his performance on the tasks described in this section.

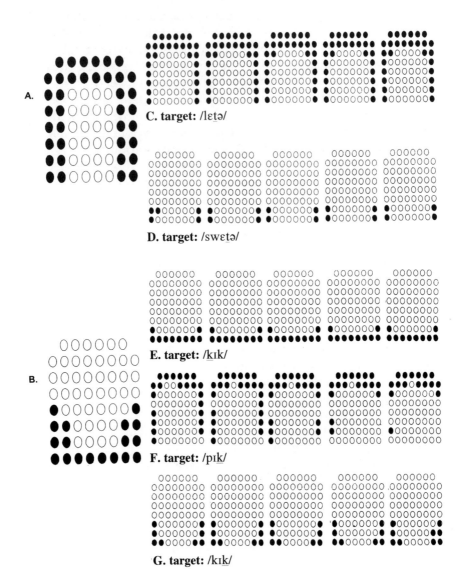

C. target: /lɛt̪ə/

D. target: /swɛt̪ə/

E. target: /k̲ɪk/

F. target: /pɪk̲/

G. target: /k̲ɪk̲/

Figure 7.14 Jonathan's realization of target /t/ and /k/ before therapy.

SPEECH PROCESSING PROFILE

Name   Comments:

Age

Date

Profiler

INPUT	OUTPUT

F

Is the child aware of the internal structure of phonological representations?

G

Can the child access accurate motor programs?

× alveolar and velar plosive targets in words in naming tasks

E

Are the child's phonological representations accurate?

× alveolar and velar plosive targets in auditory lexical decision task

H

Can the child manipulate phonological units?

D

Can the child discriminate between real words?

× RW stimuli involving alveolar and velar plosives. (S/D Discrim.)

I

Can the child articulate real words accurately?

RW REP. performance = naming performance for alveolar and velar plosives.

nb EPG data: appropriate contact patterns in word production for alveolar and velar plosives

C

Does the child have language-specific representations of word structures?

J

Can the child articulate speech without reference to lexical representations?

NW REP. problematic ++; worse than RW REP. and naming, for alveolar and velar plosives

B

Can the child discriminate speech sounds without reference to lexical representations?

× NW stimuli involving alveolar and velar plosives. (S/D Discrim.)

A

Does the child have adequate auditory perception?

K

Does the child have adequate sound production skills?

Imitation of /t/ and /k/ in isolation effortful and distorted

L

Does the child reject his/her own erroneous forms?

Figure 7.15 Jonathan's speech processing profile, for use in Activity 7.7.

ACTIVITY 7.6

Aim: to compile broad therapy aims and methods on the basis of a speech processing profile.

With reference to Jonathan's assessment results summarized in Figure 7.15, consider what your therapy aims for him might be. Write these down and then read the following.

The severity of Jonathan's difficulties throughout the speech processing profile suggested that therapy should target both input and output skills simultaneously. Jonathan could not discriminate accurately between the alveolar and velar plosives and it was hypothesized that this had led to him storing inaccurate phonological representations for words involving these sounds. It was postulated also that this would continue to impinge on Jonathan's learning of new words, which were being introduced frequently within the context of the National Curriculum. (See Popple and Wellington; and Stackhouse, this volume for further information about this curriculum.) Similarly, Jonathan could not differentiate consistently between the alveolar and velar plosives in his output. This deficit was no doubt related to his inaccurate phonological representations, which are one source of information in the construction of motor programs and therefore a basis for output. However, Jonathan's relatively poor performance on the nonword repetition task, when compared with his performance on the naming and real word repetition tasks, suggested that his output errors were also caused by a motor programming deficit, i.e. difficulty co-ordinating production of sounds for the construction of new motor programs. It was hypothesized that Jonathan's severe difficulties imitating alveolar and velar plosives in isolation were further evidence of his problems in motor programming, which might involve experimentation and rehearsal via single sound production. Consequently, there would be little to gain from focusing on either input or output in isolation since the development of one is contingent on development of the other; there would be little point in establishing accurate motor programming for new word production, if Jonathan could not first discriminate accurately the new words that he needed to produce.

Jonathan appeared to need as much information as possible about his alveolar and velar targets, in order to develop simultaneously his auditory and articulatory skills with respect to these sounds. It was hypothesized that only then would he be able to modify his incorrectly stored phonological representations and motor programs.

EPG therapy with Jonathan

Therapy employing the EPG system was therefore considered appropriate. The information about articulatory placement provided by the visual display was used as a support, along with cued articulation (Passy, 1993a), colour coding and orthography for both auditory training and articulation. A range of activities was employed, during which Jonathan was exposed to the alveolar and the velar plosives in isolation and in simple real word and nonword stimuli. Activities included the following.

(i) Teaching auditory and articulatory features
The following activity was one of several that focused on teaching these features during the initial stages of therapy. The alveolar target /t/ was discussed in terms of its EPG characteristics, (i.e. contact around the edges of the palatogram like an upside down horseshoe, with complete contact across the first two rows at the top), and Jonathan drew and coloured a schematic palatogram which was then employed throughout therapy. The alveolar was also discussed in terms of its cued articulation sign and colour code and its sound and letter names. A simple real word or nonword was then presented in written form, e.g. LIGHT; /mɪtə/, and the alveolar plosive was highlighted using the cued articulation colour code and its position in the word (i.e. beginning, middle or end) was discussed. Jonathan then listened to and watched the therapist as she produced the word and the cued articulation sign with her EPG palate in place. As she produced it, the therapist copied her contact pattern for the plosive to the right of the computer screen. Jonathan was then asked whether he had heard the /t/ sound, and to check that the palatogram on the screen was correct for the sound, the sign, the letter and the colour code. This procedure was completed for several words, to expose Jonathan to lots of examples of the alveolar plosive, in order to broaden and consolidate his knowledge about the auditory and articulatory features of the sound.

In the second part of the activity, the same procedure was repeated using the same items, but for some items the therapist produced a different sound, for example the labiodental fricative /f/, with its cued articulation sign, instead of the alveolar plosive. On these occasions, Jonathan listened and watched, and was then asked whether he had heard the /t/ sound, and to check the palatogram, sign, letter and colour code, in just the same way as for the other items. When Jonathan had noted the error, the features of the error sound and the alveolar plosive were the focus of some discussion. Again, this procedure was repeated for several words, to build on the skills taught in the first section of the activity, by contrasting /t/ with other, quite different sounds.

This activity was extended during later therapy sessions by

modifying the second part; the entire procedure was completed in exactly the same way, but this time Jonathan listened but did not watch the therapist's production and therefore did not have available the support of the cued articulation sign. The activity was also used in the same way to teach the auditory and articulatory features of the velar plosive /k/. At no point during this activity was Jonathan required to produce either target sound. The focus was the teaching of features to be employed in future discrimination and production.

(ii) Teaching motor programming of simple sequences

Because Jonathan found isolated sound production extremely difficult, and EPG analysis had revealed that he was able to produce appropriate tongue–palate contact patterns for the alveolar and the velar plosive, early production activities involved simple CV and VC words. Real word stimuli were employed before nonwords because of Jonathan's motor programming difficulties. However, the activity and items were presented in a way that would encourage Jonathan to employ motor programming and the articulatory information taught during previous activities to construct a new motor program. Again, stimuli involving the alveolar plosive /t/ were targeted first. Later, activities were repeated with stimuli involving the velar plosive /k/.

In one such activity, a CV or VC sequence was presented in written form, e.g. TIE; AT. As before, the alveolar plosive was highlighted using the cued articulation colour code and its position in the word, (i.e. beginning, middle or end) and letter and sound names were discussed. Jonathan was then asked to produce the appropriate cued articulation sign, and to find his own schematic palatogram for /t/. Only after each of these points had been covered was Jonathan asked to produce the sequence and the cued articulation sign with his EPG palate in place. He was reminded to watch the computer screen and to think about the /t/ target as he did so. His tongue–palate contact pattern during produc-tion of the plosive was copied to the right of the screen. Jonathan was then asked to compare the pattern on the screen with his schematic palatogram, and to comment on how his production had sounded. The procedure was completed for several real word CV and VC sequences. During the second part of the activity, the same procedure was repeated using nonword sequences such as /tei/; /ait/.

(iii) Practising discrimination and production skills

At a later stage of therapy, Jonathan was asked to discriminate and produce a target within words in a single activity. This was expected of him only when he had demonstrated consistent discrimination and production in words in activities focusing on one skill in isolation. Again, stimuli containing the alveolar plosive /t/ were targeted first, and those containing the velar plosive /k/ later.

In one such activity, Jonathan was involved in compiling a word-processed list of real words and nonwords. During compilation, the target plosive in each item was highlighted using the cued articulation colour code. The corresponding EPG palatogram, cued articulation sign, letter sound and name were also discussed. The therapist and Jonathan then took turns to produce one of the words and sign with their EPG palates in place, while the other listened. During production, the speaker copied her/his tongue–palate contact pattern for the plosive to the right of the computer screen. At times, the therapist made deliberate errors, replacing the target plosive with another sound and sign, as described earlier.

Initially, the listener was allowed to watch the speaker (for the support of the sign) and look at the EPG screen (for the support of the palatogram) before making a decision regarding what had been heard. In later versions of this activity, the whole procedure was repeated, first withdrawing the sign support, and second that of the palatogram.

At each stage of intervention, therapy aims and rationale were made clear to Jonathan through discussion and illustration, as his awareness of what he was learning and why it were considered an integral aspect of the therapy programme. He was actively involved in keeping a careful record of his performance during each session and in determining when he had reached the criterion level set for moving on to the next stage. Jonathan was motivated by the challenge of the criterion level, which appealed to his competitive spirit, and this helped him to focus on activities that were intrinsically very difficult for him. He also enjoyed working on the computer and completing tasks independently.

Assessment of Jonathan following EPG therapy

Following this programme of therapy, Jonathan was able to discriminate the alveolar and velar plosive targets and produce each of them much more consistently during very structured therapy activities such as those described above. However, he continued to find such tasks difficult and had to focus his attention for discrimination and monitor his output very carefully. A brief assessment was conducted of Jonathan's discrimination and production skills, which included items that had not been the focus of therapy, and during which the supports provided in therapy were absent. This revealed somewhat fewer, but nevertheless persistent, inconsistencies in both discrimination and production. It was evident that, while his performance during therapy activities suggested that Jonathan had used his new knowledge and skills to update phonological representations and motor programs for the items included in tasks, such modification had not generalized to other items not targeted in therapy. Furthermore, he was not yet able to function independently of the supports provided by therapy when processing items that had not been actively taught previously. Thus, despite some progress, Jonathan clearly had some persistent difficulties in his processing of the alveolar $\sim$ velar plosive contrast. He needed help now to transfer his new skills spontaneously to other words in his lexicon, and to become less dependent on visual support systems.

Efficacy

The detailed and objective articulatory information that the EPG system provides is useful not only during the process of therapy, but also, if recorded and analysed effectively as pre- and post-therapy measurements of performance, as an indicator of the efficacy of therapy itself. This has been demonstrated in the case studies of Paul and Jonathan. There are increasing demands on the speech and language therapy and teaching professions to account for time and financial resources by demonstrating the effectiveness of procedures selected for use with a particular client group. In this climate, computer-based techniques such as the EPG system, which can supply objective and quantifiable data and which can guarantee identical measurement across different assessment times, are particularly useful.

Summary

The following points have been raised in this chapter.

- EPG is a computer-based technique which provides a visual display of tongue contact with the hard palate during speech.
- EPG can be employed along with other procedures as an assessment tool in the compilation of speech-processing profiles.
- EPG can provide information that cannot be obtained via other, perceptually based methods of assessment and which may be crucial to accurate diagnosis and treatment planning.
- EPG can be employed during therapy at the level of motor execution to provide visual feedback of tongue placement and movement. This allows the task of learning how to produce a speech sound to be broken down into smaller steps than is possible through more traditional therapy methods.
- EPG can be employed as a visual support in therapy that targets other levels of speech processing, such as auditory discrimination and motor programming.
- EPG data recorded as pre- and post-therapy measurements of performance can be employed as an objective indicator of the efficacy of the therapy undertaken.

KEY TO ACTIVITY 7.1

The palatograms in Figure 7.4 are typically seen in the production of the following English sounds (from left to right):

top	/k/;	/i/;
middle	/s/;	/t/ or /d/;
bottom	/t/ or /d/;	/p/.

KEY TO ACTIVITY 7.2

The word is 'tactics'. The figure below presents a full printout from the EPG system of the word TACTICS produced by a normal adult speaker. The sampling interval is 10 milliseconds. The phonetic symbols for each of the sounds in the word have been supplied to the right of the corresponding palatograms.

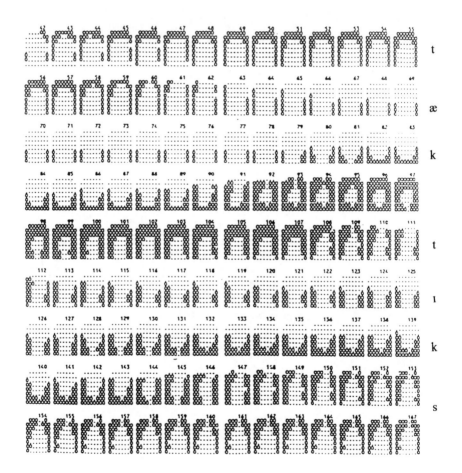

Figure 7.16 Key to Activity 7.2: TACTICS.

KEY TO ACTIVITY 7.3

Sophie's and Sam's speech processing profiles at CA 8;6 and 10;5 respectively are presented in the figure below:

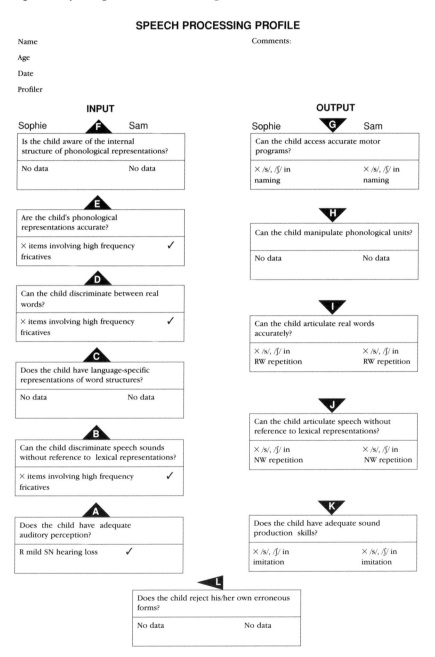

Figure 7. 17 Key to Activity 7.3: Profiles of Sophie and Sam.

KEY TO ACTIVITY 7.4

Hypotheses regarding Emily's processing of speech, modified in light of the EPG assessment data presented in Figure 7.10:

1. Emily's auditory discrimination skills and phonological representations for the contrast between alveolar and velar plosive targets are intact.
2. Emily has a specific motor execution deficit affecting her production of all alveolar plosive targets, such that her attempts at these are sometimes perceived to be inaccurate.
3. Emily's motor programs for items involving alveolar plosive targets may be inaccurate as a result of her motor execution deficit.

Acknowledgements

Part of the work described here was supported by a project grant from the UK Medical Research Council (Project No. G8912970N). Thanks are due to Bill Hardcastle and Fiona Gibbon who were principal investigators on the project, to Becky Clark who collaborated on the work described in Paul's case study and to Joy Stackhouse for her advice.

Chapter 8
Designing a Literacy Programme for a Child with a History of Speech Difficulties

LIZ NATHAN AND SARAH SIMPSON

When Luke was asked whether he liked reading, he replied:

> ...No, because...it's wasting your time...You could be doing better things, like playing; like doing fun work and things that you know...

By the end of Year 1 of primary school (CA 6;0), Luke was not only experiencing specific and significant literacy difficulties, he was also acutely aware of his problems.

The aim of this chapter is to describe the design and implementation of a literacy remediation programme that was informed by an understanding of how Luke's profile of speech processing skills and his early history of speech difficulties interacted with his development of reading and spelling. Part 1 of this chapter describes Luke's speech processing skills and emerging literacy problems from the age of 4 to 6 years in order to illustrate the unfolding nature of his literacy difficulty. His problems are discussed in the context of current research on the relationship between early speech difficulties and the development of phonological awareness and literacy ability. Part 2 of the chapter draws on literature relating speech processing development to theories of literacy acquisition, and describes how a literacy remediation programme was designed and implemented in Year 2 when Luke was aged 7 years. This part illustrates how a structured, individualized teaching programme can be directly informed by assessments of underlying speech processing ability as well as by a knowledge of how the current difficulties have emerged from an earlier stage of development.

Part 1: Tracking the Development of Emerging Literacy Difficulties between 4 and 6 Years of Age

Speech and language skills play a central role in learning to read and spell (see Book 1, Stackhouse and Wells, 1997, pp.17–22). Children who develop literacy problems often have a history of subtle or pervasive speech and/or language difficulties. Luke's history of pre-school speech difficulties suggests a causal relationship between his speech difficulties and the development of literacy problems. Figure 8.1 shows a diagram that conceptualizes the links between speech, phonological awareness and literacy development, with all three being underpinned by the speech processing system (see Book 1, pp.57–58). These links are now widely recognized and are reflected in the design of baseline assessment tests administered to children in school reception classes (i.e. at 4 and 5 years of age) which incorporate assessment of phonological awareness skills (see documentation produced by the Qualifications and Curriculum Authority, 1997).

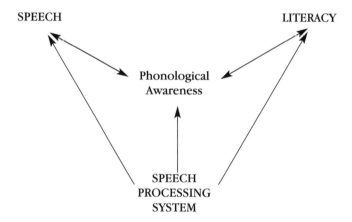

Figure 8.1: The connection between speech and literacy development (from Book 1, p.58).

Young children attending speech and language therapy because of pervasive speech and language difficulties are at increased risk of developing later literacy problems (Bishop and Adams, 1990; Catts, 1993). Several studies (Bird, Bishop and Freeman, 1995; Larrivee and Catts, 1999; Stackhouse, Nathan, Goulandris et al., 1999) have shown that young children identified as having primary speech difficulties are also more likely than children without such difficulties to have later literacy problems. However, many children with early speech difficulties do not experience later problems. A variety of factors have been identified that differentiate typical vs delayed later literacy performance; these include: severity of the speech difficulty; speech input problems; lower language scores; poor phonological awareness; and poor letter name knowledge (see Stackhouse, this volume). The influence of these factors may change with age, and having a developmental view of speech processing skills gives an important perspective from which to examine a current problem. A psycholinguistically driven assessment procedure (as presented in Book 1) structures and directs the investigation of what difficulties might make a child vulnerable for later literacy problems, or underlie a current literacy problem in any individual. In the case described in this chapter, this sort of detailed assessment procedure made two key contributions to understanding the literacy problem that Luke exhibited at the end of Year 1 at school:

1. Knowledge of Luke's past speech processing difficulties informed our understanding of his current literacy skills.
2. Detailed assessment of Luke's current speech processing skills gave us insight into his literacy difficulties.

In this case study, knowledge of both historical and current speech processing ability therefore provided information that could be directly incorporated into the management of the literacy problem. Luke's case history is particularly notable because he had neither a severe speech difficulty nor pervasive speech and language difficulties. By the time literacy difficulties had emerged, no significant speech problems were apparent and his school had no awareness that there ever had been problems. However, a detailed history of Luke's difficulties (and these are subtle rather than obvious) informed teaching practice because it alerted us to a potentially more intractable problem that required an early and intensive intervention programme rather than a wait-and-see approach. Current information enabled this remediation programme to be tightly focused around the particular strengths and weaknesses of the child.

Luke's Background

Luke was a highly personable young boy; in one-to-one situations with adults, he was always friendly and eager to co-operate. He was very chatty and liked to tell the authors funny incidents that had happened to him, his friends or family, or to chat about his favourite hobby, football (a Tottenham and England supporter). In the classroom, he was reported to be more boisterous and easily distracted with low levels of attention. He much preferred to be out in the playground playing with friends.

Detailed information about speech processing history is not usually available for most children presenting with literacy difficulties at school. However, information about Luke was available because a speech delay had prompted an earlier referral to speech and language therapy at CA 3;6. He had a history of ear infections that were treated by antibiotics and grommets (fitted in his third year and again 18 months later). He was reported to have delayed phonological processes: cluster reduction (e.g. STAMPS → [dæmps]) and voicing errors (e.g. MONKEY → [muŋgi]). However, direct intervention was not deemed appropriate and speech and language therapy consisted mainly of review appointments.

In addition to this information, extensive assessment data were available on Luke because of his involvement with a research project which collected speech, language and literacy data on children with and without speech difficulties at yearly intervals between the ages of 4 and 6 years (see Stackhouse, this volume for further details of this study). Although Luke's speech difficulties were not severe enough for him to be included in the main cohort of this study, he was still assessed annually as part of a smaller group of children with mild/resolved speech difficulties (Nimmo, 1998; Thurston, 1999; Stackhouse, 2000). Thus, Luke's speech processing development, language skills and phonological awareness ability had been charted systematically and can be examined with reference to his emerging literacy difficulties.

Luke's development was compared in two ways: first, with the study's main control group of 47 normally developing children who were also assessed between the ages of 4 and 6 years; and second, with one specific child from this control group, a boy called Terry, who was the same age and also attended Luke's school. As well as being in the same class as Luke over this time period (and therefore receiving very similar educational input in the classroom environment), Terry also obtained similar scores (also within normal limits) on two nonverbal assessments carried out at CA 4;4. Thus, the two boys shared several key factors: age, gender, school environment and nonverbal ability. Any difference in performance between them was therefore not due to these important factors; any difficulties Luke experiences with the tasks can probably be attributed to past or current speech processing skills.

Luke at 4 and 5 Years of Age

Luke's language skill at CA 4;4 and 5;5

Luke was assessed on a range of expressive and receptive language tasks. He performed within normal limits on all language tasks, and so language competence can be assumed throughout the following description of his performance (this was also the case at CA 6;5 and 7;2).

Luke's speech processing skills at CA 4;4 and 5;5

Speech Output

Luke was seen by the first author at CA 4;4. Similar phonological processing errors to those observed by the speech and language therapist when he was originally referred were observed (i.e. cluster reduction and voicing errors). In addition, difficulty with affricates (e.g. BRIDGE: [bɪdz] and WATCH: [wɒts]) were noted. However, in spite of these residual problems, Luke was perfectly intelligible and had no difficulties communicating with others. His speech output skills were formally assessed using three tasks: real word repetition, nonword repetition and naming pictures. He performed significantly less well than the normally developing control group on all three of these measures. Despite little difficulty noted in conversation and no concern expressed by family or professionals, his performance on single word assessments was below his expected age level, suggesting speech processing problems of a more subtle nature.

Luke was reassessed on these skills one year later. By 5 years of age, he performed within normal limits on the three speech tasks administered at CA 4;4. However, on a repetition task using low-frequency real words that ranged from one to five-syllable words (e.g. BRAN, SCRAPER, CHRYSANTHEMUM), Luke performed poorly compared to controls. This shows that when required to repeat challenging and less frequent words Luke still had deficits in processing and producing speech. These subtle speech deficits did not in any way compromise his ability to communicate, and went largely unnoticed.

Speech Input

Luke's performance on speech input skills at CA 4;4 fell within the normal range. He was able to discriminate similar sounding real words and nonwords, and on a lexical decision task with pictures he could judge when a word corresponding to a picture was said correctly or not. When Luke's performance on speech input tasks was reassessed a year later he still showed no difficulties in this area.

Phonological awareness

(i) Rhyme awareness: At CA 4;4, Luke's ability to produce as well as detect rhymes was assessed. On a rhyme production task, Luke was required to generate rhyme strings from six stimuli (e.g. DOG; CAT; VAN). Although he was not able to produce very long strings, 5/6 of his first responses to each word was correct. This represents a good score; the control group scored an average of 2.6 first responses correctly. On the rhyme detection task, Luke was required to identify which two out of three pictures rhymed with each other. He scored 8/12, which matched the control group's mean score. There were therefore no problems with rhyme skills at this age. At CA 5;5, again Luke performed both rhyme tasks competently; he scored above average on the rhyme production task and was able to produce long rhyming strings.

(ii) Phoneme awareness: Since many normally developing 4-year-olds have not developed phoneme awareness, Luke was tested on only one task: phoneme completion. On this task a child is shown a picture, e.g. DOG, then hears [dɒ] spoken by the tester, and is required to supply the missing (final) phoneme, i.e. /g/. Luke scored 0, but given the generally poor performance of normally developing children on this task, it could not be concluded that he had any specific deficits. One year later, Luke showed only minimal improvement on this phoneme completion task, scoring 2/8. However, again his performance was within the normal range for his age. Alliteration fluency was also tested at CA 5;5. He found producing a string of words beginning with the same sound much more difficult than generating rhyme strings. He was able to produce only one correct alliterative response for each item (compared to an average 4.5 responses for each stimulus on the rhyme production task). This performance placed him more than 1 standard deviation (SD) below the control group's mean.

ACTIVITY 8.1

Aims:
- To compare two phonological awareness tasks according to processing level, task demands and design.
- To predict Luke's performance on the second task based on his performance on the first task.

Read the description of the following two phonological awareness tasks and answer the questions below:

1. **Alliteration fluency task** (as administered to Luke at age 5 years)
The child is asked to produce a string of words beginning with a given sound. The tester provides the initial phoneme using the instruction: "Think of as many words as you can beginning with /m/" and the child is given a 20-second limit to produce as many words as possible beginning with that particular onset. Three phonemes are presented in this task /m/, /s/ and /k/.

2. **Phonological awareness: recognizing initial sounds** assessment developed by the Qualifications and Curriculum Authority (1997) for optional use in the baseline assessment scheme that is administered to children at the start of their first year at school, Reception (age 4–5 years in the UK).

The examiner shows the child sets of pictures, labels them and then asks the child to point to the picture beginning with a given sound. The instructions for the practice set state: "Say, 'duck, bird, cup'. Ask each child to listen and then to point to the object which begins with the 'b' sound. Repeat the objects again. Then say, 'Can you hear that bird begins with the 'b' sound?" The manual suggests 40–80 per cent of children would be able to recognize at least three of the initial sounds correctly in this task. The test items and instructions are as follows:

Say:
(a) CAR, FORK, BUTTON
      Which object begins with the 'c' sound?
(b) DOOR, CAT, ANT
      Which object begins with the 'a' sound?
(c) MOUSE, NEST, BOOK
      Which object begins with the 'm' sound?
(d) BROOM, HOUSE, GATE
      Which object begins with the 'h' sound?
(e) BUCKET, COMB, SOCK
      Which object begins with the 's' sound?

1. Do both assessments require the child to access lexical representations in order to complete the task?
2. What are the differences in the way in which the initial sound is presented to the child?
3. Are there any problems in choice of test items in either task?
4. Luke had some difficulty with the alliteration fluency task at age 5 years. How would you predict Luke would perform on recognizing initial sounds?

Check your answers with Key to Activity 8.1 at the end of this chapter.

Luke's literacy attainment at CA 4;4 and 5;5

Letter knowledge

Problematic phonological awareness development between 4 and 5 years of age is often associated with slow progress in alphabet

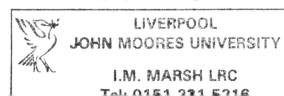

knowledge. At CA 4;4, Luke was able to name only two letters: C and W. For other letters, he produced a random letter name or number and did not know any letter sounds. He scored less well than Terry (his matched control) who already knew 10 letter names and four letter sounds. However, because there was such a huge variation in letter knowledge skills in the normally developing control group, Luke's performance fell into the 'low average' range and was not a specific deficit at this stage.

A year later, Luke showed some improvement. He knew 18 letter names, a score within the range expected for a 5-year-old and only slightly lower than Terry's score of 24, which is slightly above average for his age. However, a different story was emerging on knowledge of letter sounds. Luke had improved from a score of 0 at CA 4;4 to a score of 6 at CA 5;5 but, compared to the control group of 5-year-olds, this represents a performance of more than 1 SD below the expected level. At this stage, Terry knew 15 letter sounds.

Other literacy assessments

No standardized literacy assessments are suitable for administration to children at 4 years of age. A year later, at CA 5;5, Luke was able to read only two words accurately (THE; YOU) on a test of single word reading (Elliott, Murray and Pearson, 1983), and spelt only one word correctly (THE) on a spelling assessment (Elliott, 1992). However, it is difficult to interpret the results of standardized literacy assessments at this age because of the amount of individual variation among normally developing children.

To investigate spelling strategies further, a picture spelling task was also administered at CA 5;5. This consists of 12 pictures of animals (e.g. SPIDER, GORILLA) which are presented individually via a picture book (one picture per page). The child is asked to name each animal as it is presented and then to spell it. The tester does not name the picture or model the target word for the child, so the child's own lexical representations have to be accessed and then segmented into phonemes for spelling. The percentage of phonemes correctly represented is calculated, rather than whether the whole word was spelt accurately or not. This scoring system taps a child's ability to represent the phonemes in a word by an appropriate grapheme and shows whether phoneme-to-grapheme correspondence is developing. Luke was able to spell only 21 per cent of phonemes correctly. This score was more than 1 SD below the mean (Terry scored 30 per cent of phonemes correct).

Summary of Luke's Performance at 4 and 5 Years of Age

By age 5 years, Luke appeared to have no speech difficulties although his performance on low frequency repetition tasks indicated that subtle speech processing difficulties remained. Rhyme skills were a strength and indicated that one aspect of phonological awareness was developing well. However, performance on other phonological awareness tasks had not kept pace with this rhyming skill. He had made little improvement on phoneme completion between CA 4;4 and 5;5 and he was scoring significantly less well than the control group on alliteration fluency. His poor knowledge of letter sounds and his performance on the picture spelling task reflected emerging difficulties with phoneme-to-grapheme correspondences. Despite displaying some areas of strength, performance on these latter two tasks suggested that Luke was at risk for later literacy difficulties. The next section summarizes Luke's performance at the end of Year 1 (CA 6;5) when many children make rapid gains in their literacy development.

Luke at 6 Years of Age

Luke's speech processing skills at CA 6;5

Speech output and input

At age 6 years, Luke performed within normal limits on the repetition and articulatory naming tasks although subtle difficulties were still noted, e.g. he scored slightly below average on nonword repetition and made speech errors (though he kept appropriate rate when asked to repeat a word as fast as possible). He continued to perform age appropriately on the speech input tasks.

Phonological awareness

Luke's good performance on the rhyme tasks was still apparent at CA 6;5 and he had less difficulty with the alliteration fluency task. However, he scored 0/12 on a phoneme deletion task (e.g. "say FLY without the /f/") showing poor phoneme awareness. Thus, a persisting dissociation between the rhyme and phoneme level was observed; Luke was able to manipulate the phonological units of onset and rime very well but could not manipulate phonemic units.

Luke's literacy attainment at CA 6;5

Luke continued to be delayed in letter sound knowledge and showed minimal improvement over the year on the literacy measures. He could read only: THE; GO; ONE, and spell: ON; AND; THE; MY; DO. This lack of improvement is illustrated dramatically in the picture spelling task. Compared to Terry, whose score improved from 30 to 74 per cent between CA 5;5 and CA 6;5, Luke's score actually decreased from 21 to 12 per cent. During these assessments Luke was acutely aware that he was struggling. He would attempt to sound out the sounds he thought were in the word, repeatedly saying a string of the same sounds e.g. for DOG, he said "g-g-g-g" and eventually wrote the letter ‹k›. He was putting so much effort into isolating what he thought was the most salient sound and trying to 'hear' what that letter was, that it was often impossible for him to attempt the rest of the word. On one occasion he said, "I'm trying to sound out the letter but I can't hear it", before asking whether he could go on to the next item.

ACTIVITY 8.2

Aim: to analyse Luke's spelling errors on the picture spelling task at CA 6;5, and compare them to spellings from a child with normally developing literacy.

Examine the two sets of spelling presented in Figures 8.2 and 8.3 and answer the following questions:

1.   What are the differences between Luke and Terry's sets of spelling?
2.   What knowledge does Luke have of phoneme-to-grapheme correspondences?
3.   What sound confusions is Luke making in spelling these words?

Check your answers with Key to Activity 8.2, then read the following.

The relationship between Luke's spelling and speech

Analysis of the spelling data and comparison with Terry's attempts show that not only is Luke's performance poorer overall, but also that he makes specific errors because of difficulties with segmenting words into phonemes. In particular, Luke makes voicing errors (e.g. PIG written as ‹bk›) which mirror past speech difficulties. In this respect, he resembles the case of Zoe presented in Book 1 (Chapter 10, p.284). However, voicing spelling errors can occur in normally developing children as well as in children with dyslexia. Treiman, Broderick, Tincoff et al.,(1998a) propose that one of the reasons for this could be that a voicing contrast, e.g.[p] ~ [b] or [f] ~ [v], is more difficult for children to differentiate than other phonetic contrasts, such as place of articulation (although see Snowling, Hulme, Smith, et al., 1994).

Having been alerted to Luke's difficulties with voicing from his spelling attempts, it was important to identify the locus of the problem, i.e. whether he still had subtle difficulties in speech output with voicing, and/or whether he had auditory difficulties discriminating

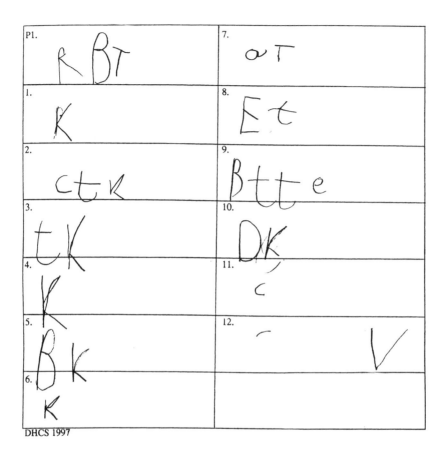

Figure 8.2: Luke's spelling from pictures, at CA 6;5. The target pictures were: (P1) RABBIT; 1. CAMEL; 2. CAT; 3. TIGER; 4. CROCODILE; 5. PIG; 6. GORILLA; 7. HEN; 8. ELEPHANT; 9. BUTTERFLY; 10. DOG; 11. SPIDER; 12. GIRAFFE.

between voice/voiceless sounds. The assessment revealed that he had both speech output and speech input difficulties. On production of voice/voiceless contrasts, Luke devoiced some sounds, e.g. /z/ was realized as [s] in his production of zoo. An auditory discrimination task was used to test out some voice/voiceless pairs of words. For the pair ZOO/SUE, Luke was required to point to a picture of a little girl named SUE or a picture of a zoo when he heard one of the words produced by the tester. He performed at chance level, showing little ability to discriminate accurately between the two words. A subsequent hearing test revealed no difficulties. Thus, his poor performance on this auditory picture discrimination task could not be attributed to a lower-level hearing difficulty.

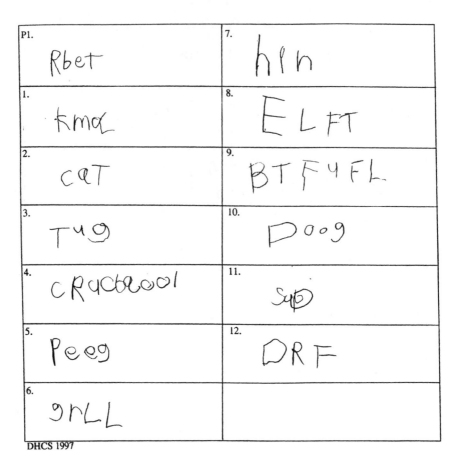

DHCS 1997

Figure 8.3: Terry's spelling from pictures, at CA 6;5. The target pictures were: (P1)RABBIT; 1. CAMEL; 2. CAT; 3. TIGER; 4. CROCODILE; 5. PIG; 6. GORILLA; 7. HEN; 8. ELEPHANT; 9. BUTTERFLY; 10. DOG; 11. SPIDER; 12. GIRAFFE.

Summary of Assessment: Ages 4–6 years

The areas of difficulty identified at each of Luke's assessments between CA 4;4 and 6;5 are summarized in Table 8.1. The speech processing profiles based on these assessments are presented in Figures 8.4, 8.5 and 8.6. These profiles show that Luke had only minor speech output deficits and that his speech processing difficulties were specific and subtle in nature. At CA 5;5 and CA 6;5, significant difficulties had emerged on phonological awareness tasks and letter knowledge. By CA 6;5, these problems were accompanied by specific literacy difficulties.

At this point, Luke was identified as having significant and specific difficulties with reading and spelling. He was also aware of his difficulties and the constant struggle to keep up was beginning to affect his confidence, behaviour and attention in the classroom. Although he appeared to have few difficulties on the initial speech output and speech input tasks administered, his spelling errors uncovered some subtle speech processing difficulties that were compromising his ability to acquire accurate phoneme-to-grapheme correspondences. Targeted investigation of the level of breakdown of these speech processing problems revealed that he had difficulties in both input and output speech processing. As Luke reached the end of Year 1 (CA 6;5) in his local primary school he was registered at Stage 1 of the *Code of Practice on the Identification and Assessment of Special Educational Needs* (DfE, 1994) (see Popple and Wellington, this volume, for further information about the *Code of Practice*).

Table 8.1: Areas of difficulty identified at each of Luke's assessments (between CA 4;4 and 6;5)

CA 4;4	CA 5;5	CA 6;5
Speech output	Speech output	Speech output (voicing)
	Letter sounds	Speech input (voicing distinctions)
	Alliteration fluency	Letter sounds
	?Reading	Phoneme deletion
	Spelling	Reading
		Spelling

Part 2: Moving from Assessment to Intervention

In Luke's first term in Year 2 (CA 6;8), his teacher aimed to address his difficulties by differentiating classwork according to his needs. However, by the second term of Year 2 (CA 7;0), it was apparent to both Luke and his teacher that he was falling further behind his peers. As he was at only Stage 1 of the Code of Practice (DfE, 1994), an individual education plan (IEP) was not considered necessary. However, because he was known to us through being a participant on a research project, he was offered literacy support by the second author. Luke's speech processing and literacy skills had been well documented over time, and his progress could therefore be viewed from a developmental perspective; but this information alone was not enough to inform an individual teaching programme. His difficulties should also be placed in the context of what is currently understood about the dynamic relationship between speech processing and phonological awareness, and should be related to theories about the processes involved in learning to be literate.

SPEECH PROCESSING PROFILE

Name   Luke   Comments:
                                               Nonverbal SS 11
Age   4;4

Date

Profiler

INPUT	OUTPUT

F

Is the child aware of the internal structure of phonological representations?
Rhyme detection chance performance

G

Can the child access accurate motor programs?	
Naming	×

E

Are the child's phonological representations accurate?	
Auditory discrimination pictures	✓

H

Can the child manipulate phonological units?	
Rhyme production	✓

D

Can the child discriminate between real words?	
Auditory discrimination real words	✓

I

Can the child articulate real words accurately?	
Word repetition	× × ×

C

Does the child have language-specific representations of word structures?
Not tested

J

Can the child articulate speech without reference to lexical representations?	
Nonword repetition	×

B

Can the child discriminate speech sounds without reference to lexical representations?	
Auditory discrimination nonwords	✓

K

Does the child have adequate sound production skills?	
Oral-motor skills	✓

A

Does the child have adequate auditory perception?	
Noise discrimination and hearing	✓

L

Does the child reject his/her own erroneous forms?
Not known

Figure 8.4: Luke's speech processing profile at CA 4;4.

SPEECH PROCESSING PROFILE

Name   Luke

Age   5;5

Date

Profiler

Comments:

Letter names ✓

Letter sounds ✗

INPUT	OUTPUT

F

Is the child aware of the internal structure of phonological representations?	
Rhyme detection	✓

G

Can the child access accurate motor programs?	
Naming	✓
Phoneme completion	✓
Alliteration fluency	✗

E

Are the child's phonological representations accurate?	
Auditory discrimination pictures	✓

H

Can the child manipulate phonological units?	
Rhyme production	✓

D

Can the child discriminate between real words?	
Auditory discrimination real words	✓

I

Can the child articulate real words accurately?	
Word repetition	✓
Low frequency word repetition	✗

C

Does the child have language-specific representations of word structures?	
Not tested	

J

Can the child articulate speech without reference to lexical representations?	
Nonword repetition	✓
Low frequency nonword repetition	✓

B

Can the child discriminate speech sounds without reference to lexical representations?	
Auditory discrimination nonwords	✓

A

Does the child have adequate auditory perception?	
Noise discrimination and hearing	✓

K

Does the child have adequate sound production skills?	
Oral-motor skills	✓

L

Does the child reject his/her own erroneous forms?	
Not known	

Figure 8.5: Luke's speech processing profile at CA 5;5.

SPEECH PROCESSING PROFILE

Name   Luke

Age   6;5

Date

Profiler

Comments:

Letter names   ✓

Letter sounds   × × ×

INPUT	OUTPUT

F

Is the child aware of the internal structure of phonological representations?
Rhyme detection   ✓

G

Can the child access accurate motor programs?
Naming   ✓ Alliteration fluency   ✓

E

Are the child's phonological representations accurate?
Auditory discrimination pictures   ✓

H

Can the child manipulate phonological units?
Rhyme production   ✓ Phoneme deletion   × ×

D

Can the child discriminate between real words?
Auditory discrimination of voicing contrasts   ×

I

Can the child articulate real words accurately?
Word repetition   ✓

C

Does the child have language-specific representations of word structures?
Not tested

J

Can the child articulate speech without reference to lexical representations?
Nonword repetition   ✓   (but below average)

B

Can the child discriminate speech sounds without reference to lexical representations?
Auditory discrimination nonwords   ✓

K

Does the child have adequate sound production skills?
Oral-motor skills   ✓

A

Does the child have adequate auditory perception?
Noise discrimination and hearing   ✓

L

Does the child reject his/her own erroneous forms?
Not known

Figure 8.6: Luke's speech procesing profile at CA 6;5.

The Relationship between Speech Processing and Phonological Awareness

A child who can demonstrate the ability to appreciate and reflect on the sound structure of language is a child who shows phonological awareness. Phonological awareness is not, however, an all-or-none skill, as Luke's speech processing assessment profile demonstrates. It comprises a number of skills, develops on a continuum moving from intuitive to explicit, and involves awareness of different levels of linguistic analysis ranging from syllables at a relatively shallow level, through onset/rime, and on to phonemes at a much deeper level of awareness (see Book 1, Chapter 3, p.55). Luke's speech processing profile indicates that his input skills have always been more secure than his output skills, and that while he demonstrates competence at the level of onset and rime, at a more demanding level of phoneme analysis, he is out-performed by his peers.

There is evidence to suggest that while pre-school and pre-literate children are able to segment words into syllables, phoneme segmentation is acquired only through exposure to literacy teaching (Liberman, Shankweiler, Fischer, et al., 1974). Fowler (1991) has proposed that the ease with which children acquire awareness at the level of the phoneme may be directly related to the quality of their stored phonological representations. She suggests that initially words are stored as whole units, but that, in order to discriminate between items in a growing vocabulary, the phonology of these holistic lexical representations becomes increasingly segmental, well specified and accessible. This gradual refinement of the lexicon, she believes, then lays the foundations for the development of phonemic awareness, which, in turn, is promoted by learning to read. Swan and Goswami (1997) also relate the accuracy and organization of a child's phonological representations to the ease with which phonemic awareness is acquired, and it would seem that in the case of Luke, a child who is failing to acquire either phonemic awareness or reading skills, it is the quality of his phonological representations that must be questioned.

It has been shown that sensitivity to the featural properties of sounds, such as place and manner of articulation and voice, has a part to play in establishing fine-grained, and readily distinguished, phonological representations (Snowling, Hulme, Smith, et al., 1994; Rack, Hulme, Snowling, et al., 1994). It has also been suggested that speech perception (Mody, Studdert-Kennedy and Brady, 1997), and early articulation quality are implicated in this process (Thomas and Senechal, 1998). Whatever the dynamics of the relationship, it is clear that Luke, with his history of early speech processing difficulties, his persisting voicing confusions and subtle output difficulties, presents with a parallel history of an unfolding difficulty in developing his phono-logical awareness to the point where it is deep (i.e. at the level of the phoneme), explicit and automatic.

The Relationship between Phonological Awareness and Literacy

The evidence for a relationship between phonological awareness and literacy is impressive and mounting, and children like Luke, whose phonological awareness is compromised in some way, must be considered at risk for difficulty in learning to read and spell. It has become increasingly apparent, however, that phonological awareness and literacy acquisition are rather more multifaceted processes than may have been previously recognized. In addition, as development progresses, their relationship may be expected to change over time, and unfortunately for the practitioner, who must translate theory into practice, the precise mechanism of their relationship remains unclear.

Phonological awareness is a relatively complex skill that develops as a result of experience and under the influence of a number of factors: therefore individual differences in children's phonological awareness are to be expected. However, regardless of these individual differences, unlike Luke, most children will come to the task of learning to read and spell with levels of phonological awareness that enable them to apply their knowledge of the structure of spoken language to written language (see Stackhouse, this volume). A number of different theories, and studies, have examined the relationship between phonological awareness and literacy, and it now seems clear that the causal connection between them, far from being unidirectional and direct, is perhaps quite interactive, mutually facilitative and complex (Wagner, Torgesen, Rashotte, et al., 1997). A child such as Luke, therefore, who comes to the task of literacy with inadequate phonological awareness skills, is not only at risk of reading and spelling difficulties, he is also unable to avail himself of the 'bootstrapping' relationship that exists, in turn, between literacy and phonological awareness.

Frith (1985) suggests that three strategies, logographic, alphabetic and orthographic, are key to the process of learning to read and write words. These develop in a series of stages, with new skills emerging from and merging with old, and reading and writing developing out of step with, but dependent on, one another. Her six-step model proposes that in the first phase of literacy acquisition phonological factors are secondary, and that the child relies on logographic strategies, so recognizing familiar words automatically on the basis of their context or salient visual features. This strategy is less useful for spelling, however, and although a child may make some attempt to write, s/he will probably be able to write only one or two well learned words such as their own name. At CA 6;5, Luke was able to recognize and read a few words and to write some high frequency words that he had been taught, and could therefore be described as showing evidence of using logographic strategies. Frith suggests that it is the gradual acquisition of alphabetic strategies for writing that allows the developing reader to move from recognizing words to analysing and recoding them. At this age, Luke was applying some rudimentary alphabetic strategies in his responses to the picture spelling task (e.g. TIGER written as ‹tk›), but was not yet applying this strategy to reading. In this phase, knowledge of phoneme–grapheme correspondence is required, and phonological factors act as a self-teaching device (Share, 1995) which enables the child to set up the print-to-meaning connections necessary for the development of orthographic strategies. These strategies are applied first to reading and allow the child to analyse words into orthographic (spelling) units that, ideally, are the equivalent of abstract, internally represented, morphemes or 'chunks' of words (e.g. -MENT, -ING, -TURE), and as they become increasingly automatic and proficient, so they become useful for spelling too. By this point, the child is in a position to apply a full range of strategies to both reading and writing. Clearly Luke, with his difficulties in speech processing and limited letter sound knowledge, was at risk of failing to advance his alphabetic strategies to a level where they could support the development of the orthographic strategies that, according to this model, are the hallmark of skilled reading and spelling.

A similar stage model, focusing more on the development of reading, has been proposed by Ehri (1992, 1995). She, like Frith (1985), makes strong claims about the centrality of phonological skills in reading acquisition and fluent reading, but also has something to say about the mechanism by which children acquire their reading skills. Ehri suggests that the developing child moves first from a *pre-alpha-betic phase*, in which arbitrary connections are made between the visual attributes of a word and its meaning, to a *partial-alphabetic phase* where systematic connections are established between some of the letters of a word, and its pronunciation (for example, ‹husband› read by a normally developing 6-year-old as "handbag"). From here, as the child learns to form complete connections between a word's letters and its pronunciation, s/he moves on to the *full alphabetic phase*, and starts to be able to decode unfamiliar words. As recurring letter patterns become consolidated units, there is a steady increase in his/her sight vocabulary (i.e. words stored in memory on the basis of their orthographic–phonological connection), and the child enters the *consolidated alphabetic phase*. In this final phase, connections are formed between a word's written form and its pronunciation and meaning, and reading becomes automatic as sight word reading takes over from decoding. According to Ehri's model, 6-year-old Luke, with his restricted sight vocabulary and notable absence of phonic knowledge, has yet to make any useful connections between the letters in a word and its pronunciation, and so is struggling to progress beyond the pre-alphabetic phase.

A theory that concentrates more on causal connections than stages in learning to read, but that also views phonological coding as having a central role, has been put forward by Goswami (1993). Unlike stage theories, with their focus on early mappings between single sounds and letters, this theory proposes that children come to the task of learning to read sensitive to sound segmentation at the level of onset and rime. It suggests that the beginning reader capitalizes on this awareness to make increasingly better specified analogies between familiar and new words, and thus, the child who can read LIGHT can, by analogy, read words like NIGHT; FIGHT. It identifies rhyming and segmentation as separate skills, suggesting that phoneme awareness develops as a result of teaching and reading experience, and claiming that it is sensitivity to the linguistic units of onset and rime that is critical for good progress with literacy. According to this theory, Luke at 6 years of age, with his relatively well developed rhyming skills, could perhaps have been expected to move smoothly through the initial stages of learning to read. However, his history of early speech difficulties, and the record of his unfolding speech processing skills, should not be forgotten; it is important to view his emerging literacy difficulties in relation to both his strengths and his weaknesses. It may be that rhyming skills, in the absence of adequate segmentation skills, are not enough to drive the process of learning to read, and that it is the relationship, and inter-action, between different phonological skills that is important.

Rhyming skills are only one factor playing a part in, and predicting, reading development. Recent studies have compared the predictive relationship of onset–rime awareness and phoneme awareness with reading development, and suggest that it is segmentation at the phonemic level that is crucial to the development of reading (Hoien, Lundberg, Stanovich, et al., 1995; Nation and Hulme, 1997; Muter, Hulme, Snowling, et al., 1998; Hatcher and Hulme, 1999; Stackhouse, Nathan, Goulandris, et al., 1999; but see Goswami, 1999 for further discussion). Furthermore, children need a certain level of cognitive development (Bruck and Treiman, 1990), and some decoding skills (Ehri and Robbins, 1992) in order to be able to use analogy strategies, i.e. they must have some letter sound skills from the outset. Letter name knowledge has been shown to be an enduring predictor of progress in learning to read (Badian, 1995), and also to facilitate the learning of letter sounds (Treiman, Tincoff, Rodriguez, et al., 1998b).

Muter, Hulme, Snowling, et al. (1998) have looked not only at the relationship between phonological processing and the early stages of reading, but also at the power of letter name knowledge as a predictor of early reading skills. Their study suggests that it is segmentation, rather than rhyming, skills that correlate with early reading and spelling development, and also that segmentation skills and letter name knowledge interact, and are predictive of later reading and spelling development. None of this is good news for Luke, who has come to the task of learning to read with poorly developed phoneme segmentation skills, rather late acquired knowledge of letter names, and limited success in abstracting letter sounds from these names. His rhyming skills alone are unlikely to provide him with the support he needs to acquire literacy skills easily or typically.

Models that consider the cause as well as the course of reading development, and can offer an explanation for individual children's literacy difficulties, fit well with recent computer simulations and connectionist models of reading (Hulme, Quinlan, Bolt, et al., 1995; Plaut, McClelland, Seidenberg, et al., 1996; Snowling, 1998). Such models perhaps reflect more accurately than stage models how children actually learn to read, and also go a long way towards accounting for the range of individual differences seen in beginning readers. These models conceptualize the process of learning to read as highly interactive, and also view it as a product of teaching and learning opportunities. They demonstrate how orthographic, phonological and language factors can exert a simultaneous influence in skilled reading, but also show how the balance of importance attributed to these factors shifts as learning progresses. In the early stages of learning, rather ominously for Luke with his speech processing difficulties, it is not phonological awareness but the quality of the stored phonological representations that determines the strength of the links that are set up between a word's written and spoken form, and drives the learning process. With experience and as learning progresses, generalizations are made between the orthography of known and unknown words, and at this point higher-level language skills (semantics; syntax) start to become more significant.

Once Luke's unfolding speech processing and literacy difficulties are set in the context of models that offer insights into the processes involved in learning to read, their implications for him as a learner become clear. This exercise also has implications for assessment and teaching, however, and suggests that if an appropriate teaching programme is to be designed for Luke, an up-to-date and theoretically driven assessment of both his speech processing skills and his literacy attainments is required. Consequently, at CA 7;2, Luke's speech processing and literacy skills were once again systematically investigated; this time with a particular focus on his development at the level of the phoneme.

Luke's Assessment at 7 Years of Age

Learning opportunities and motivation

In order to consider the interaction between cognitive and environmental factors, Luke's mother and class teacher were consulted about his literacy experience and teaching, his current interests and attitude to learning. He himself was also consulted and he was observed in class. Information from these sources, together with that from his developmental case history and current and previous speech processing assessments, was interpreted within a framework of understanding of the normal acquisition of literacy. In this way, the persistence, severity and underlying nature of Luke's difficulties were uncovered, and a profile of his strengths and weaknesses was built up.

Luke's educational history had been unremarkable. School records showed that he had settled well in his nursery. He had always been considered to be socially well integrated with his peers but was more interested in active pursuits than in tabletop activities. His mother reported that he enjoyed watching television and listening to music, in preference to looking at books or being read to. No formal reading scheme was used in Luke's school, but phonics were taught explicitly and there was a school–home reading system; spelling was taught using the *Spelling Made Easy* (Brand, 1984) scheme, and *The National Literacy Strategy* (DfEE, 1998) was implemented. Luke's teacher commented that he had yet to develop a mature attitude to learning, found it hard to sustain his attention and that he rarely worked independently. He was not perceived to be a high achiever in other areas of the curriculum, but at this time it was only his literacy that was seen as an area of concern.

Luke's speech processing skills at CA 7;2

Speech output and speech input

As at earlier assessments, Luke was asked to repeat a series of relatively complex real words and nonwords derived from these, and once again he produced both sets of words less accurately than might be expected for a child of his age. In general, his speech was no longer a cause of concern; however, his pronunciation of longer and less familiar words was often imprecise (e.g. "helicocter" for HELICOPTER). Voicing difficulties were still apparent between pairs of words such as SIP ~ ZIP; PEAR ~ BEAR. Furthermore, in connected speech, this imprecision was even more apparent and there was some evidence of difficulties accessing new or unfamiliar vocabulary. These findings suggest that, despite his apparently resolved speech difficulties, Luke was continuing to have some problems in both assembling and establishing new motor programs.

On the input side, Luke was now able to *detect* the difference between pairs of words involving voiced/voiceless contrasts. However, he was not always confident in his responses and also showed some difficulties discriminating pairs of nonwords distinguished by the sequence of sounds in a final cluster (e.g. /flɛts/ ~ /flɛst/) from the *Phonological Awareness Assessment* (North and Parker, 1993).

Phonological awareness

Luke was relatively secure in his ability to segment words into syllables. However, he performed this task mechanically and therefore this skill was not useful when attempting to spell polysyllabic words. His ability to detect and produce rhyme has consistently been found to be age appropriate, and he achieved scores well within the average range on the Alliteration and Rhyme Detection and Fluency subtests of the Phonological Assessment Battery (*PhAB*) (Frederickson, Frith and Reason, 1997). His responses, however, were often imprecise (e.g. omission of final sounds in words) and his difficulty in hearing voicing distinctions accounted for a number of his errors.

At 6 years of age, Luke had been unable to delete either initial or final phonemes in words (e.g. "say PIT without the /p/"; "say HEAP without the /p/"). At 7 years of age, he was slow to appreciate the demands of the task, and was able to delete the initial phoneme on only 1/6 trials. He was more successful in deleting the final phoneme (correct on 4/6 trials), but his final score of 5/12 remains well below that expected for a child of his age. Although phoneme deletion skills are generally taken to be predictive of concurrent and later reading development (MacDonald and Cornwall, 1995), it may also be that his performance on this test was affected by, and reflects, his current level of reading ability (Perfetti, Beck, Bell, et al., 1987; but see Goswami and Bryant, 1990, for further discussion).

Naming speed

Continuous naming tasks (as opposed to discrete naming tasks) are considered to simulate the processes involved in reading, in that they require the child to scan visually presented information while simultan-eously accessing and retrieving phonological information (Wolf, 1991). Several studies have shown that children with specific reading difficul-ties are characterized by their slow naming speed (Denckla and Rudel, 1976; Badian, 1995; Meyer, Wood, Hart, et al., 1998). Luke's naming speed on both the Picture Naming and the Digit Naming subtests of the PhAB (Frederickson, Frith and Reason, 1997) was found to be well below the average range, and on the basis that his speech rate (although not his accuracy), was consistently within the expected range, this was interpreted as further evidence for his difficulty in representing and/or accessing phonological information.

Summary of Luke's speech processing skills at CA 7;2

Luke presented with a mixed profile of speech processing skills. His ability to detect and generate strings of words that share an initial sound (alliteration) or that rhyme, was within the range expected for a child of his age. However, his subtle difficulty with voicing, his auditory discrimination, his inaccurate word and nonword repetition, his slow naming speed and his difficulty in phoneme deletion and blending tasks, suggested that he had problems in storing, accessing and manipulating phonological information. It may be that while his lexical representation of words was precise enough to support tasks requiring phonological processing at the level of syllables, onsets and rimes, they were not sufficiently accurate to support more demanding tasks such as those requiring on-line processing at the level of the phoneme. It may also be that Luke had some subtle motor program or programming difficulties, or that the links between his lexical representations and output processing skills were faulty (see Appendix 2).

It is possible to look back over earlier speech processing profiles and to view Luke's speech processing skills from a developmental perspective. It would appear that while many of his earlier deficits had resolved by CA 7;2, Luke was still struggling to make the transition between the *assembly phase* and the *metaphonological phase* of development (see Book 1, Chapter 8, pp.220–232). In view of his developmental history, it seems reasonable to suggest that his earlier difficulties may have affected the course of, and left their mark on, his developing speech processing system, and that it is the interaction between resolved and persisting difficulties that can be held to account for his current subtle speech processing difficulties. How can this history be used to inform a remediation programme?

ACTIVITY 8. 3

Aim: to integrate information provided by assessments of speech processing skills over time, and to consider how this information could be used to inform objectives for an individual teaching programme.

Look at the information about Luke's strengths and weaknesses over time presented in Table 8.2 and answer the following questions:

1. How does Luke's development of phonological awareness compare with the expected sequence of development?

2.   How might the information about the pattern of development of Luke's phonological awareness be used in designing an individual teaching programme?

3.   How might the information about the development of Luke's speech input and output skills be used in designing an individual teaching programme?

Check your answers with Key to Activity 8.3 at the end of this chapter, then read on.

Table 8.2: Luke's speech processing and literacy skills between CA 4;4 and 7;2

CA	Weakness	Strength
4;4	Speech output (real word repetition; nonword repetition; naming)	Speech input Rhyme detection and production
5;5	Speech output (subtle difficulties) Letter sounds Alliteration fluency ?Reading Spelling	Speech input Rhyme detection and production
6;5	Speech output (specific to voicing) Speech input (specific to voicing) Letter sounds Phoneme deletion Reading Spelling	Rhyme detection and production
7;2	Speech output (specific to voicing; word and nonword repetition) Speech input (specific to voicing) Naming speed Letter sounds Phoneme deletion Reading Spelling	? Rhyme detection and production ? Alliteration detection and production

Luke's literacy attainments at CA 7;2

Letter name and sound knowledge

When Luke's phonic knowledge was last assessed at CA 6;5, he knew the names of 25 of the letters, but could give a sound for only one. In the current assessment at CA 7;2, he named 24 lower case letters correctly (naming <b> as "d"; and <d> as "b"), and gave the correct sounds for 18 of the letters. His errors on this assessment reflected his <b>~<d> confusion, uncertainty over the short vowels and inadequate knowledge of the letter sounds for <x>, <y> and <c> (he gave the less common sound for <c> as in CITY).

Single word reading

Luke was able to read 11 words from the *British Ability Scale—II (BAS—II) Word Reading Test* (Elliott, Smith and McCulloch, 1996). He read the first words relatively confidently, relying on his limited sight vocabulary, and then resorted to rather laborious and not particularly successful sounding out strategies. He successfully sounded out two words (BOX; VAN) by producing each phoneme in isolation, then, rather than blending these to produce a word, he carried out a lexical check, producing a word triggered by the sounds (e.g. [b]...[ɒ] [ks] – box!'). His score was well below the range expected and placed him in the bottom 10 per cent of children his age.

Nonword reading

In nonword reading, semantic information is not available, and decoding makes heavy demands on phonological skills. On the *Graded Nonword Reading Test* (Snowling, Stothard and McClean, 1996) a child of Luke's age might be expected to read at least five to nine nonwords, but although he was able to produce sounds for all the symbols, Luke had limited success in blending the simple CVC practice items, and was unable to decode any of the more complex test items involving consonant clusters.

Prose reading

The *Individual Reading Analysis* (Vincent and de la Mare, 1990) was attempted but discontinued as, despite a relatively promising start, Luke lost heart as soon as he was unable to recognize a word and quickly resorted to sounding out words letter by letter. He appeared to make little use of the picture to provide a cue, and was unable to read enough of the text to make use of context cues. When invited to re-read a passage he had initially read successfully, he was no longer able to produce correct responses as on this second attempt he tried to sound out the words, rather than rely on his sight vocabulary.

Spelling

Spelling was formally assessed using the *BAS–II Spelling Test* (Elliott, Smith and McCulloch, 1996), and although Luke was able to spell only nine of the words, this was sufficient to give him a standardized score of 88 and placed him at the lower end of the average range (21st percentile). Two of the words he spelled correctly were high frequency words (THE, MY); the rest were regular CV, VC or CVC words which, with considerable effort, he segmented and represented sound by sound. While this was an appropriate strategy to adopt, as Luke's segmentation skills and his knowledge of sound–symbol correspondences is not yet secure it led to a number of responses that failed to reflect the sound structure of the target word (e.g. ‹yoz› for WAS; ‹Dam› for DOWN). He was able to represent both parts of the initial cluster in the word PLAY, but was unable to segment a final consonant cluster (as in OLD). It was also observed that Luke consistently adopted the strategy of using capital letters for the letters B and D, presumably to avoid the confusion over direction that he had shown on the letter knowledge task.

More informally, Luke's spelling was once again explored using the picture spelling task, and on this occasion he was able to identify and represent a number of salient sounds in words and the target word was evident in many of his attempts (e.g. ‹rabit›, ‹camol›). His score of 66.7 per cent of phonemes correct is a significant improvement on the 12 per cent he scored at CA 6;5. However, it still placed him at the lower end of the range expected for a child a year younger than himself. As in the single word spelling test, errors related to difficulty in mapping sounds to symbols (especially short vowels), together with sporadic difficulty in isolating sounds in consonant clusters, omission of unstressed syllables (e.g. CROCODILE represented as ‹codiol›), and Luke's assumption that the unstressed schwa sound can be represented by a preceding consonant (e.g. TIGER as ‹tig›; ZEBRA as ‹zbr›; BUTTERFLY as ‹btrfli›).

Luke was also observed in class during a session in which a new set of target spelling words was introduced. This involved tracing, then copying the set of words to be learned (five trials per word). Luke sat beside the classroom assistant, worked reluctantly, and clearly found the task demanding; unlike other members of his group, he did not appear to be engaged in the task or to have an interest in completing it.

Free writing

Luke was unable to produce a piece of free writing for analysis, and it was clear from the work in his exercise books that he was not yet an independent writer. Pieces of work produced in class were either short or incomplete, and drew heavily on vocabulary and spellings provided. The pieces were too short to be analysed in terms of their content, grammar or punctuation.

Handwriting

Luke is right-handed, and holds a pencil with a rather awkward three-fingered grip and a tight hold. He complained that his arm often ached when he wrote. Many letters were formed incorrectly, and he continued to show directional confusions, e.g. ‹b/d›, ‹s/z›. Motor skills were assessed using the *Beery–Buktenica Developmental Test of Visual–Motor Integration (VMI)* (Beery and Buktenica, 1997), a pencil and paper test requiring the child to copy a series of increasingly complex geometric shapes, and on this assessment Luke achieved an age-appropriate standard score of 100 (50th percentile).

ACTIVITY 8.4

Aim: to analyse Luke's responses on single word reading and spelling tests in terms of the information they provide about his use of strategies and phase of development according to the six-step model of Frith (1985), and to consider how this information may inform an individual teaching programme.

Examine the information in Table 8.3 and answer the following questions:

1. What strategies is Luke using for reading and spelling?
2. Are his phonic strategies more useful for reading or spelling at this point?
3. With reference to the six-step model (Frith, 1985), could Luke be described as following a normal sequence of development? If so, is it appropriate to describe him as developmentally delayed?
4. How does this error analysis, together with comments about Luke's prose reading, inform an individual teaching programme?

Check your answers with Key to Activity 8.4, then read on.

Luke's profile of strengths and weaknesses at CA 7;2

The nature and degree of Luke's literacy difficulties become clearer once the assessment information is drawn together and examined in

Table 8.3: Summary of Luke's performance on the single word reading and spelling tests

Read correctly	Reading errors	Spelled correctly	Spelling errors
‹the›	‹out› oo	ON	BUS ‹Brs›
‹up›	‹jump› jam	AND	BOX ‹Boz›
‹on›	‹fish› fire	THE	WAS ‹yoz›
‹go›	‹cup› camp	UP	HOME ‹hoom›
‹he›	‹said› don't know	GO	OLD ‹oD›
‹at›	‹water› don't know	BIG	DO ‹Doe›
‹you›	‹bird› don't know	SIT	PLAY ‹pla›
‹one›	‹wood› don't know	MY	BACK ‹bac›
‹box› (sounded out)	‹running› w...don't	THAT	DOWN ‹Dam›
‹van› (sounded out)	know		EAT ‹it›
			COME ‹crm›

the light of insights provided by previous assessments. This information can now be integrated with that provided by Luke's mother and teacher, and summarized to provide a profile of his current strengths and weaknesses.

Strengths

(a) Wide range of interests that can be harnessed in a learning support programme.
(b) Responds well in a one-to-one situation.
(c) Relatively determined attitude; prepared to persevere even when he finds a task difficult.
(d) His mother, while not putting pressure on him, has expressed an interest in reinforcing work at home; his class teacher is also positive about the extra support offered.
(e) Oral language skills relatively well developed; not considered at-risk for reading comprehension difficulties (Hatcher and Hulme, 1999).
(f) Speech processing profiling has consistently indicated that, apart from appreciation of voicing distinctions, speech input skills are within normal limits.
(g) Assessment of phonological awareness has consistently indicated that appreciation of rhyme is within normal limits; assessment indicates appreciation of alliteration is also now within normal limits.

(h) Has acquired a small sight vocabulary for reading.

(i) Is able to spell a few high frequency words.

(j) Has a secure knowledge of the names of the letters of the alphabet and is gaining in his knowledge of phoneme-to-grapheme correspondence.

(k) Is developing his phoneme segmentation skills and is applying this skill for spelling (able to segment and represent simple CVC words, and showing an emerging ability to segment sounds in CCVC words).

Weaknesses

(a) Does not have a natural interest in books and written language and his experiences in this area are limited.

(b) Is starting to show some anxiety in literacy-based tasks.

(c) Although language skills are well within the expected range, he is not by nature a particularly verbal child.

(d) His speech processing profile suggests that while speech is now maturing, Luke continues to have some subtle but specific difficulties in speech output and phonemic awareness tasks. It is hypothesized that he has difficulty in storing, accessing and manipulating phonological information at the level of the phoneme.

(e) In reading, Luke focuses his attention on sounding out words, rather than building a sight vocabulary and harnessing his language skills or making use of context cues.

(f) In spelling, Luke's sound segmentation skills, his knowledge of phoneme-to-grapheme correspondences and his handwriting skills are not yet secure enough to allow him to work with any degree of fluency or automaticity.

(g) Has become relatively dependent on adult support and supervision in literacy-based tasks, and lacks the confidence to work independently.

(h) Does not yet show any insight into his difficulties.

(i) Some of the strategies he is now adopting are not helping him to make progress, and he is at risk of developing atypical strategies as a compensatory device.

Luke's Teaching Programme

When Luke's profile of strengths and weaknesses was viewed in relation to the expected pattern of development, and the demands of the National Curriculum and *The National Literacy Strategy* (DfEE, 1998), it was clear that the literacy instruction he received in class was not able to meet his needs. Drawing on this profile, an individual teaching programme was therefore devised, which was to be delivered over a

10-week period in a series of one-to-one, hour long, sessions. Although intensive and individual support of this kind is not always considered the most appropriate way to meet a child's needs (Moss and Reason, 1998), for Luke at this point it was considered to be the best option. Once again there was consultation with Luke, his mother and his teacher, this time about both the content and delivery of the programme, and weekly lesson plans and evaluations were shared. The principles that underpinned the design of the programme reflect current understanding of good practice in the field of literacy remediation, and are outlined in Table 8.4.

The long-term objectives for Luke's teaching programme were devised in relation to specific skill areas (see Table 8.5), with objectives for reading and spelling being combined to ensure integration of skills.

When designing intervention programmes that can be evaluated, there is a danger of choosing targets for the ease with which they can be measured, at the expense of less readily quantified targets that are integral to a child's progress (Tod and Blamires, 1999). Thus, the long-term objectives were broken down into a series of small steps that were designed to be both specific and manageable in the time available,

Table 8.4: Principles to guide the design of a teaching programme

---

A well planned programme will:

- Be informed by a thorough and up-to-date assessment of speech processing and literacy skills
- Reflect the child's current interests and curricular needs
- Have regard to the child's levels of self-esteem and confidence
- Focus on the child's strengths as well as weaknesses
- Acknowledge the child's particular learning style
- Specify attainable and measurable targets
- Be structured and cumulative
- Offer opportunities for review and reinforcement
- Aim for automatic and fluent application of skills and strategies
- Allow for integration of targets
- Incorporate, and integrate, work at the level of the word, sentence and text
- Employ multisensory teaching and learning techniques
- Promote transfer and generalization of skills
- Promote active learning
- Facilitate the development of metacognitive skills (the ability to reflect on what is being learned)
- Involve parents, teachers and other professionals as appropriate

Table 8.5: Long-term objectives for one term (10 weeks) for Luke

Listening and speaking	Reading and spelling	Writing and composition
• Be more aware of subtle differences between speech sounds	• Be more confident in his approach to reading	• Show improved letter formation
• Be more adept at syllable segmentation	• Be more aware of the value of context cues	• Translate sounds into symbols with more confidence and fluency
• Have improved his phoneme segmentation and blending skills	• Have increased his sight vocabulary	• Hold a pencil with a more relaxed grip
• Be able to reflect on what he is learning	• Be more secure in knowledge of the alphabet sequence, letter names and sounds	• Demonstrate some knowledge of punctuation
• Be able to seek clarification as needed in one-to-one sessions	• Understand (at an explicit level) how sound segmentation skills map on to literacy skills (encoding and decoding)	• Be able to structure and dictate a sentence
• Be able to structure a sentence	• Be more aware of the link between phoneme manipulation and letter manipulation, and be able to use this knowledge in encoding and decoding words (phonological linkage)	• Be able to write to dictation
• Be able to recount a story in a structured and organized way	• Have increased the number of words he can spell by rote	

while at the same time retaining the broad functional goals of the programme (see Table 8.6). Although Luke was showing some lack of confidence and anxiety in literacy-based tasks, he was not considered to be lacking in confidence in general, therefore there were no objectives relating directly to promoting self-esteem and confidence. Instead, work to promote these aspects of his development was incorporated into many of the targets.

Methods and materials

There are as many theories about how to teach normally developing children to read and spell as there are about how children learn these skills. However, the way in which children respond to teaching will reflect their particular cognitive profile, emotional development and learning opportunities (Reason, 1998), and no one teaching method will suit all children. Good classroom practice (as reflected in *The National Literacy Strategy*, DfEE, 1998) generally suggests that a comprehensive approach to literacy teaching is taken, with the teaching of phonological skills and phonics integrated with a 'whole language' approach. There is no reason to suppose that a child with difficulties of the kind experienced by Luke will not benefit from this type of teaching. However, the difference for Luke, and children like him, is that the teaching will need to be carefully structured if it is to harness his strengths and remediate his weaknesses, and he will need to be given more time to learn, practise, consolidate and apply new skills. He will need an individual programme that reflects his individual differences.

Phonics teachers are divided over whether it is better to work from words to sounds (analytic phonics), or sounds to words (synthetic phonics). For Luke, the latter approach was taken, and his area of strength (i.e. ability to appreciate onset/rime, a relatively large sound unit) was used as a bridge to his area of weakness (i.e. appreciation of phonemes, the smallest sound unit). Teaching methods and materials that were chosen were designed to facilitate multisensory teaching and learning, and to reflect his interests and curricular needs. Explicit links were forged between sounds and symbols using plastic letters and written representations, and at all stages the teaching of phoneme awareness, spelling and reading was integrated (Hatcher, Hulme and Ellis, 1994).

There is a wealth of materials, including manuals of ideas and teachers' handbooks, currently available to support the teaching of literacy skills at all levels of development. Apart from plastic letters, coloured paper, felt tips and an array of exercises books, certain resources and techniques lent themselves well to the particular requirements of Luke's programme and these are listed at the end of this chapter.

Table 8.6: Short-term targets for one term (10 weeks) for Luke

Listening and speaking	Reading and spelling	Writing and composition
• Consolidate auditory discrimination skills between words that differ in voice/voiceless contrast (p/b, k/g, s/z,), or place of articulation of nasals (m/n)	• Be able to use context cues (title and pictures), length and print size as a guide to selecting appropriate books for paired reading (Topping, 1995)	• Be able to form letters s/z, b/d correctly and use upper and lower case appropriately
• Be able to break words into syllables and phonemes (orally)	• Be familiar with, and in the habit of, paired reading (Topping, 1995)	• Be able to represent the short vowel u correctly
• Be able to discuss the following skills involved in reading and spelling – knowing sounds of letters, blending, segmenting, using context cues, automatic reading and spelling of high-frequency words	• Have the confidence to use context cues (semantics, syntax and grapho-phonic) and make informed guesses in paired reading	• Be more confident and automatic in his knowledge of phoneme-to-grapheme correspondence where a single symbol represents a sound, and consonant digraphs th, sh, ch in word-initial position
• Have the confidence and skill to ask for help, and be specific in his request	• Read at least 10 new words relating to his interests or curricular needs	• Be able to identify the difference between a tight/comfortable grip and to relate this to his arm aching as he writes
• Be able to structure a sentence around a given word (oral)	• Spell at least five new high-use words – to include his family name, sister's name, day of lesson	• Start a sentence with a capital letter, finish with a full stop; know that capitals are used to refer to self (I), names of people, days, months
• Be familiar with simple frameworks for structuring a story and recounting an event; be able to summarize a story or recount an event using this framework	• Read (in and out of context) and spell at least 20 new high-frequency words	• Be able to structure a simple sentence around a given word
	• Distinguish between b and d (name and sound)	
	• Know the sequence of the alphabet and give the sounds of letters more automatically and confidently	

- Be able to discuss characters and events in a story read to or with him; to make predictions about outcomes; to answer literal and inference questions

- Show more awareness of the sounds of the short vowels (a, e, i, o, u) in rime units
- Be able to blend and read (decoding) specified onsets and rimes (at, am, an, ap, and, amp; et, ed, en, ent, end; un, um, up, ump; it, in, ip; ot, op)
- Be able to segment rimes (oral and written) into individual phonemes, and manipulate sounds/symbols to produce new words
- Have improved his ability to segment consonant clusters (initial clusters incorporating <s> i.e. sp, st, sk/sc, sm. sn, sw, sl and final clusters incorporating a nasal i.e. mp, nt, nd; and be able to represent these in spelling (encoding)
- Be confident in use of digraphs th, sh, ch in word initial position.
- Be aware of use of plural s as a suffix.
- Have the confidence to apply syllabification procedures, identify dominant sounds in a word and represent unfamiliar words phonically ('have a go' spelling)

- Be able to chunk a dictated sentence into meaningful pieces and write to dictation

Delivery of the programme

The ultimate responsibility for meeting the needs of a child with literacy difficulties rests with the child's local education authority (LEA). In most cases, therefore, the appropriate person to deliver an individual teaching programme will be a teacher employed by that LEA. However, in situations where a child has a history of spoken language difficulties, the speech and language therapist (traditionally employed by the Health Service) has a contribution to make. The exact form of this contribution will vary according to the age and stage of the child and may take the form of identification, intervention, training, liaison or collaboration (see Simpson, 2000). A programme such as Luke's would generally be designed and delivered by a special needs teacher who is aware of the complexity of the links between spoken and written language.

Monitoring and evaluation of the programme

The efficacy of an intervention programme is difficult to measure because distinguishing between the specific effects of teaching, and the more general effects of time and attention, is problematic (Broom and Doctor, 1995). Luke's progress was monitored on a weekly basis, and amendments were made to the programme as new information came to light (for example his difficulty in forming the letters G and E). After 10 weeks (at CA 7;5) the success of the programme was evaluated using a range of methods, which, together with their outcomes, are described here. There had been no changes in Luke's circumstances during the course of the teaching programme, and he had not received any other individual or group support.

Informal discussion and structured interview with Luke

An important objective of the programme was that Luke be able to reflect on what he was learning. In the first lesson, a Mind Map (Buzan, 1974) of the skills that underpin literacy was started, and at this point Luke was only able to suggest that 'practice' and 'getting older' would help him to become better at reading and writing. After 10 lessons Luke was able, in his own words, to refer to the following skills, and to relate them to literacy:

(a) breaking words in bits (syllable segmentation);
(b) breaking words into sounds (phoneme segmentation);
(c) putting sounds together (phoneme blending);
(d) knowing the sounds for letters, and letters for sounds (phoneme-to-grapheme correspondence);
(e) recognizing words (sight vocabulary);

(f)   sounding out (decoding);
(g)   knowing a word it looks like (reading by analogy);
(h)   looking at the picture, and thinking of the story (use of context cues);
(i)   practice.

ACTIVITY 8.5

Aim: to use interview data to evaluate progress made following a period of intervention.

A structured interview (adapted from Francis, 1982) that looked at Luke's attitudes toward reading and his awareness of reading strategies had been carried out with Luke at CA 6;5 and post-intervention at CA 7;5. Both interviews were sound and video-recorded. Table 8.7 presents Luke's responses to the questions in these two interviews. Compare these responses and write down your conclusions about any progress made.

Check your answer with Key to Activity 8.5 at the end of this chapter.

Discussion with Luke's class teacher and mother

Luke's mother maintained an interest in his work but found it hard to reinforce activities or practise with Luke between lessons. However, she observed that Luke was more interested in reading with her now that she had learned the technique of paired reading (Topping, 1995). She also commented that Luke had enjoyed the lessons and had been motivated by the success he had experienced.

Luke's class teacher was consulted before each lesson, and provided many helpful insights into him as a learner and as a member of his class. She took a keen interest in the programme and provided a supportive environment in which Luke could practise his developing skills. However, while she observed that he was growing in confidence about his ability to work alone, she had become increasingly aware of his difficulty in sustaining attention and concentrating in a group, and of his relatively immature attitude towards learning. It was apparent that mathematics had now become a source of concern, and in the Key Stage 1 Statutory Assessment Tests (SATs), Luke was assessed as a Level 1 in mathematics (i.e. below average) and W (i.e. Working towards Level 1) in English. On the basis of these results, his teacher had recommended that he be moved to stage two of the *Code of Practice* (DfE, 1994). Once Luke is registered at stage two, the school's special

Table 8.7: Summary of Luke's responses in two structured interviews at CA 6;5 and 7;5 (Questions taken from Francis, 1982)

Question	Response at 6;5	Response at 7;5
Do you like reading? What do you like about reading? What don't you like about reading?	No. Because it's ...wasting your time You could be doing better things ...	Yes. It's just fun to read for like if you're bored and you can just read for fun ... Sometimes it can get a bit boring, or sometimes it can get a bit tiring
What sort of books do you like reading?	Small ones	Chapters...RoDahl [Roald Dahl] ... stuff like that
Do you find it easy to remember words?	No	Yes
What do you do to read a word you can't remember?	Like, you break the word up and then you just add the other word up.	I just sound it out then I remember
What do you do when you come to a new word?	I just like try and guess it	I sound it out...or I leave it out and go on to the next word then... I read a line then I go back and just read it so I will know it
Do pictures help you to read? How?	Yes ... it just helps you	Yes... 'cos you can look at them, and then you can just look at them and then you can just look at the word, then you can just say it
Does 'sounding' words always work?	Yes	No. When you're on a really long word ...if you sound it out you might forget the beginning so then you need to do it all over again
Does it help if you think of another word that looks like the one you're trying to read?	Yes	Yes....cos if it's 'look' and if it's 'cook' I can just remember 'look' and put a 'c' there and then it would say 'cook'
How?	I don't know	

| Do you think reading is useful to children of your age? | Yeah. Like big children know how to read so little children should practise more often | Yes. Because it's useful for learning more words ... it's good for us 'cos we can just learn and learn and learn |
| Would you like to do more reading in school if you could? What would you like to do instead? | No. Play in the sand or play with the bricks or something fun. Or play football | No. Rounders or I'd like to work with you! |

educational needs co-ordinator (SENCo) will take responsibility for carrying out further assessment, gathering together all the relevant information, and devising an IEP. This plan will detail the nature of his difficulty, the action to be taken by the school to meet his needs, the role and responsibility of his parents, the targets to be achieved in a specified time, and the arrangements for monitoring, assessing and reviewing progress.

Reassessment on a selection of formal and informal tests; perform-ance on tasks designed to evaluate progress in achieving specific targets; and information from lesson evaluations

Despite Luke's growing confidence, he responded to the more formal situation of re-testing with anxiety and a rather defeatist attitude, indi-cating how insecure he felt about his literacy skills. Table 8.8 summarizes assessment information (quantitative and qualitative) from a range of tasks pre-intervention and post-intervention.

ACTIVITY 8.6

Aim: to evaluate progress by analysing errors on a spelling-by-sound task.

Compare the data from Luke's pre- and post-intervention performance on the picture spelling task presented in Table 8.9, and summarize the changes in his performance.

Check your answer with Key to Activity 8. 6 at the end of this chapter and then read on.

Table 8.8: Summary of Luke's pre-intervention (CA 7;2) and post-intervention (CA 7;5) assessment

Skill	Pre-intervention (CA 7;2)	Post-intervention (CA 7;5)	Comments
Speech input – voicing distinctions	Insecure performance on auditory discrimination of voicing contrasts	Consistently able to discriminate	No further concern
Speech output – voicing distinctions	Difficulty in signalling some contrasts	Aware of need to contrast s/z; p/b and can do so with effort	Consolidate this skill
Phoneme deletion	Initial: 1/6; Final: 4/6. Slow to understand task; effortful	Initial: 3/6; Final: 5/6. More automatic and confident	Continue work on segmentation (all levels) and relate this directly to spelling
Nonword reading	Unable to read even practice words (CVC)	Able to decode some practice words but no test words (CVCC; CCVC)	Starting to apply alphabetic strategies to reading, but very basic level; work on blending onset + rime
Letter name and sound knowledge	Letter names 24/26 Single sounds 18/26	Letter names 26/26 Single sounds 26/26	Consolidate direction of b/d; work for automaticity u/w/y
Single word reading	Raw score = 11 Limited sight vocabulary; mechanical letter by letter sounding out; no blending	Raw score = 13 Reliably learned 17 high-frequency words; sight vocabulary more fluent; sounding out more successful	Becomes discouraged relatively quickly; needs more work on blending (work from onset + rime level, to phoneme level)

Prose reading	Reluctant and lacking in strategies	Familiar with technique of paired reading; aware of use of context cues; less inclined to work word by word	Generally more confident; continue to encourage paired reading at home; needs more experience
Spelling	Picture spelling task (i.e. by sound) = 66.7% phonemes correct	Picture spelling task = 78.9% phonemes correct; slow acquisition of high-frequency words	Needs more opportunities for reinforcement; needs work on consonant clusters
Sentence/story structure	Unfamiliar with term 'sentence'; no awareness of story structure	Able to formulate (orally) sentence around given word	Needs work on story structure (recount and composition)
Handwriting	Tight grip; many letters incorrectly formed; directional confusions ++	More relaxed grip; forms 'e' correctly; has strategy for b/d; aware of common starting pattern for c/o/a/d/g	Slow and lacking in automaticity – needs more practice
Punctuation	Random use of capitals	Capital letter at start of sentence; full stop at end	Continue to stress purpose of capitals – not to be used within words

Table 8.9: Pre-intervention (CA 7;2) and post-intervention (CA 7;5) performance on the picture spelling task

Target	Pre-intervention (CA 7;2)	Post-intervention (CA 7;5)
RABBIT	‹raBit›	‹Rapt›
CAMEL	‹Camol›	‹Camil›
CAT	‹cat›	‹Cat›
TIGER	‹tig›	‹Tiger›
CROCODILE	‹coDiol›	‹Cokdiyl›
PIG	‹pig›	‹PiG›
GORILLA	‹gyil›	‹Giler›
HEN	‹han›	‹Han›
ELEPHANT	‹elft›	‹Elfoot›
BUTTERFLY	‹BtrFli›	‹BertFliy›
DOG	‹Dag›	‹Dog›
SPIDER	‹sbr›	‹Sbider›
GIRAFFE	‹Dyrf›	‹Derf›
phonemes correct	66.7%	78.9%

Summary of evaluation and future plans

Reassessment and evaluation of Luke's progress show that after 10 hours of individual teaching, he is growing in confidence, has more interest in reading and writing, and at a metacognitive level he has good awareness of useful strategies. However, while he has made some encouraging progress, especially in his ability to segment words into phonemes and map phonemes to graphemes, his literacy skills remain well below the expected level. In addition, he continues to have speech processing difficulties of the type that can be expected to interfere with his development of phonological representations and phonemic awareness (arguably the level of awareness that is ultimately the most important in the acquisition of literacy). The programme will therefore now need to be modified to reflect both his progress and his continuing areas of need.

As Luke's phonic skills become more functional, explicit links can be forged between phonological and orthographic information. This should serve to reinforce his lexical representations, and raise his conscious awareness of the connections between spoken and written language, thus increasing the fluency of his decoding skills. In addition, as Luke develops automaticity in segmenting words into phonemes and relating phonemes to graphemes, work on common letter strings (e.g.

-IGHT, -OUND, -TURE) and morphemic units (e.g. -ED, -ING), can be incorporated into the programme. In this way, Luke will be helped to acquire the orthographic strategies that will enable him to progress to the next phase of literacy development. Finally, if skills are to be transferred and generalized, Luke's programme will need to: work towards integrating word and sentence level work more; offer increased opportunities for practice by involving his parents more; and to include plans for integrating work into the classroom more effectively.

Once Luke has been registered at Stage two of the *Code of Practice* (DfE, 1994), an IEP will be drawn up and implemented. If his difficulties persist, he will be moved on to Stage three, and the SENCo may then decide to consult an LEA educational psychologist for further advice. The educational psychologist may, on reviewing the evidence and on the basis of the definition recommended by The British Psychological Society (BPS, 1999), be of the opinion that Luke's specific literacy difficulties can be identified as dyslexia. This definition states that,

> ...Dyslexia is evident when accurate and fluent word reading and/or spelling develops very incompletely or with great difficulty. This focuses on literacy learning at the 'word level' and implies that the problem is severe and persistent despite appropriate learning opportunities. It provides the basis for a staged process of assessment through teaching.
>
> (BPS, 1999, p.18)

This definition offers no explanation for the cause of the difficulty, but Luke's early and persisting speech processing difficulties do.

Summary

When Luke entered school his early speech problems appeared to have resolved and there was apparently nothing to indicate that he was at-risk for literacy difficulties. As a result, it was not until the end of Year 1 (CA 6;5) that it became evident that although Luke's speech may have sounded unremarkable, it was underpinned by a faulty speech processing system which was interfering with his ability to acquire early literacy skills. In Year 2 (CA 7;2), detailed assessment showed that Luke's earlier difficulties had left their mark on his speech processing system. It is suggested that, while his phonological representations were sufficiently well specified to support the development of rhyme awareness, they were not of a high enough quality to support the acquisition of phonemic awareness. Current research indicates that both of these, together with letter–sound knowledge, are necessary, although not sufficient, for fluent word decoding and encoding. Luke had entered school unable to take advantage of the learning opportunities he was offered, and now two years later his problems were exacerbated by the atypical strategies he was starting to develop and rely on (e.g. exaggerated sounding out), and his growing lack of confidence.

Single case studies of children such as Luke highlight a number of points relating to identification and intervention for children with literacy learning difficulties. These can be summarized as follows:

- The effect of a deficit in a developing system may manifest in different ways at different ages and stages of development.
- When more obvious difficulties appear to have resolved, hidden difficulties may persist.
- A speech processing system that can support the development of spoken language may not be robust or finely grained enough to support the acquisition of written language.
- Assessment and screening procedures need to be informed by current understanding of the way links between spoken and written language develop.
- Assessment and screening need to be systematic and detailed enough to uncover even relatively subtle difficulties.
- Assessment needs to be ongoing and based on multiple sources of evidence to allow the child's difficulties to be viewed in context.
- Drawing up a profile of a child's strengths and weaknesses, and being aware of their interactions, will provide insights into the nature of a child's learning difficulties.
- An individual teaching programme will reflect a child's cognitive profile, and will use strengths to support weaknesses.
- An effective teaching programme will be informed by an understanding of how children learn.
- Methods for monitoring and evaluation need to be built into a teaching programme.
- A child's parents will have an important part to play at all stages of the assessment, intervention and evaluation.
- The child should be consulted at all stages of the assessment, intervention and evaluation.
- Collaboration between a range of professionals will be important in the prevention and early identification of special educational needs; it will also facilitate the process of identifying and meeting such needs.

Resources and techniques used in Luke's programme

1. Reading and spelling objectives were supported by *Overcoming Dyslexia: A Practical Handbook for the Classroom* (Broomfield and Combley, 1997), *The National Literacy Strategy* (DfEE, 1998), *Rhyme and Analogy: A Teacher's Guide* (Goswami, 1996), *Making*

the Alphabet Work (Hardwick and Walter, 1994), *Sound Practice: Phonological Awareness in the Classroom* (Layton, Deeney and Upton, 1997), *Helping Children with Reading and Spelling* (Reason and Boote, 1994), *Teaching Reading and Spelling to Dyslexic Children* (Walton, 1998), *Phonological Awareness Training: A New Approach to Phonics* (Wilson, 1993).

2. Chapters in *Dyslexia, Speech and Language: A Practitioner's Handbook* (Snowling and Stackhouse, 1996) provided practical ideas and were a source of further references.

3. The programme recommended the use of paired reading (Topping, 1995) as a means of promoting Luke's confidence and fluency in reading, and simultaneous oral spelling (SOS) (cited in Cootes and Simpson, 1996) as a method for teaching the spelling of high-frequency words.

KEY TO ACTIVITY 8.1

1. The alliteration fluency task requires the child to access a lexical representation. As well as accessing an appropriate lexical item (i.e. one that begins with the phoneme specified), the child must also access a motor program and execute it. In the second task, recognizing initial sounds, pictures of the items are shown and the tester names them, so that the child can access the representations easily. However, this is not *necessary* for the task, i.e. the child can listen to the tester say three words that are associated with a particular picture and, without understanding the words or accessing any lexical information about them, select the item/picture beginning with the prescribed sound.

2. In the alliteration fluency task, the initial phoneme is presented to the child. In the initial sounds recognition task, the tester must ask the question, e.g. "Which object begins with the 'c' sound?" It is not specified whether 'c' is the letter <c>, pronounced [si], or the sound of the letter <c>, pronounced [kə]. This ambiguity in the instructions is problematic: if the examiner says [si], alphabetic knowledge is entailed rather than phonological awareness skills.

3. Although the alliteration fluency task has only three items, each phoneme has a different manner of articulation (nasal, fricative and plosive) and each has a different place of articulation (bilabial, alveolar and velar) ensuring that, within a short test, there is phonological differentiation between the test items. There are more items in the initial sound recognition test, but no rationale has been given for choosing the items and it seems that they are less carefully selected. First, it is unclear whether word frequency has been

considered carefully. For instance, BROOM could be regarded as quite a low frequency word in a young child's vocabulary compared to HOUSE. (However, since the child can perform this task without necessarily accessing representations, it could be argued that this would not affect performance.) Second, syllable length has not been controlled for, with test items (a) and (e) having a two-syllable word (BUTTON; BUCKET), but all of the other items being one-syllable. The importance of considering these lexical factors in designing tasks is discussed in detail in Chapter 11 of Book 1 (pp.307–309). Phonological factors are another key area to consider in test design (see Book 1, pp.310–311). In the initial sound recognition task, the rationale is unclear with regards to the phonological characteristics, e.g BROOM in item (d), is the only stimulus with an initial cluster; test item (a) uses initial /k/ in CAR and final /k/ in FORK, but other items do not follow a similar pattern; test item (b) uses the same vowel /æ / in CAT and ANT, but none of the other items share the same vowel; and test item (c) has two nasals /m/ and /n/ which are known to be particularly difficult for young children to discriminate.

4. It is likely that Luke would also have difficulty with recognizing initial sounds. To complete the task, he would have to segment the initial sound of each word and match it to the spoken stimulus. Whether the sound was presented as a letter name or a letter sound, he is likely to find it difficult to perform the manipulation even with the help of the pictures.

KEY TO ACTIVITY 8.2

1. Terry is able to supply a grapheme for most of the phonemes in a word and makes good attempts at the syllabic structure of the longer words. He is clearly reflecting upon the phoneme-to-grapheme correspondences. In contrast, Luke produces far fewer letters and in five instances writes only one letter. It would be very difficult to guess what word Luke was spelling, while Terry's attempts can often be interpreted correctly.

2. The attempts Luke makes to spell a word are not simply arbitrary guesses. He is generally best at supplying the initial grapheme; in eight out of 12 cases he supplies an appropriate grapheme to represent the initial sound, e.g. the letter ‹c› for the /s/ in SPIDER. However, he is not able to sustain this phoneme–grapheme skill throughout the whole word.

3. Luke makes voice/voiceless errors. A voiceless sound is articulated

with no vibration of the vocal folds (e.g.[p]) and a voiced sound is produced with vibration of the vocal folds (e.g [b]). [p] and [b] differ only in voicing; their place (bilabial) and manner of articulation (plosive) is the same. A failure to contrast voice/voiceless sounds therefore results in confusion, e.g. if the voicing distinction between PIG and BIG is not made in speech, then both may sound like "big" (or "pig"). Luke is sometimes not able to distinguish this voicing contrast in his spelling, e.g. the voiceless /p/ in PIG is represented with the letter ‹B› (a voiced sound), and Luke devoices the voiced /g/ in GORILLA and writes ‹K›. This type of confusion also occurs word finally in GIRAFFE when the final /f/ is represented with a ‹V›. Voicing errors in Luke's speech were indeed noted early on, at the age of 4.

KEY TO ACTIVITY 8.3

1. Table 8.2 shows that Luke's ability to detect and produce rhyme has followed a normal pattern of development, while his ability to appreciate alliteration has developed more slowly than expected. His phonemic awareness is of increasing concern.

2. A successful programme will do more than target the weakness (in this case phonemic skills). As well as considering the possible knock-on effects arising from his more slowly developing appreciation of alliteration and phonemes, it should also harness Luke's persisting strength in his appreciation of rhyme.

3. Assessment over time reveals the changing nature of Luke's speech processing difficulties. Assessments at 4 and 5 years of age had indicated that Luke's speech input skills were within the normal range and that his difficulties were confined to performance on speech output tasks. However, by 6 years of age, a more demanding auditory discrimination task uncovered subtle speech input difficulties. By 7 years of age, these input difficulties appear to have largely resolved, and Luke's remaining output difficulties are relatively subtle and specific. However, his earlier history should not be forgotten when planning his teaching programme. The programme must be sensitive to the fact that Luke may have developed some poorly specified phonological representations, and it must reflect his need to consolidate and reinforce the speech processing skills that underpin the acquisition of phonemic awareness. In addition, it will need to employ multisensory teaching methods and to make meaningful links between auditory and visual information.

KEY TO ACTIVITY 8.4

1. As Luke has read some irregular words (THE, YOU, ONE), he must be recognizing these by sight, i.e. he is using logographic strategies. With varying degrees of success he has also sounded out some words on the reading test and applied his phonic knowledge to spelling i.e. he is using alphabetic strategies.

2. Comparison of Luke's reading and spelling errors suggests that his alphabetic strategies are more useful for spelling than reading. In reading they have helped him to segment and blend two simple CVC words, but, although he pays attention to more than the initial sound in a word (e.g. ‹cup› read as "camp"; ‹jump› read as "jam"), he is not yet able to decode words involving consonant clusters or digraphs, or vowel digraphs. In spelling, however, although his weak sound–symbol knowledge and lack of orthographic knowledge lead to spelling errors (‹bac› for BACK ; ‹pla› for PLAY), he is starting to segment single-syllable words into their salient sounds relatively successfully. It is also worth noting that although Luke has spelled some irregular words correctly (e.g. THE, GO, MY) these are not interpreted as evidence for use of orthographic strategies, but are taken to represent word-specific knowledge. Orthographic strategies are evident first in reading, and develop from sophisticated alphabetic strategies (Frith, 1985); Luke's alphabetic strategies are not secure enough to be useful for reading, let alone to support the development of orthographic strategies.

3. Luke's pattern of development appears to be in line with the sequence suggested in the six-step model proposed by Frith (1985). However, he is acquiring skills at a rate well below that of his peers and appears to be having difficulty in developing useful alphabetic strategies. At his age and stage of education he could reasonably be expected to be acquiring orthographic strategies for reading and to be starting to apply these to spelling. It appears that Luke's underlying and persisting speech processing difficulties have interfered with the normal acquisition of alphabetic strategies, which, although now useful at a rudimentary level for spelling, are not yet functional for reading. Therefore, while he may be following the same developmental sequence as his normally developing peers, Luke is not mastering skills at the same rate or in the same way as they are, and may even fail to move on to the next phase of development altogether. It therefore may seem more appropriate to describe him as having a developmental disorder, rather than as being developmentally delayed.

4. Analysis of Luke's responses suggests that he needs to increase and strengthen his use of logographic strategies (i.e. sight vocabulary)

so that they can foster and support his emerging ability to use alphabetic strategies. He also needs to consolidate his knowledge of sound–symbol correspondence before his alphabetic strategies can be truly useful for spelling. In addition, reading behaviours such as his laborious sounding out, suggest that his alphabetic strategies are not yet secure enough to be applied effectively to the reading process. At this relatively basic level, phonics may be better taught and practised explicitly through spelling, although it will be important to reinforce this through reading (Foorman, Francis, Novy, et al., 1991; Hatcher, Hulme and Ellis, 1994).

KEY TO ACTIVITY 8.5

Luke's responses show a significant change in attitude towards reading over the year. At 7 years of age, he expresses himself more fully, reflecting his growing maturity and understanding of the skills and strategies involved. While at CA 6;5, he had a sense of the importance of segmentation ("you break the word up"), at CA 7;5 and after intervention, he shows a more detailed understanding of an analogy strategy in his description of how to read COOK and LOOK. However, comments such as, "sometimes it can get a bit tiring", show he continues to find reading and writing difficult. In addition, his claim to enjoy reading chapter books could be interpreted as evidence for his lack of insight into his own reading level. Also, his final comment about doing more work with the second author, in preference to more reading in school, perhaps suggests that he is not yet seeing the connection between these two activities.

KEY TO ACTIVITY 8.6

The following observations can be made about Luke's spelling strategies and knowledge at CA 7;5:

(a) aware now that the schwa sound is not part of a consonant and is using ‹er› to represent this;
(b) more syllable awareness;
(c) more successful in identifying sounds in words;
(d) less frequent use of capital ‹B› and ‹D› to avoid confusion over direction;
(e) continued confusion over medial vowel which may reflect his own imprecise/inconsistent pronunciation;

(f) some continuing voicing uncertainty of /p/ ~ /b/ in medial position (RABBIT) and in initial cluster (SPIDER), although this is a common developmental spelling error.

In addition, observation of Luke's performance revealed that he approached the task with more confidence and was more automatic in mapping sounds to letters. Overall he had made encouraging progress.

Acknowledgements

The authors warmly thank Luke, his family and school for their co-operation over the last four years. We would also like to thank the speech and language therapist who originally referred Luke to the research project and Dr Valerie Hazan, Department of Phonetics and Linguistics, University College London, for making available her speech pattern audiometry assessment (www.phon.ucl.ac.uk/home/val/ home#SPA). The longitudinal study was funded by a Research and Development Grant from North Thames Regional Health Authority to the Department of Human Communication Sciences at University College London in collaboration with the speech and language therapy services in Camden and Islington, Barnet, Enfield and the Nuffield Hearing and Speech Centre, London. Thanks are also extended to Joy Stackhouse, Nata Goulandris and Claire Jamieson.

Chapter 9
Working Together:
The Psycholinguistic
Approach Within a School
Setting

JILL POPPLE AND WENDY WELLINGTON

We are two speech and language therapists working at a school in Sheffield, in the north of England, for children with severe communication difficulties. There are 60 children in the school, all with a statement of special needs relating specifically to their severe communication or speech and language problems. The classes are made up of a maximum of 8 children in each and these are staffed by a class teacher and at least one child support assistant. All the children follow the National Curriculum at a pace according to their needs. The school has input from three speech and language therapists and other professionals, including educational psychologists and physiotherapists.

Before the Psycholinguistic Framework

In the school, the tradition was that two of the (part-time) speech and language therapists dealt with the children with speech difficulties while the other therapist dealt with the children who had language difficulties. We worked in this way to allow each therapist to keep abreast of recent research and bring this into practice within the school. However, at this time we did not work collaboratively with the teachers, although we did feed back our test results and findings to each other. Support teachers for learning difficulties and dyslexia were also based at the school, and although there was discussion among these teachers, class teachers and ourselves about specific children, we tended to keep to our own disciplines. As a result, our speech and language therapy was not linked directly to classroom practice and the National Curriculum. It was not long, however, before the team began to notice that although the children's speech output difficulties were improving, their literacy difficulties were persisting. Research at that time was linking phonological and literacy difficulties, and we wanted to know more.

299

In 1991, we attended a course at University College London on the psycholinguistic approach to children's speech and literacy difficulties. Following this, we questioned the way we were working and wondered how we could get teachers and speech and language therapists working together more effectively. In the event, this was no problem within our own school. The psycholinguistic approach gave us a common language: everyone became very excited about the prospect of changing our traditional work patterns and becoming more collaborative.

What areas did we test?

Before 1991 our routine assessment procedure for each child examined the following areas:

(1) medical background and developmental history;
(2) expressive and receptive language level;
(3) use of syntax;
(4) hearing;
(5) auditory discrimination of simple real words;
(6) oral skills including mobility, co-ordination and muscle tone and the functioning of the lips, tongue and palate;
(7) ability to repeat sounds in isolation and within syllables;
(8) ability to sequence single sounds and syllables;
(9) diadochokinetic rates (the speed and sequencing of sounds in a repeated response);
(10) naming pictures to examine sound production skills in single-syllable words and in words with increasing articulatory complexity;
(11) spontaneous speech.

If we examine these assessments now within the psycholinguistic framework, we can see that there were gaps in our knowledge about the children's input and output skills.

ACTIVITY 9.1

Aim: to identify areas not covered by our 'pre-psycholinguistic' assessment procedure.

Consider the psycholinguistic demands of assessments (4)–(11) in the above list.

1. Write the number of each assessment at the appropriate level on the speech processing profile in Figure 9.1, i.e. to mark which question will be addressed by the findings from each assessment. For

SPEECH PROCESSING PROFILE

Name   Comments:

Age

Date

Profiler

INPUT	OUTPUT

F

Is the child aware of the internal structure of phonological representations?

G

Can the child access accurate motor programs?

E

Are the child's phonological representations accurate?

H

Can the child manipulate phonological units?

D

Can the child discriminate between real words?

I

Can the child articulate real words accurately?

C

Does the child have language-specific representations of word structures?

J

Can the child articulate speech without reference to lexical representations?

B

Can the child discriminate speech sounds without reference to lexical representations?

A

Does the child have adequate auditory perception?

K

Does the child have adequate sound production skills?

L

Does the child reject his/her own erroneous forms?

Figure 9.1: Blank profile sheet.

example, (4), hearing test, goes under question A. Appendix 2, Book 1, may help you.

2. How many questions were not answered by this assessment procedure?

See Key to Activity 9.1 at the end of this chapter and then read the following summary.

In retrospect, we are surprised at these gaps. Yet this was a typical speech and language therapy assessment at that time. Indeed, as a specialist centre where we see children intensively, our assessment was viewed as comprehensive. The Key to Activity 9.1 shows that our focus was more on output (particularly lower-level articulatory skills) than on input, and that we were not investigating the children's developing lexical representations and phonological awareness. The lack of a means to collate our assessments in relation to each other also meant that we viewed each test result in isolation and did not examine the relationship between specific tests or broader areas, for example input and output processing. This segregation of tests and bias to output processing was, therefore, reflected in the therapy we used and the targets that we set for our children.

How did our therapy reflect our assessment?

Following Activity 9.1, it is not surprising that most of our therapy targets were aimed at the children's output skills. For example, for each child we would target:

(i)   one to three specific sounds for production work, not necessarily related to the child's literacy teaching;
(ii) repetition of these sounds;
(iii) syllable repetition;
(iv) blending of consonants and vowels together into nonwords;
(v)   repetitive practice of specified words with the target sounds;
(vi) repetitive practice within sentences of specified words that included the target sounds.

We would work at this level until a revised articulatory pattern for that particular sound or set of sounds had been built up. When this was achieved, we would move on to:

(vii) working at the level of spontaneous naming rather than repetition;
(viii) the production of sentences with the target words and sounds within them;

(ix) choosing key words as a focus for accurate production within the classroom setting.

We did not ignore input skills. We worked specifically on increasing the children's awareness of concepts that would link into their perception of sounds and so their production. These included work on:

(i) Long/short. This was related to the contrast between plosives and fricatives: /p/ is a short sound (plosive), /f/ is a long sound (fricative).
(ii) Loud/quiet. This was related to the contrast between voiced and voiceless sounds: /t/ is quiet (voiceless), /d/ is loud (voiced).
(iii) Minimal pairs. These incorporated the sounds that had been specifically targeted for production work.
(iv) Targeting sounds at initial, medial and final positions in the word.

This approach incorporated assumptions about how the children were storing words that contained the target sounds that were difficult for them. We were concentrating on building or adjusting their articulatory patterns for that sound and for words containing that sound. However, we were not relating this directly to the developing lexical representations. Nor were we making any links between our speech skills work and the child's literacy development, for example by introducing letters to link with the sounds targeted. Making such links was not typical of traditional speech work at that time.

How We Changed Our Working Practices

Following the course on the psycholinguistic framework, we collected articles and procedures and did a great deal of reading. This allowed us to explore further our questions about the relationships between written and spoken language development.

A sharing of expertise and knowledge

We shared our findings with the teachers, who in turn shared their knowledge of literacy development and teaching research and practice. We then selected appropriate tests for the different levels of the speech processing profile and presented these to the teachers involved. This gave us the basis for our collaborative practice. Thus we began to link our speech and language therapy directly to the teacher's literacy development practice, and vice versa.

Discussions developed with the specialist teachers as well as classroom teachers. These culminated in the setting up of joint training courses to share expertise and knowledge about the psycholinguistic approach and about the relationship between speech and language therapy and teaching methods. Initial joint training took place over a 6-week period and has continued on a regular basis.

Collaboration between professionals

Having established a close dialogue between professionals, our next task was to decide how best to collaborate to inform each other's practice for teaching and therapy. Most of the children we were dealing with at the school had some element of phonological disorder. It was therefore presumed that there would be some educational implications, particularly in the field of literacy development. This relationship between speech processing skills and literacy development provided an opportunity for discussing and implementing an integrated approach to spoken and written language development. Education staff and therapy staff carried out assessments relevant to their own professional viewpoint and pooled the results.

The speech and language therapist's assessments focused on attention and listening skills and the ability to process auditory information, both in a one-to-one situation and within the classroom. Standardized assessments were used to complete the speech processing profile, which covers input, output and storage skills, and to investigate all aspects of spoken language, i.e. comprehension, expression and functional use. Using National Curriculum guidelines, specific concepts necessary for following the curriculum were also assessed e.g. MORE/LESS for the mathematics curriculum, FIRST/LAST for written and spoken language, HEAVY/LIGHT for science and BEFORE/AFTER for history. (Further information about the National Curriculum is provided later in this chapter.)

The teacher's assessment was carried out at the same time, informally looking at each child's coping strategies, spoken and written communication in class, relationship with the peer group and self-esteem. In addition, vital knowledge was gained from the teacher on how the child was performing in all areas of the curriculum. This included detailed knowledge of a child's written language development, reading for meaning, spelling strategies, mathematics, project work and physical education, e.g. information about gross and fine motor skills. Pooling assessments and observations from different professional perspectives promotes collaborative skills (Wright and Kersner, 1998) and helped us to plan intervention for the children jointly.

Joint planning

From the pool of assessment results we could then, as a team, discuss each child's strengths and weaknesses in terms of input and output skills and how different aspects of learning may be affected. This in turn gave us an idea of what strengths, if any, could be used to compensate for weaknesses, and what strategies or support for learning would need to be employed. For many children with phonological difficulties, visual support for learning is essential, e.g. *Cued Articulation* (Passy, 1993a, b), signing, use of letters. Looking at all these things we were able to produce jointly with a teacher an individual education plan (IEP) aimed at prioritizing areas of work and achieving realistic targets. This joint approach allowed us to:

(i)   plan teaching aims and objectives
(ii)   plan therapeutic intervention for speech and language difficulties
(iii) identify areas of possible literacy and other difficulties and put strategies into place to support the child
(iv)   work on these areas together as a team so that speech and language therapy became an integral part of a child's school day
(v)   decide together which areas were a priority to work on in both classroom and therapy sessions, so that similar work was carried out by both therapist and teacher, but from a slightly different perspective.

Joint half-termly meetings were called to review and update joint objectives and plan. In this way effective collaboration was carried out. Figure 9.2. summarizes the joint planning process and highlights the roles of the professionals involved.

General Intervention Strategies

Each child's profile of strengths and weaknesses is different, and intervention has to be tailored to meet individual needs. However, we have found the following general strategies useful in our school setting. All these strategies allow the children to gain confidence in their own abilities and can easily be implemented both in the classroom and in the therapy situation.

A multidisciplinary approach

It has been very helpful to adopt a multidisciplinary approach so that all professionals are aware of relevant and recent information. This may seem obvious but cannot be stressed enough; it is essential for all professionals to combine their expertise in order to develop a complete assessment/management programme. For example, an occupational therapist's help with the sitting arrangements of a child with limb dyspraxia can facilitate work on listening and attention skills by allowing that child to sit comfortably and therefore be more focused.

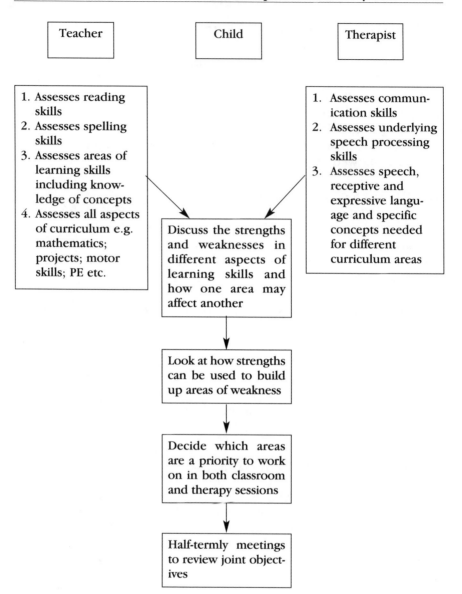

Figure 9.2: Joint planning process.

A common multisensory approach

We have found that children's phoneme–grapheme links are enhanced by using a common multisensory approach in classroom and therapy situations. This link is vitally important for spoken language and written language development. For example, both teacher and therapist use the written letter and cued articulation, and both encourage the child to write and say the word or sound.

Auditory perception

Through assessment and observation it can be seen if the child is having difficulty with auditory perception. If this is the case then visual clues can be used to back up auditory weaknesses. These may include the use of plastic or wooden letters, cued articulation, signing and Rebus symbols (1997), which help visually and physically to highlight the concepts involved in tasks, e.g. marking the beginning or end of words.

Word retrieval and storage

Children with phonological difficulties often have problems with word retrieval and storage (see Constable, this volume). It is therefore important that all concerned with the child take care when teaching new vocabulary. The sound structure of the word is emphasized with all new vocabulary, to allow the child to develop an accurate motor program that the child can store for future use. This is linked with as much semantic information about the word as possible. For example, the teacher and therapist look together at the vocabulary needed for a particular subject area and develop the child's awareness of the number of syllables, sequence of sounds, awareness of any rhyming patterns and the meaning and semantic links with the word, e.g. PYRAMID has three beats, starts with /p/, the sequence of onset sounds is /p/, /r/, /m/, the last sound is /d/ and it is a large, stone monument, built thousands of years ago in Egypt.

Use of signing and symbols

Children's general understanding of speech and language can be backed up by signing and Rebus symbols if necessary. For example, if teaching the mathematical concept of MORE in the classroom, the teacher or therapist would sign MORE and show the symbol, to reinforce this visually.

Personal dictionaries

Personal dictionaries can be made by linking onset grapheme to Rebus symbols, thus making access to these words simpler, e.g. the /p/ page would contain the symbols for PIG, PEN, PENCIL etc. Further words are added as and when required. This helps children to begin to write and spell more independently and thus enhances their self-esteem. A sample page is shown in Figure 9.3.

A common vocabulary

Therapists and teachers need to agree on a common vocabulary when working with a child and communicating with one another. This is not always as straightforward as it seems.

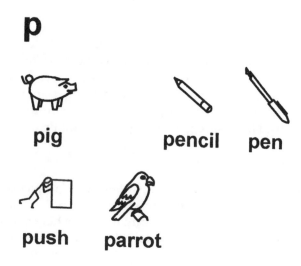

Figure 9.3: Example of a personal dictionary.

> ... A problem for the multidisciplinary team is not just to understand each other's jargon, but to realise that the same terminology may be used differently by different professions. (Stackhouse, 1993)

For example, the term PHONOLOGY may be interpreted differently by a speech and language therapist, teacher, and psychologist (see Book 1, Stackhouse and Wells, 1997, pp.7–8 for further discussion of this terminology).

ACTIVITY 9.2

Aim: to find out how terms are used by different professionals

Write down your definition of the following terms:

    (a) phonological awareness;
    (b) high-frequency word;
    (c) blend;
    (d) digraph;
    (e) numeracy.

Now ask your colleagues in different professional groups for their definitions. Add other terms to the list that are pertinent to your work. How close are the definitions?

See Key to Activity 9.2 at the end of this chapter for possible responses.

This activity demonstrates the importance of checking what you and your colleagues understand by terms in popular usage. It is easy to assume that by sharing the same terminology we also share the same understanding. In a recent survey of training needs for pre-school workers (Wood, Wright and Stackhouse, 1999), 53 per cent thought they knew what the term PHONOLOGICAL AWARENESS meant, but only 5 per cent of these defined it accurately when compared with the definition in *The National Literacy Strategy* (see Key to Activity 9.2 at the end of this chapter).

Confusion also arises when professionals use different words for the same meaning. This is explored in the next activity.

ACTIVITY 9.3

Aim: to find out the range of vocabulary used by different professionals.

Ask your colleagues what they would call the examples underlined in the following when working with their children:

> (a) FLOWER, STRIPE.
> (b) CAT; FLAT; SPLAT
> (c) MUG; TENT; LAMPS
> (d) PO-TA-TO

Check your answer with Key to Activities 9.3 at the end of this chapter and then read the following.

It is important that the meaning of terminology is discussed between the team and that there is agreement on the vocabulary to be used before work commences. The same terms should then be used consistently with the children and their carers to avoid any confusion. A failure to do this will result in confusion for the children; also the collaborative process will be jeopardized because of communication difficulties between the professionals and carers involved.

How Does the Psycholinguistic Approach Link with the National Curriculum?

The National Curriculum is a document produced by the Department for Education and Employment, which covers all the subjects required to be taught in schools. The curriculum is divided into four key stages of chronological age bands:

Key Stage 1: 5–7 years;
Key Stage 2: 8–11 years;
Key Stage 3: 12–14 years;
Key Stage 4: 15–16 years.

In England the following subjects are included in the National Curriculum:

Key Stages 1 and 2: English, mathematics, science, technology (design and technology and information technology), history, geography, art, music and physical education.
Key Stage 3: The same as Key Stages 1 and 2 plus a modern foreign language.
Key Stage 4: English, mathematics and science, physical education, technology (design and technology and information technology) and a modern foreign language.

Programmes of study include what should be taught for each subject in each key stage, and attainment targets for the expected standard of pupils' performance are set. The children in our school have specific special needs and so work within the National Curriculum at a pace according to their needs. If we look in particular at Key Stages 1 and 2, we can see how working within a psycholinguistic approach can integrate well with the statements of the National Curriculum.

English

One of the fundamental aims of the general requirements for English states that it "should develop pupils' abilities to communicate effectively in speech and writing and to listen with understanding". Further, "all pupils are, therefore, entitled to a full range of opportunities necessary to enable them to develop competence in standard English"; and they "should be given opportunities to develop their understanding and use of standard English". Recognition of how grammatical features should be formed is also required. Such features are present in spoken and written forms. With this in mind, we can see that the psycholinguistic approach provides us with 'opportunities' for understanding why children are having difficulties and allows us to develop their skills both in speech and literacy development.

Reading

Examining the more specific aims for reading in Key Stage 1, we see that the children "should be taught the alphabet, and be made aware of the sounds of spoken language in order to develop phonological awareness. They should also be taught to use various approaches to word identification and recognition". Under the heading of 'phonic knowledge', the National Curriculum talks specifically about focusing on the relationships between print and sound patterns and goes on to specify alliteration, rhyme, syllables, initial and final sounds in words, identifying sounds and blends and looking at the link to their formation in words. Children with speech and language difficulties, have problems with these phonological skills and need to be taught them specifically. They are generally able to reach a stage in reading development where they can learn and retain a number of printed words as whole chunks, but cannot use their phonological skills in order to move on to the next stage of reading development, which uses that knowledge to read new words and to spell (see Nathan and Simpson, this volume, for discussion of stage models of literacy development). In order to cope with the National Curriculum, children need to have appropriate *input* skills in order to discriminate and develop an awareness of sounds and sound patterns; have the correct *storage* of these words within the lexicon; and also have consistent *output* skills in order to produce, rehearse and manipulate sounds in words. However, studies have shown that teaching these skills in isolation from literacy instruction will not promote reading and spelling development (Bradley and Bryant, 1983; Hatcher, Hulme and Ellis, 1994). This is particularly true of phonological awareness teaching (see Stackhouse, this volume).

Writing

When writing at the Key Stage 1 level, the children need to be taught to "understand the connections between speech and writing" and to be able to use that knowledge. They also need to be able to "break long and complex words into more manageable units, by using their knowledge of meaning and word structure". Without knowledge and awareness of sounds and sound patterns, children will have difficulties accessing initial and subsequent sounds/letters at Key Stage 2 when they are expected to use dictionaries, glossaries and thesauruses to help them check spellings and meanings of words.

Mathematics

In the mathematics curriculum, children are expected to understand and use the "language of number, properties of shapes and comparatives". For the child who has difficulty in comparing and contrasting similar sounding words, pairs of numbers like 13 and 30, 14 and 40, or 13 and 14 will be easily confused (see Wells and Peppé, this volume). For example, children may start to count correctly but when they get to 13 they move directly to 31 because of the confusion between the similar sounding 13 and 30. This is typical of young children learning to count but persists in children with speech and language difficulties.

Shape names are taught in mathematics and are not only complex words to say but are also often similar in sound and difficult to distinguish, e.g. PENTAGON, HEXAGON, OCTAGON. In order to break these words into manageable chunks for accurate lexical storage and easy access, children need good phonological awareness and production skills for rehearsal and generation. Comparatives are also crucial to the development of mathematical skills and pose particular problems for a child who has difficulty in perceiving final sounds and sound patterns, since s/he cannot pick up on the key feature of the word that marks comparative vs superlative, e.g. BIGGER, BIGGEST. Vocabulary that compares and contrasts by using different morphological markers at the end of the word is not specific to mathematics but runs through all subjects in the curriculum.

Science

Like mathematics, science requires children to learn complex vocabulary. Words often have similar sound patterns, e.g. FRICTION, FRACTION. Precise input skills are required to analyse the subtle differences between such words if the vocabulary is to be correctly stored in the lexicon. This storage requires that the word is not only analysed in terms of its phonology, semantics, grammar, motoric properties and orthography but also that the appropriate connections are made between these (see Constable, this volume). Without these, children's understanding of the task and their ability to follow instructions is hampered. The result is inaccurate and/or slow performance on tasks that are difficult to remember.

Throughout the curriculum children are being confronted by new vocabulary which they need to learn quickly. Difficulty with word storage and retrieval affects the ability and speed to accommodate and use vocabulary. This is a major difficulty, since it affects children's learning of all subjects and is a major contributor to slow educational progress. In order to meet the children's need to access the appropriate vocabulary and concepts for the current curriculum, collaborative planning and working is a necessary part of any intervention programme. The following description of David's therapy and teaching is an illustration of how we have tried to address this in our school.

David, CA 9;0

At 6 years of age David had had unintelligible speech and had been making very little progress with his literacy skills. By the age of 9 years, his literacy had improved and he was intelligible in most situations. However, his speech still deteriorated in multisyllabic words and when producing sentences. He also had a significant word finding difficulty that affected all areas of the curriculum. He had particular difficulties retaining, producing and using new vocabulary at a time when the amount of vocabulary being introduced in the curriculum was increasing. This resulted in obvious attention and memory problems as David's processing energy was taken up in trying to retrieve and identify vocabulary rather than in using it to access the curriculum.

The vocabulary targeted in his intervention programme was very specific and focused on words required for various topics and subjects in the National Curriculum. It was used within therapy and teaching situations. Where possible it was taught before a topic was introduced to the class so that he would have prior knowledge of the lexical items. Our intervention took into account the nature of lexical representations, discussed in Book 1 (pp.9–10, 157). For each word, we targeted the following:

(a) Semantic representation – what the word means. This could be a definition, or a description of the word, e.g. what size is it, what is it used for, what is it made of, any words associated with it.
(b) Phonological representation – phonological information about the word, e.g.:

> how many syllables in the word
> initial phoneme of each syllable
> final phoneme of each syllable
> sequence of phonemes within the word
> whether the word rhymes with any other words.

(c) Orthographic representation – the sequence of graphemes within the word that allows the child to recognize the written word.
(d) Motor program – the sequence of motor movements necessary to say the word. This can be supported by:

> teacher's model;
> cued articulation;
> visual support via graphemes.

(e) Orthographic program – the ability to write or type the letters in the correct sequence to denote the word.
(f) Grammatical representation – the positioning of the word within a sentence and the grammatical function of the word.

These aspects of the lexical representation are not discrete: it is important to link them systematically to aid the efficient and effective storage and retrieval of new vocabulary.

ACTIVITY 9.4

Aim: to plan teaching/therapy activities that develop target words.

WEATHER is one of our National Curriculum topics. With reference to the above description of how we try to target the different aspects of the lexical representations and the links between them, think of appropriate activities that could be carried out with David to help him understand and use appropriately the target word HURRICANE.
Jot your ideas down under the following headings and try and show how you would make links between them:

(a) Semantic representation;
(b) Phonological representation;
(c) Orthographic representation;
(d) Motor program;
(e) Orthographic program;
(f) Grammatical representation.

Compare your ideas with the following account of what we did with David.

A typical session for David was to take several of the words identified by the teacher and therapist and to work through these in a very structured way. When working on the topic, WEATHER, and in particular the word HURRICANE, we targeted the lexical representations in the following way.

(a) Semantic representation

Signing and Rebus symbols had already been introduced to the whole class. Pictures of a HURRICANE were presented and a brief description of the word was given (e.g. "a violent windy storm") and discussed. Semantic networking activities were carried out. Figure 9.4 shows how a semantic network might be presented, incorporating signing and symbols as well as the written word.

(b) Phonological representation

The teacher/therapist produced the word HURRICANE for David (with or without cued articulation) and asked him:

(i) to identify the number of syllables (here, three). This may be done by clapping, placing counters on a board or whatever is appropriate for the child;

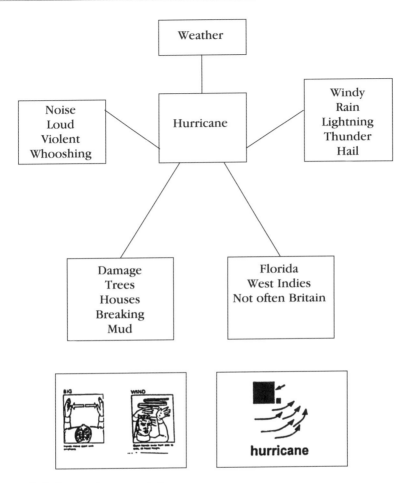

Figure 9.4: Semantic network for HURRICANE.

(ii) to identify the initial phoneme of each syllable, /h/, /r/, /k/;
(iii) to identify the final sound, /n/;
(iv) if the word rhymed with anything.

(c) Orthographic representation

David and his teacher linked the phonemes and graphemes by:

(i)   identifying the corresponding grapheme for the initial phonemes of each syllable (this was sometimes aided by cued articulation);
(ii) identifying the corresponding grapheme for the final phoneme;
(iii) grouping words alphabetically in a topic dictionary with a Rebus symbol used if necessary to aid retrieval;
(iv) displaying key topic words in the classroom so they become familiar, as in Figure 9.5.

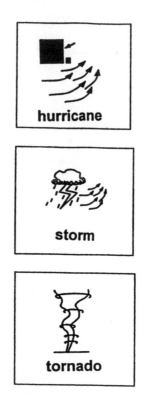

Figure 9.5: Pictures depicting key topic words.

(d) Motor program

As David placed each grapheme in the appropriate order the teacher said the word using cued articulation and emphasizing the order of sounds. David also touched each letter as he said the word to establish the correct order of the sounds as he said them. The target word(s) were practised in the classroom to develop motor programming skills.

(e) Orthographic program

David was encouraged to copy the target word(s), concentrating on the spelling of the word and thus developing his sight vocabulary. The topic words were grouped in a dictionary so he could spell them independently when needed. This dictionary was illustrated with Rebus symbols if necessary.

(f) Grammatical representation

The target word(s) were put into written exercises and cloze procedure activities where David had to fill in the missing word were carried out.

This task is used with the more able children and helps storage and retrieval of words.

All of these activities need to be linked together. A dictionary produced for each topic area outlining these activities has been useful for this (see Figure 9.7 later in this chapter for a sample page from such a dictionary that we used for another topic).

We have found that by working together in this way, David and children like him have benefited greatly. Although David's word-finding difficulties are still apparent, he has developed strategies to deal with them and has learnt vocabulary that is specific and useful to his classroom needs.

Code of Practice

The *Code of Practice* (DfE, 1994b) is a document produced by the UK Department for Education to give practical guidance on the identification and assessment of children with special educational needs. The *Code of Practice* recommends a five-stage model:

Stage 1: The class or subject teacher identifies the child's special educational needs and informs the special educational needs co-ordinator (SENCo).

Stage 2: The school's SENCo takes the lead responsibility for gathering information about the child and for co-ordinating any special education that the child needs, while working with the child's teacher.

Stage 3: Teachers and the SENCo are supported by specialists from outside the school, e.g. speech and language therapists, educational psychologists.

Stage 4: The local education authority (LEA) considers the need for a statutory assessment and may make a multidisciplinary assessment, if it seems appropriate.

Stage 5: The LEA considers the need for a statement of special educational needs. If it is appropriate, a statement listing these needs is made and the provision is arranged, monitored and reviewed.

The first three stages are based in school. The school will, if necessary, call upon help of external specialists. At stages 4 and 5 the LEA share responsibility with schools for providing for these special needs.

As stated in the *Code of Practice* (Speech and Language Difficulties, section 3:85), many of the children with speech and language difficulties have been identified as having specific special needs in this area early on in their development. They are often known to the speech and language therapy service before they start school. Ideally, when a child starts school, the speech and language therapist working with that child will have made contact with the education staff. In addition, the therapist may have contributed to the multidisciplinary assessment that led to the statement of special educational needs, when the need for specialized teaching or schooling was considered.

From stage 1 of the *Code of Practice* a child's teacher and SENCo collect information in order to identify and assess what the child's special needs are and how they can best be met within a mainstream school. The information drawn from a psycholinguistic assessment helps the teaching and therapy team to identify very specific areas of strengths and difficulties in the underlying phonological skills of the child. These skills are the building blocks for literacy development and as such can provide a good basis for the advice and support of the child at this and subsequent stages of the *Code of Practice*. If, at this early stage, there is a joint planning strategy between speech and language therapists and teaching staff, the goals and aims for these children can be more individually tailored to give a co-ordinated approach to remediation, which can be part of a child's individual education plan (IEP). Figure 9.6 gives an example of an IEP showing this co-ordinated approach to planning.

For children with specific speech and language difficulties, particularly the type of children who then go on to need special school provision such as an integrated unit or a segregated school, their difficulties are likely to affect access to the curriculum in many or all areas, particularly literacy (Bishop and Adams, 1990; Stackhouse and Wells, 1993; Hewitt, 1996). In section 3:86 of the *Code of Practice*, there is specific reference to the kind of discrepancies often seen between the expectations that the teaching staff have of a child and the child's actual attainment. Reference is made to receptive and expressive language skills (section 3:86 iii) being significantly below those of the majority of children of the same age; although specific reference is not made to 'speech' disorders we can consider these as being within that remit. If we look back to the skills expected of the child at Key Stage 1 of the National Curriculum we can see that the child with poor speech patterns and underlying difficulties in phonological awareness is also going to have significant difficulties in literacy development.

Within our school we are working with children who have been identified as having a need for a "special educational provision which cannot reasonably be provided within the resources normally available to mainstream schools in the area" (section 3:88 point 3). Our integrated team approach to planning and providing appropriate intervention is essential if we are to meet the special needs of these children. The psycholinguistic approach links well with this. It provides a useful focus for a large part of our discussions about remediation and education.

CHILD'S NAME: H.R.   DATE : SEPT. 93
NATURE OF CHILD'S LEARNING DIFFICULTIES : Severe speech disorder

TEACHER/KEY WORKER : S.C./S.J.   THERAPIST : J.P.

COMMUNICATION AIMS

1. Attention and listening skills   2. Vocabulary   3. Concepts   4. Language
5. Social use of language   6. Grammar   7. Phonological awareness

1. Attention and listening skills – to develop a set routine as a strategy to focus attention
2. Vocabulary – using Rebus and signing to aid learning
3. Concepts – continue to use visual support to aid learning
4. Language – work to be more specifically linked to expressive language using signing and rebus to help with listener's understanding and enhance H's broad communication skills
5. Social use of language – not specifically targeted
6. Grammar not targeted at this time
7. Phonological awareness – (a) rhythm; (b) discrimination of non-speech sounds; (c) discriminating onset of CV structures of specified sounds; (d) speech production of specified sound onset using CV structures and cued articulation as visual support

TEACHING AND THERAPY APPROACHES AND MATERIALS

1. Attention – Make sure he   (a) has stopped what he is doing
                                (b) is looking
                                (c) waits until the end of the instruction before responding

2. Vocabulary   (a) Work from topic vocabulary
                                (b) Have specific everyday words that he needs on cards on a key ring for him to use if not understood
                                (c) Reading vocabulary - using Rebus cards to aid learning

7. (a) Rhythm – work using musical instruments for general rhythm awareness
                                (i)   Give visual clues to help with auditory memory – long/short blocks to demonstrate long/short sounds
                                (ii) Focusing on left to right working
                                (iii) Teach contrast of long/short beats
                                (iv) Begin to relate to syllables
(b) Discrimination of non-speech sounds – using sound lotto tapes etc
(c) Discrimination of specific onset sounds – p b m. Link in with grapheme
(d) Production work on specified sounds using cued articulation as visual support – p b m. Link in with grapheme. Use Sheffield structured materials.

COMMENTS / ASSESSMENT
Strengths   Difficulties
1. Can imitate a wide range of sounds   1. Very difficult to understand
2. He has good oral skills   2. Not yet using much gesture
3. His language is developing well   3. Fluctuating hearing loss in right ear (40/50dB)
4. Awareness of rhyme beginning to develop   4. Unaware that he is difficult to understand
5. Better perception of contrasts using   5. Very specific difficulties with input skills
   someone else's speech model   6. Very severe output difficulties at all levels of
6. Keen communicator   profile
7. Receptive to signing and using Rebus to   7. Difficulties with auditory memory
   aid intelligibility   8. Great difficulties in working from left to right
8. Good use of visual strategies   and at all levels of sequencing skills

Figure 9.6: An individual education plan (IEP).

Service Delivery

Adopting the psycholinguistic approach has helped us to clarify when to see children individually and when to see them in a group situation. Further, examination of our children's speech processing strengths and weaknesses has led to a more effective grouping of our children for their therapy and teaching activities.

Individual therapy

Children are seen individually to work on specific areas of speech processing. Their strengths are used to support their weaknesses, e.g. intact visual processing skills can be used to support any auditory perceptual weaknesses. When specific sounds are chosen for therapy, they are targeted jointly by the teacher and therapist. Further, our increased knowledge of a child's speech processing skills allows us to teach phonemes in an order that best suits the individual child rather than adopt an accepted order throughout the school. Much of the work done in these individual sessions is backed up within the classroom in the literacy session, and in return we are able to use the strategies taught within the classroom in therapy sessions, e.g. multisensory teaching.

Individual programmes within a group setting

When children are placed together in a group for therapy we are now able to work at a level that suits the individual child, rather than choosing a middle pathway. In this way a specific area can be chosen to work on which benefits all of the children in the group, but it can be tailored to suit individuals' needs. For example, if the group were working on final sound discrimination and production of /s/, one child may need the teacher or therapist's speech model with cued articulation, plus the picture and written word, plus the movement of wooden letters to the final position in the word. In contrast, another child in the group may be able to work perfectly well from his/her own speech production to discriminate the correct final sound. However, both of these children can enjoy being part of the same activity within the group.

Linking group and classroom work

The work done in these therapy groups needs to be linked explicitly to academic work carried out in the classroom. The development of joint IEPs has helped to ensure that teachers and therapists work together through a structured approach to develop communication, literacy and educational skills (see Figure 9.6). As discussed earlier in this chapter, many children with word-finding difficulties have real problems storing, accessing and learning the new vocabulary needed for the topic or subject areas being studied. By using information from the children's psycholinguistic profiles we can present key vocabulary to the children prior to their lessons in such a way as to integrate phonological knowledge with semantic knowledge and relate it to classroom topics. One way of working on this is to make word finding dictionaries for the whole class to use. For example, one of the projects in the curriculum is THE EGYPTIANS and a target word in this project is CAMEL. Figure 9.7 presents a word finding dictionary page that was designed to help a child learn the word CAMEL. Current topic vocabulary is also used for other activities, e.g. work on phonological awareness. Thus, if a child is working on the EGYPTIANS in class, words such as CAMEL; PYRAMID; OASIS; TUTANKHAMUN may be used for segmentation activities in small group or individual sessions, ensuring that therapy activities are relevant and useful for the classroom.

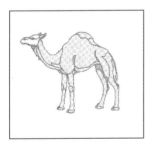

CAMEL

A camel is a large animal with humps on its back

What sound does it start with?	/k/
What sound does it end with?	/l/
How many beats are there?	2
Does it rhyme with anything?	MAMMAL
What words go with it?	SAND, EGYPT, OASIS

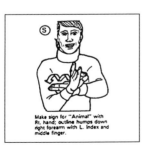

Make sign for "Animal" with Rt. hand; outline humps down right forearm with L. index and middle finger.

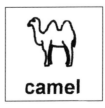

camel

Figure 9.7: Page for CAMEL from a word-finding dictionary.

Teaching groups

By using the psycholinguistic profile as well as literacy testing and observations, staff at the school have been able to group the children in a more effective way for literacy teaching. For example, if the children are working on rhyme, one group might focus on developing an awareness of rhyme judgement, e.g. "Which of these two pictures rhyme: CAT/BAT; CAT/DOG?" Another group may be working on a more complex task of rhyme detection, e.g. "Which of these pictures rhyme": CAT/ PIG/ BAT/ LION?" These activities can be done with or without add-itional visual support, e.g. the written word. Literacy work and therapy parallel each other. Therapy activities are used not only to build up the prerequisites for speech but also for literacy work; in turn, literacy development aids speech by supporting the child visually.

The children come into the first class of our school at 5 or 6 years of age and often have persisting and severe speech problems. We can therefore assume that the likelihood of literacy difficulties is high (Bishop and Adams, 1990; Bird, Bishop and Freeman, 1995; see also Stackhouse, this volume). The psycholinguistic approach allows us as a team to look carefully at each child's processing strengths and weak-nesses, target the prerequisites necessary for literacy development and so scaffold their learning appropriately. The National Curriculum and *The National Literacy Strategy* (DfEE, 1998) require a child at reception level to recognize initial consonant sounds and short vowels, to identify and write correct initial letters in response to letter sound, word, object or picture. Obviously, for some reception children this is a very difficult task.

By using the profile the teacher can group children so that one group can carry out quite complex tasks that require an increased memory load, while another tackles a much simpler task with little memory load and a lot of visual support. For example, in Group 1 we have children with relatively good input skills who are able to detect some onset phonemes and who can produce words consistently. Children in this group work on the detection of a range of phonemes with little visual support. The activities include relying on their own production, sometimes with cued articulation; pictures, and writing the phoneme or word. In Group 2 we have children who have relatively poor input skills, which require visual support to aid learning. Their own production of words may be inconsistent and they benefit from the support of a consist-ent adult model. A goal may be to detect just one or two phonemes (e.g. /p/ /s/) using the following: adult model; cued articulation; picture; grapheme; manipulation of wooden or plastic letters.

As the children get older, information from their speech processing profiles is used to group the children for other literacy activities. For example, one class has recently been working on the spelling of multisyllabic words. This has been carried out by placing the children into two groups according to their psycholinguistic needs. In the first group, the children have relatively good input skills, including segmentation skills, and are able to say words with a consistent production pattern. The children are encouraged to do the following activities, cued articulation being used only when necessary:

(i)   segment the words into syllables from their own speech model;
(ii) detect the onset phoneme for each syllable;
(iii) write the word.

The second group comprises children in need of more multisensory support. Their production of sounds within words is inconsistent, especially in multisyllabic words. Input skills are also relatively poor and segmentation skills are at an early stage of development. Cued articulation is used in the activities, which include:

(i)   beating out the number of syllables in the word from the teacher's model;
(ii) the teacher gives the model for each syllable and cues the initial phoneme;
(iii) the child finds wooden letters for each syllable onset and places them in order, using the teacher's spoken model;
(iv) the child attempts to say the word as s/he touches each letter;
(v)   the child attempts to write the word.

The work in the second group is an obvious precursor for the more independent work carried out by the children in the first group. This careful structuring allows the child to work within a group but at their own level, ensuring that each child's potential is realized.

Teachers' Perspectives on Using the Psycholinguistic Approach

All the teachers in the school have some experience of working with the psycholinguistic approach as a basis for discussing children's strengths and difficulties and for developing joint teacher/therapy objectives. Some of the teachers have been using the approach since we first went on the course in 1991, whereas for others their experience is more recent. Discussions about using the psycholinguistic approach in school has centred around five main areas:

• How the psycholinguistic approach has informed our knowledge of the links between speech and literacy development.

- The speech processing profile itself.
- How the profile has promoted discussions about individual children.
- How the profile has influenced planning for individual children.
- Evaluating how useful the profile has been.

The links between speech and literacy development

Staff at the school felt that the psycholinguistic approach had had a significant influence on our knowledge and awareness of the speech/literacy link; not just at the level of phoneme–grapheme correspondence but beyond that. It gave the teachers the information they wanted and in enough detail. It was regarded as being helpful as an indication for future teaching points to be included in each child's literacy programme. The teachers felt that the psycholinguistic framework had enabled them to develop their awareness of speech perception, storage and production and that they would find it helpful to develop their knowledge of these areas further. They felt that the collaborative working and sharing of expertise with the speech and language therapists had been a useful channel to develop the team's skills in working with children with all types of communication disorders, for instance children with pragmatic language impairments or on the autistic spectrum, as well as those with more obvious speech problems. One of the aspects that was highlighted in discussions about developing collaborative work on phonological awareness, phonics, reading and spelling was that explicit links needed to be made between these skills throughout the teaching and therapy programme in order to promote overall literacy performance.

The speech processing profile

The teachers felt that the profile was a useful tool for providing a clear explanation of why their pupils had difficulty with reading. It not only examines a child's phonological difficulties, but also highlights the child's strengths and what other skills may need to be targeted in a teaching programme. The profile had been helpful in looking at the underlying skills of children with a range of disorders including those with speech disorders, language disorders, word-finding difficulties, literacy difficulties and also for some of the children on the autistic spectrum.

Promotion of joint discussions

All the teachers felt that the psycholinguistic approach had provided a good basis for joint discussions about the children on a regular basis and resulted in more effective management. It had promoted specialized knowledge regarding children with speech and language disorders and led to a greater understanding of why some children had been unable to develop a particular aspect of their literacy skills. It had promoted regular discussions to prioritize and review the stages of the children's development. It was stressed how important the framework had been in promoting joint planning, working and feedback about the children's progress.

Individual planning

Using the psycholinguistic profile provides a teaching structure, not just a mark or a score. It has promoted joint working strategies and, therefore, more specific objectives and short-term targets have been developed. It has also provided a structure for looking at longer-term goals. It has helped to make objectives more appropriate and to allow the team to take smaller, more effective steps. The approach, and subsequently the objectives set, have allowed different aspects of work to be more integrated into classroom learning and, therefore, to become more meaningful for the child.

Evaluating the usefulness of the profile

The framework has been useful for all children but maybe for different reasons. It has promoted a lot of discussion within school and has been generally well received. It was felt that in an ideal world teachers and therapists would meet to integrate all aspects of language-based curriculum (including number and other curriculum areas). The opinion of the teaching staff in our school would suggest that the framework has provided a very positive start to the development of this ideal situation.

Summary

In this chapter we have attempted to demonstrate the changes that the psycholinguistic approach has brought about in our own working practice as speech and language therapists, and the impact it has had on our teacher colleagues. A major outcome of sharing a common framework and terminology for practice has been a more effective collaboration between speech and language therapists and teachers working with children with speech, language and literacy difficulties.

The main points about using the psycholinguistic framework in a school setting are as follows:

• It allows investigation of possible breakdown at all levels of speech processing skills and thus the subsequent effect this may have on learning.

- It allows us to appreciate the child's strengths and use these to support any difficulties.
- It has changed our therapy approach from one that focused mainly on speech output processes to one that incorporates speech input, storage and output skills, as well as the links between them.
- It has changed our service delivery, enabling a more effective grouping of children for both teaching and therapy.
- It is useful for a range of communication difficulties, not just to look at the overt signs of the disorder but also at what may underlie these and related difficulties, e.g. with literacy.
- It helps to develop therapists' awareness of literacy development, teachers' awareness of speech and language skills and the links between the two.
- As a useful tool for both therapy and teaching it can be used as a basis for collaborative practice between education and speech and language therapy staff.
- It links well to the objectives of the National Curriculum.
- It provides a focus for discussion between all professionals involved with the child .
- It enables teachers and therapists to use a common vocabulary.
- It allows teachers and therapists to prioritize areas for working together.
- It enables jointly planned, specific and individualized IEPs.

KEY TO ACTIVITY 9.1

1. See Figure 9.8, for the profile we could assemble for each child based on our 'pre-psycholinguistic' assessment procedure.
2. Eight questions were not addressed by this assessment.

SPEECH PROCESSING PROFILE

Name   Comments:

Age   d.o.b

Date

Profiler

INPUT	OUTPUT
F	**G**
Is the child aware of the internal structure of phonological representations?	Can the child access accurate motor programs?
	10, 11
E	**H**
Are the child's phonological representations accurate?	Can the child manipulate phonological units?
D	**I**
Can the child discriminate between real words?	Can the child articulate real words accurately?
5	
C	**J**
Does the child have language-specific representations of word structures?	Can the child articulate speech without reference to lexical representations?
Not tested	
B	
Can the child discriminate speech sounds without reference to lexical representations?	
A	**K**
Does the child have adequate auditory perception?	Does the child have adequate sound production skills?
4	**6, 7, 8, 9**

L

Does the child reject his/her own erroneous forms?

Figure 9.8: Key to Activity 9.1: 'Pre-psycholinguistic assessment'.

KEY TO ACTIVITY 9.2

(a) Phonological awareness

Definition in National Literacy Strategy: awareness of sounds within words – demonstrated, for example, in the ability to generate rhyme and alliteration and in segmenting and blending component sounds.

Speech and Language Therapist: the child's underlying ability to perceive the sounds and sound patterns within words.

Teacher: may see phonological awareness as being much more related to written language (e.g. phonics).

(b) High-frequency word

Speech and Language Therapist: it may mean that the sounds within the word are of a high frequency pitch such as /s/, /f/ etc.

Teacher: high-frequency may mean that the word occurs frequently.

(c) Blend

Speech and Language Therapist: blend may refer to more than one consonant together in a spoken word, e.g. /str/ in STRING.

Teacher: blend may mean to synthesize two sounds or to join two or more sounds together.

(d) Digraph

Speech and Language Therapist: diphthong.

Teacher: two letters together to make one sound e.g. ‹t›+‹h› = ‹th› (consonant digraph), or ‹ee› = /i/ (vowel digraph).

(e) Numeracy

Speech and Language Therapist: numeracy may mean all aspects of mathematics.

Teacher: specific work with numbers.

KEY TO ACTIVITY 9.3

We have found the following terms used for the examples underlined:

(a) FLOwer, STRIPE

blend; onset blend; cluster; onset cluster; cluster at the beginning of the word.

(b) CAT; FLAT; SPLAT

onset; beginning; start; initial sounds, consonant string.

(c) MUG; TENT; LAMPS

coda; final sound; end sound; final consonant; final blend.

(d) PO-TA-TO

beat; syllable; chunk.

Chapter 10
A Psycholinguistic Approach to Word-finding Difficulties

ALISON CONSTABLE

> "octopus...no.....I know it.....long neck.....big legs......eagle?"
> Michael aged 7 looking for the word OSTRICH

Vocabulary development is a complex, ongoing process which is prone to disruption in children with language and learning difficulties. Word-finding difficulties are a sign that something is going wrong with this process. They are an important component of language and learning problems for two main reasons. First, they cause communication breakdown when children are unable to convey their intended messages. Second, the underlying problems that give rise to word-finding difficulties can seriously affect classroom learning, which is dependent upon children's ability to learn and use new words quickly and easily.

This chapter will provide an overview of current theoretical issues relating to word-finding difficulties in children, and the implications of a psycholinguistic approach for assessment and teaching/therapy will be considered. The following questions will be addressed in this chapter:

- what is a word-finding difficulty?
- what causes word-finding difficulties?
- what are the implications for assessment?
- what constitutes effective intervention?

What is a Word-finding Difficulty?

A word-finding difficulty occurs when a target word is present in a child's receptive vocabulary but the child is unable to produce that word quickly and easily on demand. It is not an isolated disorder but a sign that something is going wrong with the underlying mechanisms responsible for learning and using words (or *lexical items*). In order to explore the nature of this complex problem, the presenting features (the *linguistic* evidence) will be examined before delving deeper into the underlying nature of the problem (the *psycholinguistic* aspects).

Typically, children are said to have word-finding difficulties when their expressive language contains word selection errors such as those in the OSTRICH example at the start of this chapter. Analysis of these errors usually reveals semantic and/or phonological mechanisms at work. In the OSTRICH example, Michael may have produced the word "octopus" because of the phonological similarity with the target (shared initial phoneme). Additionally, both of the items are within the same broad semantic category of living things. This would therefore be described as a *mixed phonological and semantic error*. His guess of "eagle" is a *semantic error* because it shares semantic, but not phonological, features with the target. A *phonological error* might be the selection of a similar sounding item that is not related in meaning, e.g. "basket" for BISCUIT. An alternative type of phonological error occurs when a child selects the correct target word, but seems to be groping around for the accurate structure e.g. DRILL → "rill brill" [ɹɪl bɹɪl].

Analysing the number and type of speech errors is useful for three reasons.

(i)   It provides a means of identifying word-finding difficulties. This can be achieved either through informal observation and analysis, or by comparing a child's performance with normative data on a standardized naming test. The latter gives additional information about degree of severity.

(ii) It provides a baseline measure for therapy and teaching programmes so that progress can be evaluated.

(iii) The type of error may provide clues about possible underlying difficulties in a child's lexical processing system.

ACTIVITY 10.1

Aim: to describe and categorize word-finding behaviours.

Look at these examples of naming errors that occurred on a picture-naming task.

Picture: *Response:*

1. OSTRICH   "octopus...no...I know it.....long neck.....big
                         legs......eagle?"
2. SCREWDRIVER "tool"
3. ACORN   "nut"

4. ESCALATOR   " a lift... yes a sort of lift... it takes you up or down
                    shopping"
5. FLAMINGO   "eagle...igloo"
6. SADDLE   "handle... horse...a handle... don't know"
7. MOUSTACHE   [bɪjəʔstaʃ bʌ'staʃ bɪjə bɪjəd stas bʌ'stas bʌ'stas]
8. OCTOPUS   {'ɜtəpəs 'ɒstəpas}
9. BINOCULARS   ['nɒkənɛz   'nɒkəmɪlɑz]
10. HAMMOCK   "a net where you sleep on"

Allocate the above examples of picture-naming difficulties into the
following categories by writing the number of the example by the
appropriate category:

(a) Semantic error.
(b) Phonological error.
(c) Mixed phonological/semantic error.
(d) Circumlocution (a description of the meaning).

Check your answer against Key to Activity 10.1 at the end of this chapter,
and then read the next section.

Response 1 is a mixed error already discussed above. Responses 2
and 3 are semantic errors, because the child has substituted a word that
is linked in meaning to the target (in both of these cases the responses
are superordinate terms or category labels). Responses 4 and 10 are
examples of circumlocution where the child tries to explain the
meaning of the word (you could argue that response 4 also includes a
semantic association: "lift").
    Responses 5, 6 and 7 can all be interpreted as mixed errors. In 5,
FLAMINGO, the child seems to have accessed a word from the correct
semantic category ("eagle" – a bird) which has triggered the further
response "igloo" which is semantically unrelated to the target, but
shares common phonological features with both the target and the first
response "eagle". In 6, SADDLE, it could be argued that "horse", which is
semantically related to the target, has been accessed, and is somehow
interfering with the retrieval of SADDLE resulting in the phonologically
related word "handle" being produced. Similarly, response 7 illustrates
how the phonological structures of two words of similar meaning
(BEARD and MOUSTACHE) have become inextricably entwined. Responses
8 and 9 are phonological errors as they involve several unsuccessful
attempts to produce the correct target word accurately.
    Attempts both to avoid and recover from word selection problems
like these can lead to repetitions, false starts, reformulations, pauses
and fillers (such as "um" and "er"). Sometimes children are unable to

attempt the desired word at all and they may give up on what they were trying to say. Alternatively, they may attempt to describe the meaning of the target as Michael did in the OSTRICH example ("no...I know it...long neck.....big legs"). Some children with word-finding difficulties are talkative and their problems are immediately apparent, while others are more reluctant to engage in conversation because of their problems.

There is a lot of variability in how word-finding difficulties manifest themselves, not only between different children, but also within the same child. Teaching and therapy techniques that work for one child may not work for another. The main reason for this is that word-finding difficulties are usually part of a complex speech and language problem. There are likely to be different underlying mechanisms contributing to the problem, and each child brings a different profile of strengths and weaknesses. In order to plan intervention for a child it is therefore necessary to carry out further psycholinguistic investigations to explore the underlying causes of the word-finding difficulties.

What Causes Word-finding Difficulties?

As yet there is no single theory of causation. However, through research, the mechanisms underlying lexical processing in children are becoming better understood and a clearer picture is emerging.

The storage and retrieval debate

Most of the relevant research in the 1980s used an experimental methodology and group designs to explore whether developmental word-finding difficulties were caused by problems in the *storage* of information in the lexicon, or in the *retrieval* of lexical items during speech. (e.g. Leonard, Nippold, Kail, et al., 1983; Kail, Hale, Leonard, et al., 1984; Dollaghan, 1987). This distinction between storage and retrieval has been made in the study of adults with acquired language problems (dysphasia) following a stroke or head injury. However, an important difference between adults and children is that adults normally have an intact lexicon at the onset of their dysphasia. In contrast, children are still engaged in the complex process of lexical development, and their word-finding difficulties evolve gradually as part of a developmental speech and/or language difficulty. Words that are stored inaccurately during development are also likely to be hard to retrieve, leading to problems in *both* storage and retrieval, which are difficult to disentangle in group experimental designs.

Psycholinguistic investigations

An alternative strategy, which enables us to take a developmental perspective on word-finding difficulties, is to use a psycholinguistic approach in order to find out what is going on underneath the surface word-finding behaviours (Constable, Stackhouse and Wells, 1997). In this way we can try to answer two questions:

1. How does a word-finding difficulty arise during lexical development?
2. What causes particular words to be hard to find, i.e. how does the lexical processing system operate in a child with word-finding difficulties?

The remainder of this chapter will focus on how a psycholinguistic approach to assessment and intervention can help us to answer these questions.

Taking a look beneath the surface at the mechanisms that underpin word-finding difficulties, we come first of all to the lexicon itself and the information stored there. As described in Book 1 (Stackhouse and Wells, 1997, p.57), information about lexical items is stored in the form of *lexical representations* which comprise several different types of information:

- what the word means (semantic representation);
- what it sounds like (phonological representation);
- how to produce it in speech (motor program);
- how to use it in a sentence (grammatical representation);
- how to recognize and produce the written form (orthographic representation).

The lexicon can be thought of as a highly complex database with intricate cross-referencing systems between items. Entries and connections are constantly being reorganized and refined as new items are added. Lexical development is gradual and open-ended, since we are constantly extending and elaborating our lexical representations even as adults.

Lexical information has to be stored accurately and organized efficiently if children are to learn and access words as quickly as they do. This process of lexical acquisition is dependent upon intact input and output speech and language processing skills: auditory discrimination, segmentation, rehearsal and memory of the new sound pattern, along with the integration of semantic, syntactic and pragmatic information from context. When things go wrong with one or more of these skills, the implications for lexical development are significant. Phonological processing in particular seems to have a pivotal role to play in lexical development and lexical disorders (Gathercole and Baddeley, 1990; Stackhouse, 1993; McGregor, 1994; Constable, Stackhouse and Wells, 1997), and yet this area is only just beginning to feature in assessment and intervention with these children.

The psycholinguistic framework as presented in Book 1 enables us to identify phonological and lexical processing difficulties in children. This approach works well with children with word-finding difficulties, particularly when the framework is extended to incorporate the interface with semantic processing that occurs early on in the process of producing a word.

To extend the psycholinguistic framework we need to isolate the processing route for word production, and identify possible levels of breakdown which can then be tested. When a child attempts to name a picture of a familiar item on a picture-naming task, the first thing that happens is that the picture activates the semantic representation for that word and the picture is recognized. Once the semantic representation is activated, this in turn activates the corresponding motor program, which then provides the instructions for the articulators at the motor execution level to move appropriately to produce the spoken word (see Figure 10.1).

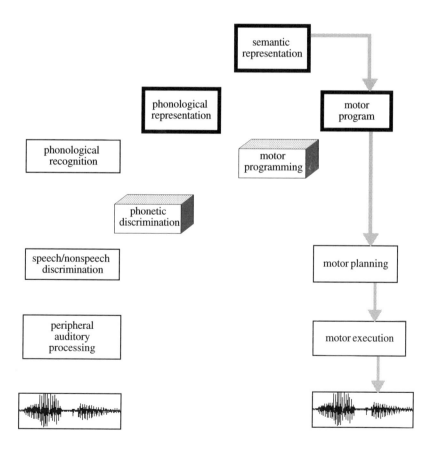

Figure 10.1: Processing route for naming.

In a single word-naming task, problems could therefore occur at one or more of these levels:

(i)   in the semantic representation;
(ii) in the motor program;
(iii) in motor execution.

The following case study (from Constable, Stackhouse and Wells, 1997) illustrates how a psycholinguistic approach can be used to systematically explore the underlying reasons for word-finding difficulties, by focusing in particular on these three levels.

Michael

Michael was first suspected of having communication difficulties at the age of 18 months and he was referred to speech and language therapy at CA 2;6. At CA 5;6 he moved from his mainstream nursery to a residential school for children with severe communication problems. At 7 years of age he presented with obvious word-finding difficulties as part of his persisting developmental language disorder. He was friendly and determined to make himself understood, but he was acutely aware of his speech and language problems, which caused him to be unintelligible at times. Michael had some persisting gross and fine motor co-ordination problems, otherwise his developmental milestones were reached normally. He had a history of fluctuating hearing loss related to repeated middle ear infections. There was also a family history of speech and literacy difficulties. Michael's nonverbal skills were described as being in the low average range; however, he was capable of functioning at a much higher level when given help in organizing his approach to tasks. He also demonstrated auditory short-term memory difficulties.

Michael's assessment will be presented in two stages:

1. using available tests;
2. further psycholinguistic investigation.

Stage 1 — Using available tests

Michael's word-finding difficulties had already been identified, so the next step was to investigate the nature of the difficulty and to try to deduce how the problem had arisen. The first stage of this investigation involved using available test materials to begin to fill in a speech processing profile (see Figure 10.2). Two specific questions to address were:

SPEECH PROCESSING PROFILE

Name   Comments:

Age

Date

Profiler

INPUT	OUTPUT
F	**G**
Is the child aware of the internal structure of phonological representations?	Can the child access accurate motor programs?
E	**H**
Are the child's phonological representations accurate?	Can the child manipulate phonological units?
D	**I**
Can the child discriminate between real words?	Can the child articulate real words accurately?
C	**J**
Does the child have language-specific representations of word structures?	Can the child articulate speech without reference to lexical representations?
B	**K**
Can the child discriminate speech sounds without reference to lexical representations?	Does the child have adequate sound production skills?
A	
Does the child have adequate auditory perception?	

L

Does the child reject his/her own erroneous forms?

Figure 10.2: Blank profile.

- Is there evidence of phonological processing difficulties?
- Is there evidence of semantic processing difficulties?

Receptive language and vocabulary

At CA 6;9, Michael's verbal comprehension was fine for everyday conversations, but he displayed some difficulty comprehending complex sentences on the *Test for Reception of Grammar (TROG)* (Bishop, 1989). His standard score was 77 with a CA equivalent of 4;6. On *The British Picture Vocabulary Scales (BPVS)* (Dunn, Dunn, Whetton, et al., 1982) at CA 7;3 he performed at the 6;0 year level, with a standard score of 88, placing him at the low end of the average range for receptive vocabulary.

Expressive language and speech

Michael's expressive language was characterized by sentence formulation problems, which could be attributed to his word-finding difficulty. There were frequent hesitations, omissions of words, false starts and circumlocutions. He had considerable variability in his speech output, with examples of phonological trial and error behaviour, e.g. GIRAFFE → {hɛfɑ gɛfɑ ɑ fɑɛɑʊ} ("hafrar gafrar rar frarow").

Speech and language therapy had focused on establishing the full range of speech sounds and increasing his articulatory accuracy. Michael was able to imitate all speech sounds in isolation and could copy sequences of sounds such as /p t k p t k/. Residual difficulty lay with clusters and multi-syllabic words.

Literacy

No formal test results were available; however, Michael's teachers reported that he had considerable literacy problems affecting both reading and spelling.

Performance on the Test of Word-finding (TWF) (German, 1989)

Michael's standard score was more than 2 standard deviations (SD) below the mean (the lowest z-score possible). Although the American items in this test could affect the accuracy of the standardization information, this very low score indicated that Michael had a severe word-finding difficulty. This contrasts with his standard score of 88 on the *BPVS*, which is within 1 SD of the mean, and therefore considered to be within normal limits, if towards the low side (both tests have a mean of 100 and an SD of 15).

Initial observation of the *TWF* responses revealed a mixed profile. Some items were named rapidly and accurately, while others were responded to with circumlocution and/or articulatory trial and error, for example:

CROWN	→	[kɹaun] ("crown")
DOMINO	→	"yes I know..oh I play....they...you put it...oh..too hard......when you want to play snap and you want to you put it round something....dominoes"
DRILL	→	[ɹɪl bɹɪl] ("rill brill").

Semantic processing (single words)

Three assessments were selected to assess Michael's ability to make associations between single lexical items on the basis of semantic information.

(i) *Pyramids and Palm Trees* (Howard and Patterson, 1992). Although designed for adults with dysphasia, this task is useful for investigating semantic association skills in older children. Each page of the test consists of three pictures, one above and two below, for example PYRAMID (above), PALM TREE and PINE TREE (below). Michael was required to decide which of the two lower pictures went best with the main picture above. The answer in this example is PALM TREE. The test was presented nonverbally, so Michael had to access his own semantic representations to be able to complete the task. Michael scored 22 out of 24, giving no indication of a difficulty in making semantic associations.

(ii) *Clinical Evaluation of Language Fundamentals – Revised* (*CELF-R*) (Semel, Wiig and Secord, 1987).
(a) *Word classes subtest:* This subtest requires a child to remember four words presented orally, and decide which two go together (e.g. TIGER, LION, TREE, BABY). Michael's score of zero on this test might at first glance suggest a semantic association problem, however this was not the case. When Michael was given help to remember the items he could easily make the semantic associations. His problem with this task was not his ability to make semantic associations, but rather his restricted auditory short-term memory.
(b) *Word associations subtest:* This subtest assesses a child's ability to produce the names of as many items as they can from three given categories (animals, modes of transport and occupations). Michael performed surprisingly well on this subtest (percentile rank 90). His strategy was to produce closely linked items that related to his own

particular interests, for example, OCCUPATIONS: "making toys, making steam trains, making electric trains". His responses were fluent and accurate, suggesting that the lexical representations for those items were well established and easily retrieved. Additionally, the items were produced as a list of single words and short phrases, which is easier in terms of processing demands than producing words within a narrative structure or a conversation. This is an example of how word-finding ability can be affected by task demands and also by the child's personal interests and experience, which have a direct impact on the development of the lexicon.

Auditory discrimination

On the Bridgeman and Snowling (1988) auditory discrimination task, Michael had to decide if a pair of words or nonwords spoken by the tester were the same or different. Half of the items were simple CVC combinations while the other half included clusters (CVCC). He made same/different judgements about matched pairs of simple and complex words (e.g. LOSS/LOT and LOST/LOTS) and simple nonwords (e.g. VOSS/VOT) perfectly well. The few errors that he did make on this task were all on the complex nonwords (e.g. VOST/VOTS). When younger, Michael had had more marked auditory discrimination difficulties. These results suggested a relatively subtle residual auditory processing problem, which revealed itself only when complex stimuli were used.

Rhyme production

A set of target words and nonwords was read out to Michael (from Lane, 1993) and he was asked to produce as many rhyming words as he could for each item. Michael produced only two rhyming responses (normally developing 5-year-olds produced an average of 125 rhyming responses on this task). He tended to produce predominantly semantic responses (e.g. COW – "moo", HAY – "hey dood") and he demonstrated no concept of rhyme.

Table 10.1 summarizes the test results from Stage 1 of Michael's assessment.

Assembling a speech processing profile

Once this preliminary information had been collected it was possible to begin a speech processing profile for Michael.

ACTIVITY 10.2

Aim: to begin a speech processing profile for Michael on the basis of information gained from the Stage 1 investigations.

Consider the processing demands of each assessment in Table 10.1 and summarize Michael's results so far on the speech processing profile sheet in Figure 10.2 by adding ticks or crosses at the appropriate levels. Appendix 2, Book 1, may help you (nb the profile will not be complete at this stage).

Check your answers with Key to Activity 10.2 at the end of the chapter, then read the following.

Table 10.1: Results from Stage 1 of Michael's assessment at CA 7;3

Test	Age equivalent	Score	Ranking
Input:			
Receptive vocabulary			
The British Picture Vocabulary Scales (Dunn, Dunn, Whetton, et al., 1982)	6;0	Standard score 88	
Receptive language			
Test for Reception of Grammar (Bishop, 1989)(at CA 6;9)	4;6	Standard score 77	5th percentile
Auditory discrimination			
Auditory Discrimination Test (Bridgeman and Snowling, 1988)		Raw score 51/60	
Semantic judgement (nonverbal)			
Pyramids and Palm Trees (Howard and Patterson, 1992)		Raw score 22/24	
Semantic judgement (verbal)			
Clinical Evaluation of Language Fundamentals – Revised *Word Classes subtest*		Raw score 0	
Output:			
Expressive vocabulary			
German Test of Word-finding		Standard score < –2	<2nd percentile
Clinical Evaluation of Language Fundamentals – Revised Word Association subtest		Standard score 15	90th percentile
Phonological awareness			
Rhyme production (Lane, 1993)		Raw score 2	

Working through the profile from A to L, you should have a tick under question A because there is no current evidence of a hearing acuity problem. However, you should note here that Michael has had a history of fluctuating hearing loss. There is one cross at question B because although Michael could discriminate between simple nonwords on the Bridgeman and Snowling test, he was consistently poor at discriminating between the complex nonwords, suggesting a subtle residual difficulty in auditory discrimination, probably related to his limited short-term auditory memory. There are no data for level C as this was not considered a priority for assessment at this point. Michael could successfully discriminate between real words on the Bridgeman and Snowling test so level D gets a tick. So far we have no data for levels E or F.

On the output side, there is not a lot of information yet. Although we suspect output problems because of Michael's obvious expressive difficulties, we cannot say at this point whereabouts in the processing system the problem is arising. However, we do have information for level H, where you could have put as many as three crosses because Michael was unable to generate rhyming words (compare controls). For level K we know that Michael can produce all speech sounds in isolation, but he has had a lot of therapy in this area and has a history of articulatory difficulties. He continues to have difficulty producing multisyllabic words. To be cautious, a tick and a question mark were written at level K. For level L there is a tick because Michael spends a lot of his time self-correcting, or at least trying to.

ACTIVITY 10.3

Aim: to draw conclusions from the Stage 1 test results (see Table 10.1).

Answer the following questions on the basis of the test results so far:

(1) Does Michael have underlying semantic processing problems?
(2) Does Michael have underlying phonological processing problems?

Check your answers with Key to Activity 10.3 at the end of this chapter and then read on.

Question 1. Does Michael have semantic processing problems?

The three tests of semantic processing used in the Stage 1 assessment do not constitute a thorough semantic investigation, but the results were enough to suggest that Michael's primary problem was not one of semantic processing per se. There was no evidence of semantic association problems on the *Pyramids and Palm Trees* test, and the difficulties he presented on the *CELF-R* Word Classes assessment could be explained by auditory memory factors. His variable performance on the *CELF-R* Word Associations suggested that where words were particularly well established in his lexicon, it was easy for him to make rapid associations within a category.

Question 2. Does Michael have phonological processing problems?

At the end of Stage 1, we can conclude that Michael has phonological rather than semantic processing problems. His subtle auditory discrimination problems suggested difficulties with the temporary storage and/or segmentation of complex and unfamiliar spoken material. This was likely to be a residual difficulty from a time earlier in his life when his problems in this area were more severe. Michael's problems with rhyme production suggested a difficulty with phonological awareness, contrasting sharply with his ability to produce semantically associated word strings on the *CELF-R* Word Associations subtest. However, it was unclear how these problems were contributing to his word-finding difficulties, and further investigations were carried out.

Stage 2 – Further psycholinguistic investigation

The following mini-battery of tasks forms the basis for further psycholinguistic investigation of the underlying causes of word-finding difficulties:

(1) picture naming;
(2) auditory lexical decision;
(3) real word repetition;
(4) nonword repetition;
(5) comprehension check;
(6) further semantic assessment.

Although most of these tasks already have a place in a general psycholinguistic assessment battery, it is particularly important for children with word-finding difficulties that a single core word list is used, so that naming performance can be compared with performance on tasks that tap the accuracy of the underlying phonological representations for the same items.

Selecting a core word list

It is important to select a set of words (a minimum of 10) that is challenging to the child. If very familiar words are selected, the representations and links between items will be relatively well established and the processing difficulties that may affect more complex items will not be uncovered. If therapy and teaching goals are being set on the basis of these assessment results, the word list should comprise words that are currently important for the child to know. For example, they may be functionally useful words in an everyday sense, or they may be related to a current or future class topic. Teachers and therapists can collaborate when designing word lists to ensure that the list is appropriate in terms of classroom learning (see Popple and Wellington, this volume).

The next step is to devise a matched set of nonwords to use for two assessments: nonword repetition and auditory lexical decision. There are a number of factors to take into account when designing nonwords (see Book 1, Chapter 11, especially p.317 on matching sets of stimuli and general points about test design). For Michael's Stage 2 assessment procedures, a set of very closely matched real and nonword stimuli was made by systematically changing only one or two features of the real words. For example, in the following stimuli two segments have been swapped over:

HOSPITAL → /ˈhɒstɪpəl/ ("hostipal")
ESCALATOR → /ˈɛstəleikə/ ("estalaker").

Picture-naming test

The naming test (using pictures of the words on the list) should be carried out first of all to avoid possible priming effects from the other tasks. This enables you to see how efficient and accurate the child is at producing the words on demand. This information begins to address question G on the profile (*can the child access accurate motor programs?*).

If a child names a picture correctly, s/he must have an accurate enough semantic representation to be able to recognize the picture and access its semantic representation, which in turn activates the motor program for the target lexical item. If the word is produced without any errors, the child's lower-level articulatory skills must be intact. We could therefore put a tick in levels G, I and K (nb some words may be well established and named easily while others cause problems). However, if a child is unable to name a picture, the problem could be arising at any of the stages of the process and it is not clear what to write at level G until further assessments have been completed for comparison.

Auditory lexical decision

An auditory lexical decision task is needed to investigate the accuracy of the phonological representations for the target words (question E.).

A typical procedure is for the child to be presented with a picture, e.g. of a FISH, and then asked by the tester "Is this a FISH?; Is this a PISH?; Is this a TISH?; Is this a FIT?" One way of carrying out your own tailor-made version of this task is to record your set of real words and matched nonwords on to an audio-tape in random order. This can then be played to the child, who has to indicate whether s/he thinks each word is real or not. (You will need to train the child with some practice items first, and you can choose whatever concept of real and nonword that the child relates to best, e.g. right and wrong or silly.) Although this task might seem difficult, normally developing children aged 4–5 years have performed well on it (Constable, Stackhouse and Wells, 1997; and see Stackhouse this volume).

Two predictions can be made about children's performance on the auditory lexical task:

(i) If the phonological representation is accurate, a child will reject even closely matched nonwords.

(ii) If the phonological representation is inaccurate, a child will find closely matched nonwords acceptable when compared to his/her own inaccurate representation.

Real word repetition

The aim of this task is to establish if a child's output is better, the same, or worse when s/he is given a model to copy. The procedure involves presenting a target word from the core list, either live or on tape, for the child to repeat.

Nonword repetition

The list of nonwords is presented in the same way as the real words are for real word repetition. Repeating nonwords makes more demands on input processing (segmentation and memory) and involves the building of new motor programs (see Book 1, pp.40–41 and pp.45–48, for further discussion of speech repetition tasks).

Five predictions can be made about children's performance on the speech repetition tasks:

(i) Spontaneous production (naming) is the same as real word repetition. This suggests there is an output processing problem which affects word production, regardless of how the word is generated.

(ii) Naming is worse than real word repetition. This suggests that the motor program is inaccurate and cannot be relied upon for spontaneous naming, but lower-level skills are intact enough to result in an accurate production when a model is copied.

(iii) Real word repetition is better than nonword repetition. This suggests a difficulty in input processing and/or assembling new motor programs.

(iv) Real word repetition and nonword repetition reveal the same errors, suggesting a lower-level motor execution problem which affects output regardless of how the word was generated.

(v) No difficulty with either task suggests that input, motor programming, and lower-level output skills are intact.

Comprehension check

A picture-pointing comprehension task needs to be carried out to check that the child does have the target words in his/her vocabulary, e.g. by presenting a choice of three or four pictures from which the child chooses the one named by the tester.

Further semantic assessment

No further assessment of Michael's semantic system was carried out at Stage 2. To date, we have relatively few tools for detailed assessments of semantic processing in children, and even more importantly we have limited information about normal semantic development (see Crystal, 1987 and 1998 for persuasive accounts of why further research is needed; also Landells, 1995 for more assessment ideas). Further investigation of the integrity of the semantic representations for the core words might include the following:

(i)   Asking for definitions of the meaning of words.

(ii) Within-category games of various kinds, e.g. generating or sorting items within specific categories, or according to function, or other semantic features.

(iii) Making yes/no judgements about the accuracy of semantic information (McGregor and Waxman, 1998), e.g. picture of MONKEY, tester says "this is an animal" or "this lives on a farm" and the child has to respond "yes" or "no".

(iv) Matching semantically related pictures e.g. *Semantic Links* assessment (Bigland and Speake, 1992).

Michael's Results from Stage 2 of the assessment

Naming

Michael correctly named six out of 10 items. This score was significantly worse than control groups of age- and vocabulary-matched children. His errors were similar to those observed in his spontaneous speech, and fell into three categories:

Phonological	e.g. BINOCULARS	[ˈnɒkənɛz ˈnɒkəmɪlɑz]
Circumlocution	e.g. ESCALATOR	" a lift...yes a sort of lift...it takes you up or down shopping"
No response	e.g. MICROPHONE.	

Auditory lexical decision

Michael identified the real words with 100 per cent accuracy. For the nonwords he had more difficulty, scoring only 60 per cent correct, which was significantly worse than the control children. Inspection of the items he could not name revealed that these were also the items for which he had difficulty rejecting the nonwords. An example is the item BINOCULARS, which he produced in the naming task as [ˈnɒkənɛz ˈnɒkəmɪlɑz]: Michael accepted both {bɪˈnɒkjunəz} and {bɪˈlɒkjunəz} as correct on the auditory lexical decision task. Conversely, when he named a word quickly and accurately, he was also able to reject the closely matched nonwords for that item.

Real word repetition

Michael repeated 20 per cent of real words accurately.

Nonword repetition

Michael repeated 10 per cent of nonwords accurately.

Comprehension

Michael correctly identified all 10 items on the comprehension task.

ACTIVITY 10.4

Aim: to complete Michael's speech processing profile.

Add a summary of the new information arising from Stage 2 of the assessment to the speech processing profile in Figure 10.2 (used for Activity 10.2). Again, Appendix 2, Book 1 may help you.

Check your answers against the Key to Activity 10.4 at the end of this chapter and then read the following explanation.

Michael's speech processing profile

On the input side (question E) we now know that Michael has imprecise phonological representations for those words that he cannot name. There is a link here with question G and you could draw an arrow between levels E and G to mark it.

By comparing the results of the naming and lexical decision tasks, we have learned that Michael's naming errors arise because he is attempting to access motor programs that are built on inaccurate phonological representations. For these items, he has inadequate information stored in the motor programs, which makes them difficult to access accurately.

We also have evidence from the nature of the naming errors that there is a problem arising at the level of the motor programs, i.e.:

(i)   When circumlocution occurs, sufficient semantic information has been stored in the lexicon to be able to describe the features of the target word, but for some reason it is not possible to locate and/or activate even part of the appropriate motor program. e.g. ESCALATOR "a lift...yes a sort of lift...it takes you up or down shopping". One likely explanation is that the target motor program is stored inaccurately and so cannot be located and activated in the normal way.

(ii) Mixed phonological and semantic errors. Where part of a motor program is accessed, along with part of another, this suggests that the motor programs are not stored accurately enough for one to be clearly more appropriate and activated more strongly than its neighbours. e.g. MOUSTACHE → {b jɛ? stɑs ʊ stɑs b jɛ b jɛd stɑs stɑs bʊstɑs]. The motor programs of two semantically related lexical items – in this case MOUSTACHE, BEARD – have been activated simultaneously and Michael is unable to inhibit one or the other.

Thus, the answer to question G is two crosses: he cannot access *accurate* motor programs.

Two crosses have also been placed underneath question I because Michael demonstrated poor real word repetition. There are three crosses underneath question J because Michael found nonword repetition harder than real word repetition. See Figure 10.3 for Michael's completed profile from Stage 1 and Stage 2 of the assessment.

Figure 10.3 shows that Michael has pervasive difficulties, affecting both input and output speech processing skills, but with more severe difficulties on the output side. In addition to his auditory discrimination and his lexical difficulties, particularly with phonological representations and stored motor programs, he also has lower-level output problems. This is evident from his poor real and nonword repetition. He has specific problems in manipulating phonological units and in building new motor programs, as is evident from the nonword repetition performance. The remaining gaps on the profile were not targeted in this assessment.

SPEECH PROCESSING PROFILE

Name   Michael

Age

Date

Profiler

Comments:

INPUT

F

Is the child aware of the internal structure of phonological representations?

–

E

Are the child's phonological representations accurate?

×

D

Can the child discriminate between real words?

✓

C

Does the child have language-specific representations of word structures?

–

B

Can the child discriminate speech sounds without reference to lexical representations?

×

A

Does the child have adequate auditory perception?

✓

OUTPUT

G

Can the child access accurate motor programs?

× ×

H

Can the child manipulate phonological units?

× ×

I

Can the child articulate real words accurately?

× ×

J

Can the child articulate speech without reference to lexical representations?

× × ×

K

Does the child have adequate sound production skills?

? ✓

L

Does the child reject his/her own erroneous forms?

✓

Figure 10.3: Michael's profile from Stages 1 and 2.

ACTIVITY 10.5

Aim: to use all the available assessment information to identify levels of breakdown in the word production process and causal factors arising in lexical development.

Answer the following questions posed earlier in the chapter and then read the next section:

1. Where are the levels of breakdown in Michael's word production system:

(i)   in the semantic representations?
(ii) in the motor programs?
(iii) in motor execution?

2. How could these problems have arisen during the course of Michael's lexical development?

---

1. Where are the levels of breakdown in Michael's word production system?

(i) In the semantic representations? Michael showed no evidence of general semantic processing difficulties in the Stage 1 tasks. In Stage 2 he correctly identified the 10 target items, which tells us that he had at least enough semantic information stored about those items to select them correctly from the distracters. This evidence suggests that a primary semantic difficulty is not at the root of Michael's difficulty. However, the possibility remains that his semantic representations are not as well organized and detailed as those of a normally developing child due to the secondary consequences of his other difficulties (see question 2 below).

(ii) In the motor programs? In Stage 2, the comparison between Michael's performance on the naming task and the auditory lexical decision tasks revealed that for the words he *could* name, he was also able to reject the closely matched nonwords, suggesting that his phonological representations and therefore his motor programs for those items were intact. However for the items he *could not* name, he also could not reject the matched nonwords, indicating that his phonological representations for those items were inaccurate or 'fuzzy'. Such inaccurate phonological representations are likely to have knock-on effects throughout the lexical processing system, leading in particular to the formation of motor programs that are imprecise. There are also likely to be faulty links between semantic and phonological information.

(iii) In motor execution? Michael continues to have mild motor execution difficulties as demonstrated in the real word repetition task. This difficulty cannot in itself explain the word-finding difficulty, otherwise all children with articulatory difficulties would be having the same kind of problem. However, the presence of the ongoing motor execution difficulty makes it hard for him to update his lexical representations, as we shall see below.

2. How have these problems arisen during the course of his lexical development?

Looking at Michael's speech processing profile in Figure 10.3, we can speculate how these problems have interacted during his development. Phonological representations and motor programs may have been laid down inaccurately as a consequence of a faulty auditory processing system in the first instance. This was then compounded by articulatory difficulties which caused newly learned items to be rehearsed inaccurately and imprecise or variable information was feeding back into the system via the auditory and kinesthetic routes. As his lexicon has grown, more and more inaccurate information has been incorporated and it is possible to imagine how disorganized and inadequate the lexical representations and the links between them have become.

At the age of 7 years, his problems are being maintained because of his continuing input and output processing difficulties. Also, by this age, children are using their exposure to print as an additional means of consolidating and building their lexicons. Michael's literacy difficulties prevent him from using this source of information.

In spite of his problems, Michael has a number of strengths which need to be kept in mind when moving on to the next stage: planning intervention. He is a determined and lively communicator with good coping strategies. He spontaneously uses techniques that serve to keep the listener's attention: fillers, to let the listener know that he has not finished his turn; and circumlocution, which enables him to explain his meaning when the target word eludes him. Michael responds well to phonological cues provided by the listener, and he could be encouraged to use these spontaneously. Michael also has islands of strength within his lexicon, where certain items related to his personal interests and main pastimes are represented well and easily accessed.

This case study has demonstrated the role of phonological processing in Michael's word-finding difficulties. Evidence is growing that phonological processing is important for some if not all children presenting with this problem (Chiat and Hunt, 1993; McGregor, 1994, 1997). Although a primary problem may be arising at the phonological level, or at the semantic level, these two types of information are fundamentally linked within the lexicon and the lexical access system, and so there are likely to be knock-on effects from one to the other.

What are the Implications for Assessment?

Word-finding difficulties are relatively easy to identify using a combination of clinical observations and naming tests, so why carry out such detailed investigation when time is limited? The most important reason is that each child is different. Effective therapy relies on knowing as much as possible about an individual child's lexical representations and lexical processing skills. The issue for the therapist and teacher is to find out what the child is having difficulty learning, and why, so that weaknesses can be linked with strengths in a child's intervention programme.

It is essential that assessment has a broad base. Information about a child's word-learning and phonological and semantic processing skills needs to be placed within the context of their overall speech and language profile, together with knowledge about personality, learning style, hobbies, preferences and habits. Word-finding difficulties are usually evident in spontaneous speech, and this is where the search should begin for clues about the nature of the difficulty. It is important to observe children's spontaneous language for word-finding behaviours rather than relying solely on naming test results. This is because the testing environment creates a false context where the constraints of spontaneous communication have been removed, but the pressure of being tested has been added (Martin and Miller, 1996, p.7).

Thus, identification of word-finding difficulties can begin informally through observation of the child in different communicative contexts, noting word-finding behaviours such as those described above. A picture-naming task may be administered; either informally or by using a standardized test procedure e.g. the *Word Finding Vocabulary Test* (Renfrew, 1995); the *TWF* (German, 1989); the *Graded Naming Test* (Snowling and Stothard, unpublished). Poor performance on a naming task can be a good indicator of word-finding difficulties. However, it is important to remember that when a child cannot name a picture, it could be for a number of reasons which need to be explored so that intervention can be suitably targeted. In other words, the picture-naming procedure is only the beginning of the investigation, and caution should be used when basing a diagnosis of a word-finding difficulty on poor picture-naming performance alone (see Book 1, pp.100–101 for further discussion).

As well as assessing naming skills, it is important to evaluate the child's receptive vocabulary development in order to distinguish between a word-finding problem (where an item is present in receptive vocabulary but the child has difficulty using that word on demand) and a generally limited vocabulary (where the items present in receptive vocabulary are easily used, but limited in number). These two problems are not always distinct but can co-exist. Children with word-finding difficulties may have vocabularies of limited size. Likewise, it is possible for children with limited vocabularies to exhibit word-finding difficulties as they learn new words. Whatever the nature of the vocabulary problem, it is important to establish the underlying cause(s) so that intervention can be tailored appropriately.

Receptive vocabulary can be assessed using a receptive vocabulary test, e.g. *BPVS–II* (Dunn, Dunn, Whetton, et al., 1997). Following this, a specific comprehension check should be carried out of the items on the naming test that the child could not name. If a child cannot identify the target word from an array of pictures when given the name verbally, it is likely that the item is not yet in their lexicon. Some tests come with a comprehension check built in (e.g. German, 1989). If a naming test does not have a comprehension test built in, the naming test pictures can be used for an informal comprehension check.

An assessment procedure

1. Identifying a word-finding difficulty

- Collect observational data of spontaneous language and interaction in the classroom, playground, with several different communication partners.
- Collect reports from home and school.
- Carry out a range of speech and language assessments as appropriate, in particular a test of receptive vocabulary (e.g. *BPVS–II*).
- If available, carry out a standardized naming test (e.g. German, 1989; Renfrew, 1995; Snowling and Stothard, unpublished) as a baseline measure and to provide more error data.

2. Further investigation

- Carry out an error analysis of spontaneous data and naming test data.
- Look for phonological and semantic components of word selection errors.
- Look for other compensatory behaviours and strategies.
- Compare word selection errors and compensatory behaviour in single word-naming and discourse contexts.
- Use the error analysis data as a baseline measure against which to measure future progress.

At the end of this you should have information about a range of aspects of the child's speech and language abilities. You should know whether the problem is a word-finding difficulty as opposed to a more general problem of limited vocabulary size. You should be able to identify the types of errors (semantic, phonological or mixed). You should also be able to identify whether or not the child has a picture-naming difficulty in relation to other children of the same age. You should know what strategies the child is using to compensate for his or her difficulties in spontaneous speech.

3. Identifying the underlying cause of the word-finding difficulty

- Design a core word list.
- Carry out the mini-battery of psycholinguistic assessments described in Michael's case study.
- Supplement this with other psycholinguistic assessments to complete the speech processing profile.
- Identify whether the problems are arising at one or more of the following levels:

(i)   the semantic representation;
(ii) the phonological representation;
(iii) the motor program;
(iv) motor execution.

- Identify the factors in the child's development that are most likely to have contributed to the problem. Are they persisting, or have they resolved?
- Identify any coping strategies such as self-cueing, conversation management, that are being used, or which could be used.

Once you have all this information, you are ready to plan intervention. Taking a psycholinguistic approach to assessment moves us forward from simply being able to identify a word-finding difficulty, to being able to form hypotheses about how that word-finding difficulty came about, and what is currently going on for the child in terms of lexical processing and lexical representations. This more thorough understanding of the child, coupled with our awareness of classroom learning issues and the need for close collaboration between teachers, speech and language therapists and parents, equips us for intervention better than ever before. However, it is often difficult to know how to design the most effective intervention programme.

What Constitutes Effective Intervention?

Using a psycholinguistic approach is not about throwing out everything we used to do and starting again. It is about using techniques (new and old) in a systematic way, with a strong theoretical rationale, and with clear individual needs in mind. Evidence from single case studies like that of Michael highlights the fact that children's underlying processing difficulties and compensatory behaviours can be very different, even when surface behaviours and naming test scores appear to be similar (Constable, 1993). It is therefore inappropriate to apply a single therapy approach to all children presenting with a word-finding difficulty. Where this has been done, for example in therapy studies involving groups of children, results have been inconclusive; the individual variation across the group averages out any progress certain individuals might make.

Because each child is different, it is impossible to outline a model intervention programme. However, some general principles can be used to guide programme design. Depending on the outcome of detailed assessment, and the overall speech and language profile for the child, teaching and therapy targets generally fall into four main areas:

(1) Underlying input and output processing skills;
(2) Memory;
(3) Lexical updating – improving the accuracy of the following stored information:

  • phonological representations
  • motor programs
  • semantic representations;

(4) compensatory strategies to improve coping behaviour.

Elements from each area can be incorporated into an individual teaching/therapy programme for the child, which ideally will be designed collaboratively by the teacher and the speech and language therapist. Baseline measures should have been obtained during the assessment period and assessments can be repeated to measure maintenance of skills and knowledge after the end of the programme.

The sequence of work within the programme is flexible, and depends on the current needs of the child. It may be difficult to work on improving the accuracy of stored information until processing skills are improved. However, the curriculum does not stop and wait for new skills to be thoroughly established! Lexical reinforcement and targeted new word learning will need to happen in parallel with skills teaching. Ideally, lexical and processing skill work is combined, e.g. a core vocabulary can be used for phonological awareness or auditory discrimination or articulation work (whatever is necessary). This in turn will strengthen the phonological representations and motor programs for those lexical items.

1. Underlying input and output processing skills

It is important to target persisting input processing difficulties (such as auditory discrimination problems) and output processing difficulties (such as motor programming and motor execution problems) as soon as possible, so that information reaching a child's lexical representations via the auditory and kinesthetic routes can be as accurate as possible. For the same reason, phonological awareness and literacy difficulties are a priority so that the visual/orthographic route can support lexical updating and new word learning.

2. Memory

Children with word-learning and word-finding difficulties often have problems with both short- and long-term memory. Conceptual and lexical difficulties are compounded by difficulty storing and integrating information efficiently.

For example, Colin, a 7-year-old boy with word-finding difficulties and other speech and language processing problems took part in a school trip to the Natural History Museum in London. This was related to a class project on the EARTH focusing specifically on ROCKS, VOLCANOES, EROSION and THE WEATHER. One day later, he had very limited recall of the details of the visit. The only exception to this was a strong memory of a display cabinet filled with stuffed birds from around the world, which was completely unconnected to the exhibition that the class had gone to see. Colin was not able to use the preparatory work done in the classroom before the trip to help him to structure his experience at the museum, and he was unable to store useful information that would help him with the topic in class on his return. Instead, his eye was caught by something that related to a personal interest of his (birds and animals) which he could talk about at length.

This example illustrates the importance of incorporating activities into teaching and therapy that will help children to maximize their memories of experiences in order to elaborate and strengthen their concepts and lexical representations. Essential topic work needs to be pitched at the child's lexical level, with selection and teaching of appropriate core vocabulary and concepts linked to meaningful hands-on experiences that the child is later helped to remember. There needs to be plenty of repetition in different contexts. Discussion is essential for practising the vocabulary and strengthening links between items, and also for consolidating memories of relevant events. Most importantly, it should not be assumed that a lexical item has been integrated into a child's lexicon just because the child has been exposed to it. This is a characteristically slow process and there needs to be careful checking for learning and maintenance over time. Memory maps and narratives are useful tools. Merritt and Culatta (1998) and Naresmore, Densmore and Harman (1995) offer helpful suggestions about collaborative working using memory strategies.

3. Lexical updating: improving the accuracy of stored information

Word-finding difficulties are most likely to decrease when lexical items are stored accurately, and their retrieval and use is well practised. Lexical elaboration is a daunting prospect for the therapist and teacher, given the size of a typical child's lexicon. Traditionally, this kind of intervention has focused on strengthening semantic knowledge, but with the increasing awareness of the role of phonological processing, phonological elaboration is becoming more popular.

A relatively small number of intervention studies have been carried out in the area of word-finding difficulties. Generally speaking, the therapy techniques have not been selected on the basis of detailed psycholinguistic assessment. The main line of enquiry has been whether semantic therapy or phonological therapy is the most effective for children with word-finding difficulties, with some recent interest in a combination of the two target areas. Some studies tried to make a direct comparison between the two approaches to see which one was most effective (e.g. Wing, 1990; Hyde Wright, Gorrie, et al., 1993). Other studies have evaluated just one approach (e.g. semantic: Haynes, 1992; phonological: McGregor, 1994). More recent studies have looked at combining the two approaches to see whether this is effective (Wittman, 1996; Easton, Sheach and Easton, 1997). Conflicting results have emerged from these studies because the research methodologies varied widely in terms of numbers and ages of children studied, individual differences among the children, and variations in the therapy methods used. However, it is possible to abstract information about the usefulness of different approaches.

Is semantic therapy effective?

It seems logical to focus on building semantic knowledge in therapy when children present with word-finding difficulties, especially when the predominant type of word selection error is semantic. However, Haynes (1992) found little progress in two language-impaired boys aged 10 and 11 years after a month of semantic therapy focusing on semantic elaboration of target words. On the face of it, this might suggest that semantic therapy of this kind is not effective. Haynes points out that this was a small-scale study and many factors could have affected the outcome of the therapy. Vocabulary items were numerous (60), they were selected in a naturalistic rather than a systematic way, and the number of exposures to the words was not controlled. This may be fine for children learning language normally, but children having problems learning new words may need more explicit and structured help to organize and store semantic information for fewer items at a time (see Crystal, 1987 and 1998 for useful discussion of vocabulary teaching).

Another problem is that the therapy was not targeted at the underlying reasons *why* the boys were having word-finding difficulties. Flooding a child with a lot of semantic information is unlikely to help when he is already demonstrating that he cannot learn effectively from naturalistic contexts. It is possible that the two boys had underlying phonological processing problems that were not being addressed by this approach.

Is phonological therapy effective?

McGregor (1994) examined the effect of phonological therapy alone, and found it to be successful in reducing *semantic* word-finding errors in two boys aged 5;0 and 4;9. McGregor began with a psycholinguistic hypothesis about the naming process, based on Caramazza's (1988) work with adult clients. She predicted that a semantic representation will activate all *phonological* representations (motor programs) in the lexicon in proportion to the degree of semantic similarity each has to the target (McGregor, 1994, p.1382). Therefore, when a target item is unavailable because its motor program is underspecified, semantically related items will be competing for activation. If any of those have more accurately specified motor programs, they will be activated and named instead of the target, resulting in a semantic error.

McGregor set out to check this prediction by using phonological elaboration therapy with the two boys to see if strengthening the motor programs (what McGregor calls the phonological output lexicon) would reduce the number of semantic errors. The therapy involved two techniques. First, work was carried out to elaborate the phonological information stored in the motor program. This was achieved by helping the boys to produce both the first sound of each target word, and also the number of syllables in each. Second, retrieval of the items using picture cards was practised. If the boys were unable to name an item, they were encouraged to think of the first sound or the length of the word as a self-cueing strategy. If they could not do this, they were given the information as a cue.

When McGregor reassessed the naming skills of the children after this period of therapy, she found that both the phonological and semantic errors had decreased. McGregor proposed that her therapy was successful because the motor programs were enhanced by the therapy, so target words were more easily activated, and this enhancement caused the activation levels of competing items to be reduced.

In summary, the effectiveness of phonological therapy for a child with word-finding difficulties will depend on the nature of the underlying processing difficulties. McGregor states that her findings show that children with word-finding difficulties may have hidden phonological processing deficits that can respond to therapy. However, she does not advocate that phonological therapy is the only answer. Instead she recommends that children should be helped to "store rich and varied information about target words" (p.1391). Phonological therapy is seen as part of this.

Does a combined semantic and phonological approach to therapy work?

Wittman (1996) used semantic and phonological elaboration techniques to help Martin, a boy aged 9;11 with word-finding difficulties. Although she did not carry out detailed psycholinguistic assessment, she began with psycholinguistic hypotheses, having observed that Martin made semantic errors and used circumlocutions. Problems with semantic representations and the links between these and the motor programs were predicted. Martin also had phonological processing problems in the form of difficulties with rhyme, so both phonological and semantic processing was targeted in therapy.

Two half-hour sessions of semantic therapy and one of phonological therapy were carried out each week. The phonological therapy techniques were similar to those used by McGregor (1994) with games to encourage the child to think about the structure of target words (e.g. number of syllables, initial sound, whether it is long or short). These were also used as cues when the child was trying to name words. For the semantic therapy, target words were discussed according to various semantic features such as word family, function, location and appearance. Guessing games were played whereby the child had to use semantic clues to guess the target word. A strong theme in Wittman's therapy programme was to build Martin's awareness of his difficulties and to encourage him to use the self-cueing strategies available to him. A useful brainstorm of 'what can I do to help myself find the word that I have forgotten' was carried out. There was also close collaboration between parents, teachers and the therapist so that everyone, including Martin, was aware of the objectives for therapy, and regular practice was possible.

After 8 weeks of therapy, Martin had improved by 65 per cent on naming of target words, and by 50 per cent on control (non-targeted) words. However, maintenance of progress over time was inconsistent. This was accounted for by Martin's inability to retain new information without reinforcement. Of particular interest was Martin's ability to retain the semantic cues about the target words, but not the phono-logical cues, again reinforcing the view that phonological processing problems are implicated in word-finding difficulties, even when semantic errors are present. In designing an intervention programme for a child like Martin, it is important to target the underlying phono-logical processing *skills* as well as the lexical representations to try to alleviate the underlying causal factors that are contributing to his problem.

Easton, Sheach and Easton (1997) also carried out a study to evaluate a mixed semantic and phonological therapy programme, this time with four 10-year-old children with word-finding difficulties. They used a standard procedure for therapy for all the children, with a list of 80 words: 40 controls and 40 for treatment. After a pre-therapy naming test of all 80 items, they then carried out two sessions of therapy per week (one with the teacher and the therapist, one with only the teacher) for 5 weeks. The therapy comprised a series of games using cue cards designed to encourage the child to consider the semantic or phonological features of the words being learned (p.31). The children were retested at the end of the 5-week period and again nine weeks after that to examine maintenance of any progress. All four children made progress on the naming tests, with most progress being on the taught items, and less progress and worse maintenance on the control items. As in the study by Wittman above, performance slipped after therapy stopped, but after a further burst of intervention, self-cueing improved. Thus, a mixed semantic and phonological approach to inter-vention can be successful, but ongoing work on maintenance of newly taught information seems crucial for long-term benefit to the child.

4. Compensatory strategies to improve coping behaviour

Cueing strategies

A cue can be the initial sound of a word, or information about the structure of the word such as the number of syllables, or it could be semantic information about the word. A cue can be given as a func-tional aid in a spontaneous interaction when the target is known, or as a therapy tool as a way to enable a child to practise accessing a target word, thereby strengthening the motor program and the ease of retrieval of the word.

Teaching children to use a cueing strategy spontaneously to cue themselves in to the word that they are trying to produce is an important goal in therapy. However, this is only part of an integrated psycholinguistic approach and should take place alongside work targeting the underlying reasons for the word-finding difficulty, particu-larly the accuracy of stored information.

Conversation management

Children with word-finding difficulties can be encouraged to use strategies in conversation that help them to keep the listener's attention while they search for their chosen words. Such strategies include delaying tactics such as the use of phrases like "I'm just thinking of the word I want....", which can be coupled with non-verbal techniques such as maintaining eye contact and not withdrawing physically from the conversation. The child can also be encouraged to try explaining the meaning of the word, or to think of an alternative way of explaining their message. Some children are able to cue themselves into the word they want by thinking of the initial sound of the word, and the number of syllables it contains. This information in itself can help the listener to guess the target. The aim is that such strategies cease to be needed as a child's speech and language processing system becomes more efficient.

Summary

The psycholinguistic approach to assessment and therapy can inform our understanding of word-finding difficulties in children. Recent research has highlighted the role of phonological processing in word-learning and word-finding difficulties. The psycholinguistic approach can be used to guide assessment, to design individually tailored teaching and therapy and to evaluate progress. It can also form the basis for single case studies and intervention studies that will enable us to discover more about the nature of communication disorders in children; in particular how early in a child's development can lexical difficulties be identified, and how and when to provide the most effective intervention.

In this chapter it has been proposed that:

- Word-finding difficulties are not an isolated disorder to be approached separately from the rest of a child's speech and language disorder.
- Word-finding difficulties are a surface manifestation of underlying phonological and/or semantic processing difficulties.
- Word-finding difficulties may be a long-term consequence of phonological processing difficulties, which have knock-on effects throughout the lexicon, as faulty connections are made between different types of information and between different items.
- Children with the same low score on a naming test may have different underlying processing problems.
- Psycholinguistic investigation of speech and language processing provides a way to explore lexical processing abilities in children.

- Effective intervention can be designed on the basis of the individual profile of a child's processing strengths and weaknesses.
- Intervention should aim to improve underlying input and output processing skills, improve memory skills, update the accuracy of lexical representations and encourage use of compensatory strategies to improve coping behaviour.
- Ongoing maintenance of newly learned lexical information via the use of memory strategies, reinforcement and collaboration between carers and professionals is essential for the child to progress in the long term.

KEY TO ACTIVITY 10.1

1, c; 2, a; 3, a; 4, d; 5, c; 6, c; 7, c; 8, b; 9, b; 10, d.

KEY TO ACTIVITY 10.2

SPEECH PROCESSING PROFILE

Name   Michael

Age

Date

Profiler

Comments:

INPUT	OUTPUT

F

Is the child aware of the internal structure of phonological representations?

–

G

Can the child access accurate motor programs?

E

Are the child's phonological representations accurate?

–

H

Can the child manipulate phonological units?

Rhyme Production   × × ×

D

Can the child discriminate between real words?

Bridgeman and Snowling   ✓

I

Can the child articulate real words accurately?

C

Does the child have language-specific representations of word structures?

–

J

Can the child articulate speech without reference to lexical representations?

B

Can the child discriminate speech sounds without reference to lexical representations?

Complex nonwords   ×
(simple nonwords ✓)

A

Does the child have adequate auditory perception?

Hearing acuity   ✓
(NB fluctuating hearing loss)

K

Does the child have adequate sound production skills?

Sounds in isolation   ✓

L

Does the child reject his/her own erroneous forms?

Self corrects   ✓

Figure 10.4: Key to Activity 10.2: Michael's profile after Stage 1 assessments.

KEY TO ACTIVITY 10.3

(1) Does Michael have underlying semantic processing problems? No — at least not uncovered as yet.
(2) Does Michael have underlying phonological processing problems? Yes.

KEY TO ACTIVITY 10.4

SPEECH PROCESSING PROFILE

Name   Michael

Comments:

Age

Date

Profiler

INPUT	OUTPUT

F

Is the child aware of the internal structure of phonological representations?

G

Can the child access accurate motor programs?

(Inaccurate phonological representations and motor programs)   × ×

E

Are the child's phonological representations accurate?

(No – on words he can't name)   ×

H

Can the child manipulate phonological units?

D

Can the child discriminate between real words?

I

Can the child articulate real words accurately?

(Real word repetition)   × ×

C

Does the child have language-specific representations of word structures?

J

Can the child articulate speech without reference to lexical representations?

(Nonword repetition)   × × ×

B

Can the child discriminate speech sounds without reference to lexical representations?

A

Does the child have adequate auditory perception?

K

Does the child have adequate sound production skills?

L

Does the child reject his/her own erroneous forms?

Figure 10.5: Key to Activity 10.4: Michael's profile after Stage 2 of the assessment.

Chapter 11
Intonation Within a Psycholinguistic Framework

BILL WELLS AND SUE PEPPÉ

The main focus of the framework presented in Book 1 (Stackhouse and Wells, 1997) is children's phonological difficulties at the segmental level, and the links between underlying processing deficits and literacy development. However, there is more to phonological development than the development of segmental systems and structures. Prosodic systems and structures also play a key role in spoken language: as part of the phonology, they mediate between the phonetic substance of speech on the one hand, and on the other a wide range of lexical, grammatical and pragmatic functions. Prosody is used here to refer to systems realized by means of variations in pitch, loudness, duration, rhythm, tempo and silence.

In this chapter, we shall present data from two 8-year-old boys, Jonathan and Robin, and compare their pattern of performance on various prosodic tasks against data from a recent normative study of supralexical prosodic development (Wells and Peppé, 1999). Both children have been identified as having language difficulties serious enough to warrant special educational provision. Both met the criteria for inclusion in our study of prosodic ability in children with speech and language difficulties:

(a) age 8;0–8;11;
(b) English the first language and the language of the home;
(c) no behavioural/learning or hearing difficulties;
(d) speech/language problems identified on either the *Test for the Reception of Grammar* (*TROG*; Bishop, 1989) or the *Clinical Evaluation of Language Fundamentals – Revised* (*CELF-R*; Semel, Wiig and Secord, 1987).

Unusual prosodic output was not in itself a requirement for selection to the study, since the aim was to investigate whether prosodic deficits, either of output or of input, are present in children who have been diagnosed as having speech and/or language impairments by conventional criteria.

366

Jonathan: Background Information

Jonathan lives in London. He was delayed in his early language development, beginning to use expressive language only around 5 years of age. Now, however, Jonathan's speech and language therapist reports that, at CA 8;11, he is very chatty and communicative: he is able to talk about past and future, his own experiences, to ask questions, and to interact well with other children. While he has no obvious segmental speech errors, he makes grammatical errors, e.g. in past tense formation, pronouns, prepositions. He also has problems with comprehension. His attention can be very good in a small group, but he experiences difficulties in larger groups. Jonathan's recent performance on standard assessments is summarized in Table 11.1.

Table 11.1: Assessment results for Jonathan at 8;4 – 8;11

Assessment	CA	Results
Test for the Reception of Grammar (Bishop, 1989)	8;4	Raw score:11 Centile: 5 Age-equivalent: 5;6
Renfrew Action Picture Test (Renfrew, 1989)	8;4	*Content*: age-appropriate *Grammar*: age-equivalent 5
Weschter Intelligence Scales block design	8;11	Raw score: 16; Scaled score: 6
Clinical Evaluation of Language Fundamentals – *Revised*: Sentence formulation (Semel, Wiig and Secord, 1987)	8;11	Raw score: 1 Centile: 2
Renfrew Word-finding Vocabulary Scale (Renfrew, 1972)	8;4	Age-equivalent: 6

In Transcript 11.1 is an impressionistic prosodic transcription of Jonathan (J) in free conversation with the researcher (S). See Appendix 1, Book 1 for conventions of prosodic notation.

The following observations were made of Jonathan's prosody, compared to normally developing children of a similar age:

(i)   many syllables are unusually loud;
(ii) English speakers normally use on-syllable pitch movements, at the end of utterances; Jonathan more often has level pitch (e.g. "likes it"), or moves rapidly from one level to another ("nice"; "fishcake");
(iii) his speech is slow overall;
(iv) he lengthens vowels very noticeably in the final syllables of his utterances.

Transcript 11.1: Jonathan

```
S:    right
```

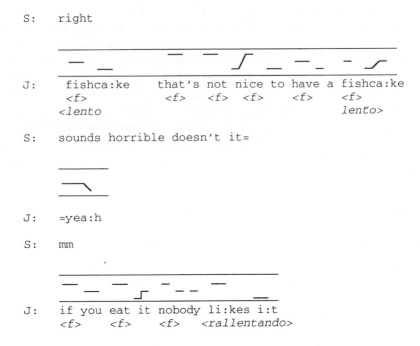

```
J:    fishca:ke      that's not nice to have a fishca:ke
      <f>            <f>  <f>  <f>     <f>     <f>
      <lento                                  lento>

S:    sounds horrible doesn't it=
```

```
J:    =yea:h

S:    mm
```

```
J:    if you eat it nobody li:kes i:t
      <f>     <f>    <f>       <rallentando>
```

Jonathan's speech has a 'sing-song' character, deriving from his pervasive use of level pitch, as well as sustained vowels in some positions (as opposed to dynamic falls and rises). This intonation was regarded as unusual by his parents, as well as by professionals and others outside the family. They noted that this feature started some time after his seventh birthday, and had become increasingly evident.

Robin: Background Information

Robin lives in Kent, in the south east of England. At CA 8;4, his speech and language therapist describes him as having a severe-moderate language disorder, but notes that he has made significant progress over the preceding 12 months, making crucial steps in developing an understanding of the use and importance of language; during the last year he has made an average of 12 months, progress on key measures of language. He has no obvious segmental speech difficulties. The therapist's main concern now is with his social skills: he finds activities such as turn-taking, requesting and compromising very difficult, possibly as a result of his growing awareness of his own language difficulties.

Table 11.2: Assessment results for Robin at age CA 8;1–8;4

Assessment	CA	Results
Test for the Reception of Grammar (Bishop, 1989)	8;1	Raw score:11 Centile: 5 Age-equivalent: 5;6
Renfrew Action Picture Test (Renfrew, 1989)	8;1	*Content*: age-equivalent 5;6. *Grammar*: age-equivalent 4;6
Weschter Intelligence Scales block design	8;4	Raw score: 21 Scaled score: 8
Clinical Evaluation of Language Fundamentals — *Revised*: Sentence formulation (Semel, Wiig and Secord, 1987)	8;4	Raw score: 20 Centile: 2
British Picture Vocabulary Scales (Dunn, Dunn, Whetton, et al., 1982)	8;4	Centile: 9

An impressionistic prosodic transcription from Robin (R) retelling the *Bus Story* (Renfrew, 1991) is presented in Transcript 11.2.

In Robin's speech there are no strikingly unusual prosodic features. For instance, the main falling pitch movements coincide with a loudness peak and occur on the word containing new information, towards the end of the utterance. e.g. "tired", "fence", "cow". This is typical for speakers of his variety of southern British English. With syntax and vocabulary he has problems of formulation, e.g. use of "through" in the last line – but the prosody appears to be done appropriately.

The features we have noted were typical of the conversational speech of each child at this point in time. Our description of their prosody gives rise to various questions. For example: why does Jonathan sound as he does? why do Jonathan and Robin sound so different, given their comparable performance on other language assessments?

We can formulate our questions in more psycholinguistic terms:

(a) In a child like Jonathan, with overtly atypical prosody, where might the 'deficit' be? Input? Representation? Output? If at Output (for example) – at what level on the speech processing framework?

(b) In the case of children like Robin who do not have overtly atypical prosody – could there be underlying intonational difficulties that might be linked to their receptive language deficits?

In order to investigate these questions, we adopt a systematic approach that parallels the assessment framework for lexical-segmental phonology presented in Book 1.

Transcript 11.2: Robin

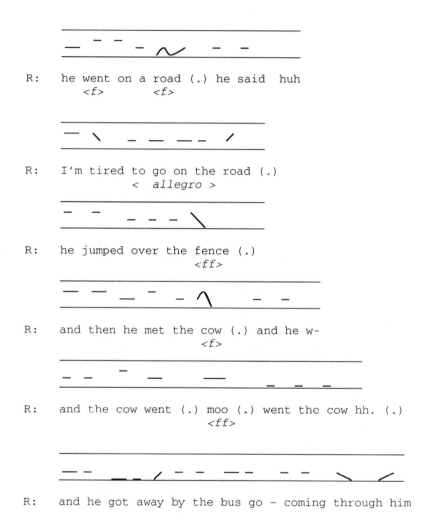

R: he went on a road (.) he said   huh
          <f>   <f>

R: I'm tired to go on the road (.)
                < allegro >

R: he jumped over the fence (.)
                            <ff>

R: and then he met the cow (.) and he w–
                        <f>

R: and the cow went (.) moo (.) went the cow hh. (.)
                            <ff>

R: and he got away by the bus go – coming through him

Theoretical Background

In order to identify the role of prosody in language development and elucidate the ways in which it may be implicated in children's speech and language difficulties, it is helpful to make a broad distinction between *lexical* and *supralexical* prosody. Supralexical prosody is used here to refer to intonational and accentual structures and systems operating at a domain greater than the word. Their phonetic exponents principally involve pitch, loudness, duration, rhythm, tempo and silence. Supralexical prosody is distinct from lexical prosodic systems such as word stress and tone, in terms of its domain, though not always in terms of its exponents. For example, word stress in English, like supralexical accentuation, is realized by means of prominence of pitch, loudness and duration, along with other features such as vowel quality. This overlap of exponency can give rise to analytical problems in distinguishing between lexical and supralexical prosodic systems, particularly when studying speakers other than typical adults, such as young children, and people with speech and/or language difficulties.

From a practical point of view, there is a lack of procedures available to researchers and practitioners for assessing children's supralexical prosodic development in comparison to their normally developing peers. This is an unfortunate gap. On the input side, in any test of spoken language comprehension, the items have to be presented with intonation patterns of some kind. While this is self-evident, it has to be said that intonation is rarely controlled for in test administration in a systematic, linguistically informed way. It is conceivable that some children fail on tests of grammatical comprehension because of difficulties in processing prosodic aspects of the input. This would be predicted by the prosodic bootstrapping hypothesis, which proposes that prosodic factors, particularly the prosodic processing of spoken language input, may be crucial to the development of other levels of linguistic organization, such as syntax and morphology, in normally developing children (Morgan and Demuth, 1996).

Apart from grammar, tests have been devised to target comprehension of more pragmatic aspects of language, such as discourse cohesion, narrative, inference and interactional aspects, and it has been shown that some children with language difficulties have particular problems with comprehension at this level (Bishop, 1997, Chapters 7 and 8). However, there are, to the best of our knowledge, no published tests that can be administered to see whether some children have a specific prosodic deficit that might, in turn, be implicated in more general pragmatic or grammatical comprehension difficulties.

Outside the test situation, a child's difficulties in interpreting intonation can be predicted to give rise to problems in social interaction – for example:

(a) in knowing whether the other speaker is finishing or projecting further talk;
(b) in interpreting a speaker's emotional meaning (Courtright and Courtright, 1983);

c)   in identifying the word in the utterance that is being emphasized or topicalized (Highnam and Morris, 1987; Wells, Peppé and Vance, 1995).

It is therefore important to establish whether or not a child has difficulties in making sense of intonation.

Turning now to production, it can be predicted that expressive prosodic difficulties may give rise to pragmatic difficulties in conversation and other forms of spoken interaction, given that the functions of prosody, particularly intonation, include the conveying of interactional and affective meaning. Unusual supralexical prosody has been described in people with a range of developmental disorders, including: autism (Baltaxe and Simmons, 1985; Local and Wootton, 1995); specific delays or disorders in speech and language development (Hargrove and Sheran, 1989; Wells and Local, 1993; Wells, 1994; Wells, Peppé and Vance, 1995; Shriberg, Aram and Kwiatowski, 1997); developmental learning disorders such as Down's syndrome (Heselwood, Bray and Crookston, 1995), and in prelingual deafness (Parker and Rose, 1990). A more detailed understanding of atypical development of supralexical prosody may open the way to more effective speech and language therapy and educational provision for such children. One of the obstacles to this is the lack of systematic data about normal intonational development. Several important studies have looked at particular aspects (Cruttenden, 1985; Cutler and Swinney, 1987; Snow, 1998) – but we lack the bigger picture.

PEPS-C: An Assessment Package for Prosodic Development

In order to make progress in our understanding of these issues, particularly in relation to school-age children with communication difficulties, we have devised a set of tasks for assessing children's intonation. The battery, PEPS-C, has been developed from a procedure for testing adults: Profiling Elements of Prosodic Systems — PEPS (Peppé, 1998; Peppé, Maxim and Wells, in press). The assessment package is constructed in terms of a psycholinguistic framework along the lines of the one presented in Book 1. It incorporates the following two dimensions:

Input (perception / comprehension) vs Output (generation / production).
Form (referring to bottom-up, phonetic processing, where meaning is not involved) vs Function (involving top-down processing, drawing on stored knowledge, relating phonetic form to meaning).

These are displayed in Figure 11.1, which parallels Figure 1.7 from Chapter 1 of this volume.

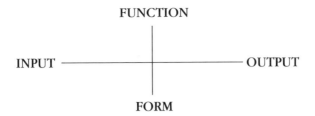

Figure 11.1: Dimensions of the PEPS-C psycholinguistic framework.

Supralexical prosody is involved in a wide range of more or less well defined *communicative areas*; for PEPS-C, we selected four communicative areas where intonation is generally agreed to have an important role.

1. Chunking

'Chunking' refers to prosodic delimitation of the utterance into units for grammatical, semantic or pragmatic purposes. This distinction can be appreciated by reading the following pair of utterances aloud, emphasizing the syllables underlined:

/CHOCOLATE-CAKE /AND HONEY/ vs /CHOCOLATE/ CAKE /AND HONEY/.

2. Affect

As an instantiation of the use of prosody to convey affective or attitudinal meaning, we use the distinction between expressing strong liking as opposed to reservation. This distinction can be expressed with the syllable "MM", by using rise-fall (∧) vs fall–rise (∨) pitch movement respectively:

/ ∧ MM/ vs / ∨ MM/.

3. Interaction

In order to assess the role of prosody in interaction, we have chosen the prosodic opposition between a low fall (0), meaning "yes I understand"; as opposed to a high rise (′), meaning "no I didn't understand, please repeat".

/ 0 CAKE / vs / ′ CAKE /.

This distinction between confirming an understanding vs checking an understanding is a rather specific, well-attested instantiation of the broad (but often inaccurate) generalization that statements are realized with falling pitch and questions with rising pitch.

4. Focus

Focus refers to the speaker's use of phonetic prominence to indicate which item is most important in an utterance. The distinction can be appreciated by reading the following pair of phrases aloud, emphasizing the syllables underlined:

/CHOCOLATE AND HONEY/ vs /CHOCOLATE AND HONEY/.

Figure 11.2 summarizes the structure of the PEPS assessment battery. Each of the four communicative areas is tested for both Input and Output, with different assessments for Form and for Function. This gives a total of 16 subtests.

The performance of Jonathan and Robin on PEPS-C will be compared to the performance of two groups of children: 30 5-year-olds (mean CA 5;6) and 30 8-year-olds (mean CA 8;7), taken from a study of prosodic ability in school-age children (Wells and Peppé, 1998). The children had no behavioural, learning or hearing difficulties, no identified speech and language problems and had English as their first language and the language of the home.

All children were tested on the following:

(a) PEPS-C: for prosody;
(b) *TROG*: for grammatical comprehension;
(c) *CELF-R* sentence formulation: for expressive language.

COMMUNICATIVE AREA	PROCESSING LEVEL	INPUT	OUTPUT
Chunking	Function Form		
Affect	Function Form		
Interaction	Function Form		
Focus	Function Form		

Figure 11.2: Structure of PEPS-C assessment battery.

The procedure consisted of individual tape-recorded interviews, each session lasting generally no longer than 30 minutes; with a maximum of three sessions per participant. Stimuli for the input subtests had been pre-recorded on digital audio-tape (DAT) in a recording studio. The stimuli were presented to participants via tape-recorder in free field, and responses were recorded on DAT. Practice items were given for all tasks, and a check was made that the child knew the vocabulary used in PEPS-C.

In this section, the tasks are grouped according to the two dimensions of the PEPS-C psycholinguistic framework (see Figure 11.1). We present results for Jonathan and Robin, and from the 5-year-olds and the 8-year-olds from the normative study. We then interpret the results in terms of the processing framework.

Input Form

The Input Form task for each of the four communicative areas comprises a 'same–different' test consisting of 16 test items. Each stimulus pair derives from the functional contrast associated with the particular communicative area, as already described. However, instead of hearing the intonation contour associated with an intelligible phrase (as above), the child is presented with stimuli in a form where the lexical and grammatical information is not audible. The stimuli in fact consist of the laryngograph signal only, from pairs of spoken utterances. Pitch, loudness and length variations are preserved: the result is a 'buzz' – not dissimilar to listening to a speaker in an adjacent room, where the intonation is audible but not the content of the utterance.

Chunking

The reader can gain an idea of what the stimuli sound like, in this case for Chunking, by humming the following pairs of utterances, emphasizing the portions underlined:

A 'different' pair:
/CHOCOLATE-CAKE /AND HONEY/
/CHOCOLATE/ CAKE /AND HONEY/.

A 'same' pair:
/CHOCOLATE-CAKE /AND HONEY/
/CHOCOLATE-CAKE /AND HONEY/.

ACTIVITY 11.1

Aim: to analyse the processing skills demanded by the PEPS-C Input Form tasks.

Identify the speech processing skills that the child needs in order to succeed on the Chunking Input Form task that has just been described. Referring to the speech processing profile in Appendix 1, identify which of the questions A – L on the profile sheet is being addressed by this task. Check your answer against Key to Activity 11.1 at the end of the chapter, then read on.

You may have decided that the task addresses *question A: Does the child have adequate auditory perception?* on the grounds that the stimuli are not linguistic. However, the stimuli, though non-linguistic in the sense of having no lexical or grammatical content, are linguistic in that they incorporate prosodic patterns that are specific to language. In fact, they are specific to English, since intonation systems differ from language to language. A purer prosodic test for question A might involve non-linguistic stimuli that tap into pitch discrimination, duration discrimination or loudness discrimination, as in a test of musical abilities.

The Chunking Input Form task is more appropriately assigned to *question B: Can the child discriminate speech sounds without reference to lexical representations?* This is because the contrast of prosodic contours is a contrast of 'speech sounds' in the same way as the contrast between, for example, voiced and voiceless plosives in a non-word discrimination task (cf. Book 1, pp.35–37).

The Input Form tasks for the remaining three communicative areas are very similar, in that they are all same–different tasks, and all use stimulus pairs consisting of laryngograph signals, producing a 'buzz' without any discernible words.

Affect

The contrast is between rise–fall vs fall–rise pitch on a monosyllable. Pairs of stimuli may be the same (both rise–fall, both fall–rise); or different (rise–fall followed by fall–rise, or vice versa).

Interaction

The contrast is between low fall vs high rise pitch, each pitch pattern being realized on a single syllable. Pairs of stimuli may be the same (both low fall, both high rise); or different (low fall followed by high rise, or vice versa).

Focus

In the 'different' pairs, the variable is the position of the main prosodic prominence. You can get an idea of the stimuli by humming the following, emphasizing the syllables underlined:

/CHOCOLATE AND HONEY/ vs /CHOCOLATE AND HONEY/.

One difference between the four Input Form tasks is stimulus length. Each item for Chunking consists of four to six syllables, for Focus four or five syllables, but for Affect and Interaction, each pair item is just one syllable in length. The Chunking and Focus tasks, while addressing the same level of processing as the Affect and Interaction tasks, will thus put greater demands on the child's working memory (cf. Book 1, p.36).

A further difference is in the phonetic contrast that is being targeted. The Chunking task contrasts the number of accents (points of prosodic prominence) in an utterance; the Focus task contrasts different accent locations; while the Affect task contrasts different types of complex pitch movement and the Interaction task contrasts types of simple pitch movement (rise vs. fall) combined with pitch height (high vs low). The differences are analogous to the differences between various segmental nonword auditory discrimination tasks that have been devised: one task may focus on sequential ordering across syllable position, e.g. 'IKIBUS vs. 'IBIKUS (Book 1, pp.29–30); another might focus on sequential ordering within syllable position e.g. VOST vs VOTS (Bridgeman and Snowling, 1988); yet another might focus on contrasts between similar clusters, or on contrasts between single vowels or consonants (e.g. VOSS vs VOT).

Results of performance on the Input Form tasks

Table 11.3 presents results for the four Input Form tasks. There were 16 items in the task; in this and subsequent tables of results, all scores are converted to percentages. In addition to results from Jonathan and Robin, there are the results from the group of 8-year-old normally developing children, including means, standard deviations (SD) and ranges. These are the data against which Jonathan and Robin are compared, to ascertain whether they have age-appropriate ability. We take a score of 1.5 SD below the mean as a cut-off point, and this score is also presented in the table. We consider a child to be below age-appropriate ability if the child's score is less than this; such scores are marked *. A score of more than 2.5 SD below the mean is indicated by **. As Robin's and Jonathan's receptive language levels are equivalent to normally developing 5-year olds (see Tables 11.1 and 11.2 above), we also present PEPS data from the 5-year-old normally developing group, so that one can see whether Robin and Jonathan are more in line with 'language age' peers, rather than chronological age peers.

Table 11.3: Performance of Jonathan and Robin on Input Form tasks, compared to controls (see text for explanation)

Task	Mean (5yr)	SD (5yr)	Range (5yr)	1.5 SD (5yr)	Mean (8yr)	SD (8yr)	Range (8yr)	1.5 SD (8yr)	Jonathan	Robin
Chunking	71.1	18	25–100	44.1	88.3	10.7	62.5–100	72.25	62.5*	87.5
Affect	63.7	21.8	31.3–100	31	78.3	19.3	37.5–100	49.4	68.8	100
Interaction	65.3	20.3	25–100	34.85	79.8	18.8	37.5–100	51.6	75	87.5
Focus	66.3	15.0	43.8–100	43.8	86.4	13.5	56.3–100	66.15	68.8	81.3

Jonathan

The only communicative area that causes Jonathan difficulties is Chunking. This may be due to stimulus length, or to his not understanding input form tasks immediately: Chunking was the first input form task that he was presented with. Initially it appeared that he had no idea what to do, but after 10 items he tuned in. Thereafter he scored within normal limits and seemed to enjoy the tasks, even though these are in some respects the most demanding of the PEPS-C battery, requiring a good deal of attention and concentration.

Robin

Robin scored within normal limits on all four tasks. This suggests that he does not have specific difficulty with discriminating prosodic patterns without reference to higher-level linguistic knowledge.

Input Function

Function tasks, unlike the Form tasks, explicitly involve meaning. They are designed as identification tasks: the child hears a spoken stimulus, and has to assign it to one of two meaning categories.

Chunking

In the Chunking task, the instructions are as follows (again, the underlined syllables are emphasized):

> "Listen to this. This sounds like two pictures: [TAPE: FRUIT-SALAD AND MILK]. This sounds like three pictures: [TAPE: FRUIT, SALAD AND MILK]. You'll hear some more lists like that. If you think a list sounds like three pictures, say 'Three'. If you think it sounds like two pictures, say 'Two' "

ACTIVITY 11.2

Aim: to analyse the processing skills demanded by the PEPS-C Input Function tasks.

Identify the speech processing skills that the child needs in order to succeed on the Chunking Input Function task that has just been described. Referring to the speech processing profile in Appendix 1, identify which of the questions A – L on the profile sheet is being addressed by this task. Check your answer against Key to Activity 11.2 at the end of the chapter, then read on.

The child has to decode the segmental phonological information (Phonological Recognition) and map it on to appropriate lexical items and the appropriate *number* of lexical items, using intonation. The first two words may form separate nouns with two separate accents (CHOCOLATE, BISCUITS...) or they may make up a compound noun with a single accent (CHOCOLATE-BISCUITS). To do this successfully, the child needs to have prior language-specific knowledge of how accentuation is used for lexical/grammatical chunking; and s/he needs to be able to access that knowledge appropriately in response to the spoken stimuli. This corresponds to question E on the profile: *Are the child's phono-logical representations accurate?* For example, without an accurate prosodic phonological representation of CHOCOLATE-BISCUITS, the child may mistake it for the string CHOCOLATE, BISCUITS... .

The Input Function tasks for the other three communicative areas resemble the Chunking task in that they require the child to associate the utterance heard with the correct one of two alternative meanings. However, the type of stored knowledge that needs to be accessed is rather different.

Affect

In the Affect task, the child has to map the pitch contour on to the appropriate affective meaning (i.e. 'liking' vs 'reservation') without any lexical involvement, as the tones are carried on the syllable MM. Liking is conveyed by a rise–fall pitch, reservation by a fall-rise. In this task a soft toy seal serves as a prop. The instructions are as follows. The child is shown two pictures:

> "Here's a smiley face and a doubtful face: somebody really enjoying himself and somebody who's not too sure if he's enjoying himself. Now, we want to find out what Seal likes. She's quite unusual for a seal, because she eats lots of the same kind of food that we eat. Look at these pictures and tell me what you see on the first one (CAKE). Seal really likes cake, so she makes a noise like this [Tape: ∧ M]. She never goes 'ugh', [done with low falling pitch] as if she hates it, but sometimes she sounds as though she doesn't *really* like it. Say the next picture (TEA). She doesn't *really* like tea so she goes like this [Tape: ∨ M]. You go through the pictures, one by one, saying what there is, and as you say each one, Seal will make a noise to show whether she likes it or not really. If you think she likes it, give me the picture of the smiley face here. If you think she doesn't *really* like it, give me the doubtful face."

Interaction

The prosodic distinction for Interaction is between a low fall, meaning "yes I understood, go on to the next one"; or a high rise, meaning "no

I didn't understand, please repeat". In the Interaction Input Function task, the child is given a set of pictures, bound together, each depicting a single object, e.g. CUP, KEY. The tester has a small folder to use as a screen. The instructions are as follows:

> "Now you're going to tell me what you see in these pictures and this time you have to listen to what I say. If I sound as though I heard what you said, you go on to the next picture. If I sound as though I didn't hear you, or as though I want you to say it again, you say it again. You don't go on to the next picture until you hear me sound quite certain. You may have to say some pictures quite a few times before I sound as though I want you to go on to the next. I'm going to put this screen up so you can't see from my face if I look as though I heard what you said.
> Let's start with the book with the cup on it. You say what you see."
> Child says " Cup". Tester repeats the word with a low falling pitch: "Cup". Child goes to next picture: " Key" . Tester repeats with high rising pitch: "Key?" Child repeats: "Key".

Focus

The Focus task taps into a pragmatic use of accentuation. The tester has two puppets, a seal and a mouse. There is also a set of pictures, each representing two items of food. The instructions are as follows:

> "Look at those two pictures [on the first card]. Seal wanted these two things to eat [STRAWBERRIES and CREAM] and Mouse went to get them. Mouse forgot to bring one of the things, and Seal said this:
> Play tape: 'I WANTED STRAWBERRIES AND CREAM'
> That means Mouse forgot the strawberries. He went away and tried again, but again he forgot one thing, and Seal said this:
> Play: 'I WANTED STRAWBERRIES AND CREAM'
> That means he'd forgotten the cream.
> [similar demonstration with the next card (CHOCOLATE AND CAKE)]."

Prosodic prominence serves to focus on the item of food that the imagined interlocutor had forgotten, possibly in order to initiate a repair. The child has to be able to identify which of the two food items is being made phonetically prominent, then map it on to the meaning of accentuation in this context, which is to draw attention to a specific item in the utterance.

Results of performance on the Input Function tasks

Table 11.4 summarizes the performance of Jonathan and Robin on the Input Function tasks, compared to the two control groups. The conventions used are as for Table 11.3.

Table 11.4: Performance of Jonathan and Robin on Input Function tasks, compared to controls

Task	Mean (5yr)	SD (5yr)	Range (5yr)	1.5 SD (5yr)	Mean (8yr)	SD (8yr)	Range (8yr)	1.5 SD (8yr)	Jonathan	Robin
Chunking	75	14.5	43.8–94	53.25	82.5	13.2	50–100	62.7	56.3*	87.5
Affect	85.9	17.9	37.5–100	59.05	94.6	8	62.5–100	82.6	93.8	75*
Interaction	70	23.2	31.3–100	35.2	90.2	17.3	31.3–100	64.25	62.5*	37.5**
Focus	49.7	14.0	31.3–93.8	28.7	67.6	19.3	37.5–100	38.65	56.3	31.3*

Jonathan

Jonathan fell below 1.5 SD on the Chunking and Interaction tasks, but was within normal limits on Affect and Focus. There is no obvious explanation for this dissociation, which will be discussed later in the context of his overall profile.

Robin

Robin fell below 1.5 SD on Affect, Interaction and Focus, but was within normal limits for Chunking. Chunking is the most grammatical use of intonation in PEPS-C: the other three areas relate more to pragmatics. This pattern of results on the Input Function tasks suggests that Robin may be having difficulty in interpreting the pragmatic meanings of intonation. This is unlikely to be due to difficulties at the perceptual level, as we have already seen that he was successful on all four Input Form tasks.

One of the characteristics of intonational phonology is 'one-to-many' mapping: an intonational pattern, such as fall–rise pitch movement (used here in the Affect task) has the potential to take on a range of different meanings according to context. This is equally true of accentuation in the Focus task; and fall vs rising pitch in the Interaction task. The nuances of meaning may be acquired only gradually – a hypothesis that is supported by the results of our normative study, which shows that some aspects of intonation continue to develop at least to age 11 years (Wells and Peppé, 1998); and also by other research (e.g. Cruttenden, 1985). In this respect, the development of intonation resembles that of vocabulary: the various meanings or nuances of meaning of a single word are learnt gradually.

Output Function

Each output task consists of twelve items. On the Output side, as for Input, the Function tasks explicitly involve meaning.

Chunking

In the Chunking tasks, pictures are used: the child has a pile of picture strips, each of which depicts either two items of food (e.g. FRUIT-SALAD, MILK) or three items (e.g. FRUIT, SALAD, MILK). The child picks up one picture strip, unseen by the tester, and tells the tester what is on it. The tester notes down whether the child sounded as though s/he was talking about two items of food or three, and then checks by looking at the picture strip. When scoring, the tester compares what the response sounded like with the contents of the picture strip itself; thus the child is assessed on whether or not s/he can realize his/her communicative intention.

ACTIVITY 11.3

Aim: to analyse the processing skills demanded by the PEPS-C Output Function tasks.

Identify the speech processing skills that the child needs in order to succeed on the Chunking Output Function task that has just been described. Referring to the speech processing profile in Appendix 1, identify which of the questions A – L on the profile sheet is being addressed by this task. Check your answer against Key to Activity 11.3 at the end of the chapter, then read on.

The child has to access the correct lexical items (either two or three, depending on the card) and select the appropriate intonational contour from his/her store of contours – e.g. for FRUIT-SALAD AND MILK, a contour that includes an accent for FRUIT-SALAD and another for MILK; then map the contour on to the words appropriately, so that the accents are correctly positioned (on -SALAD and on MILK). The child then needs to implement the appropriate motor commands to ensure that both the segmental string and the prosodic contour are realized accurately and integrated in terms of their timing.

In terms of the speech processing profile, the task addresses *question G: Can the child access accurate motor programs?* The programs here include both segmental and prosodic aspects, i.e. the specification for the accentual pattern of FRUIT-SALAD. The other three Function Output tasks aim to tap into a similar processing level.

Affect

In the Affect task the child has two choice cards (smiley face and doubtful face). The instructions are as follows:

> "Now I want to know what food you like and what you're not too keen on. I'm going to read out things one by one like you did, and if you really like it, go '∧ MM' like Seal did and give me the smiley face card. If you're not too keen, go '∨ MM' and give me the doubtful face card. Here's the first one: BANANAS."

To succeed on this task, having decided whether or not s/he likes bananas, the child has to access the appropriate contour (rise–fall or fall–rise) from his/her intonation store; and then realize it on the syllable MM. The tester has access to the child's intention because the child has to hand over either a smiley face or a doubtful face. In this way the child's ability to realize his/her communicative intention via intonation can be assessed. The items in the intonation store can be thought of as pre-learnt motor programs for intonation, equivalent to the motor programs for words described in Book 1 (p.162).

Interaction

In the Interaction task, the child hears a list of words and is required to repeat the word with an appropriate intonation. A given word may be familiar, e.g. CARROT, in which case the child repeats the word in such a way as to acknowledge that it has been understood, e.g. with a falling pitch contour. Alternatively, the word may be unfamiliar, e.g. PARGLE, in which case the child should query it – for example by using a rising intonation. As in the Affect task, the child has to access the appropriate contour, and realize it.

Focus

The Focus task taps into the child's ability to use accent placement in order to focus on a specific item in the utterance for the purposes of repair. It takes the form of a lotto game, in which the child is offered a picture that does not match the ones s/he has; the child asks for a different picture, emphasizing the thing that differentiates the picture the child wants from the one that had been offered. The instructions are as follows:

"Here is a card with four pictures on it. I can't see which pictures they are, but I'm going to offer you ones that might match them. How about A GREEN CAR? Now you've got a green car so you say 'Oh I want a green car'. Now you take it and put it face down on your green car, so it's covered up.
How about A GREEN BIKE?
You haven't got a green bike but you've got a bike in another colour, so you say
'Oh, I want a white bike'.
And I give you a white bike and you put it on your picture.
Then I might say How about A BLACK BOAT? (showing them one).
Now you haven't got a black boat but you've got something else black, a bus, so you say
'Oh I want a black bus' and I'll give you a black bus.
Now you try it."

The child's response is scored as correct if the main point of prosodic prominence in his/her response coincides with the new information, as in the above examples.

Results of performance on the Output Function tasks

Table 11.5 summarizes the performance of Jonathan and Robin on the Output Function tasks, compared to the two control groups. The conventions used are as for Table 11.3.

Jonathan

Jonathan fell below 1.5 SD on the Chunking, Focus and Interaction tasks, but was within normal limits on Affect – in fact he was at ceiling on this task. This discrepancy may be related to the fact that in the Affect task, the response does not involve any lexical material: the pitch has to be produced on the syllable 'mm'. This suggests that Jonathan's difficulties with Output Function may in part stem from a difficulty in mapping the prosodic tune on to the segmental text.

Robin

Robin fell below 1.5 SD on the Interaction task, but was within normal limits on Chunking, Focus and Affect. This suggests that he has an appropriate store of prosodic contours, and is able to access them and realize them appropriately. It is interesting to note that for Affect and Focus, he was within normal limits on the Output Function subtest, but not on the equivalent Input Function subtest. This indicates that he may be able to function appropriately enough in terms of his own speech output, but that this may conceal his imperfect understanding of what the intonation of his interlocutors means.

Output Form

The Output Form tasks involve repetition. The instructions for all four tasks are: "You'll hear some words on the tape, and I want you to copy them, saying them in exactly the same way as you heard them said on tape". For the Form tasks, digits were used, since their semantic representations, motor programs and articulatory routines at the segmental level were assumed to be familiar to children. It was assumed that there would therefore be less semantic and segmental phonological interference in the task.

Chunking

For Chunking, each item is a string of digits, e.g. FORTY, TWO, ONE; or: FORTY-TWO, ONE. In terms of the prosodic phrasing involved, these correspond to Function task items such as /CHOCOLATE/ CAKE /AND HONEY/ or /CHOCOLATE-CAKE /AND HONEY/.

Table 11.5: Results of Output Function tasks

Task	Mean (5yr)	SD (5yr)	Range (5yr)	1.5 SD (5yr)	Mean (8yr)	SD (8yr)	Range (8yr)	1.5 SD (8yr)	Jonathan	Robin
Chunking	81	15.3	45.8–100	58.05	78.1	13.4	54.2–100	58	54.2*	83.3
Affect	71.8	24.8	16.7–100	34.6	84.7	18.1	50–100	57.55	100	95.8
Interaction	68.3	20	25–100	38.3	85.8	17.9	29.2–100	58.95	54.2*	29.2**
Focus	83.6	9.5	62.5–100	69.35	88.0	8.6	70.8–100	75.1	41.7**	83.3

ACTIVITY 11.4

Aim: to analyse the processing skills demanded by the PEPS-C Output Form tasks.

Identify the speech processing skills that the child needs in order to succeed on the Chunking Output Form task that has just been described. Referring to the speech processing profile in Appendix 1, identify which of the questions A – L on the profile sheet is being addressed by this task.

Check your answer against Key to Activity 11.4 at the end of the chapter, then read on.

The Output Form tasks parallel real word repetition (as discussed in Book 1, p.41): the child may, but does not have to, access lexical representations and intonational representations in order to produce an accurate response. It thus addresses *question I: Can the child articulate real words accurately?* with the proviso that 'real words' should be modified to 'real utterances'.

Affect

The Affect task requires the child to repeat a single word (e.g. GOOD; OH) with a fall–rise or a rise–fall.

Interaction

The Interaction task is similar, except the intonation is either a rise or a fall.

Focus

In the Focus task, the child repeats a string of three digits. Different items have different accentual patterns, i.e. a different digit is made prominent, e.g. THREE TWO ONE; or THREE TWO ONE.

Results of performance on the Output Form tasks

Table 11.6 summarizes the performance of Jonathan and Robin on the Output Form tasks, compared to the two control groups. The conventions used are as for Table 11.3.

Table 11.6: Results of Output Form tasks

Task	Mean (5yr)	SD (5yr)	Range (5yr)	1.5 SD (5yr)	Mean (8yr)	SD (8yr)	Range (8yr)	1.5 SD (8yr)	Jonathan	Robin
Chunking	76.9	20.7	43.8–94	45.9	93.3	13.5	50–100	73.05	50**	50**
Affect	64.8	23.1	20.8–100	30.15	86.3	16.3	33.3–100	61.85	58.3*	58.3*
Interaction	76.2	18.3	41.7–100	48.75	85.8	17	37.5–100	60.3	58.3*	70.8
Focus	94.7	7.3	79.2–100	83.75	91.2	7.3	75–100	80.25	87.5	70.8**

Jonathan

Jonathan fell below 1.5 SD on Chunking, Affect and Interaction. This is not particularly surprising, given the unusual prosodic patterning in his spontaneous speech. It suggests that, in part at least, his unusual prosodic output may be due to lower-level difficulties in controlling prosody. However, this evidence is not completely conclusive. The Form Output tasks involve *linguistic* forms (numbers), so it is possible that deficits in higher-level knowledge (evident in the Function tasks) are interfering with his performance on this Form task. In order to identify a deficit at the level of motor execution, it would be necessary to test imitation of non-linguistic pitch features.

Jonathan failed to use lengthening and pausing in the Chunking Output Form task to convey the difference between such number sequences as TWENTY, NINE, TWO and TWENTY-NINE, TWO. His speech in this task demonstrated clearly his tendency to syllable-timing and how it obliterates the function of differential syllable-length. When no use is made of pause between utterances the problem is exaggerated and is enough to explain his poor performance on the Chunking Output Function task reported earlier.

Robin

Robin fell below 1.5 SD on Chunking, Affect and Focus. This is unexpected, given that he scored within normal limits on the equivalent Output Function tasks, since the phonetic demands of the Output Form tasks are just the same as for the Output Function tasks. One possible explanation is the 'off-line' nature of the Form task. By requiring the child to listen and imitate what he hears, the tasks may be drawing attention to aspects of linguistic and phonetic form, bringing them to conscious awareness in such a way as to interfere with performance. If this is the case, then Robin's difficulties with this task may be attributable to a deficit in metaprosodic awareness rather than in motor execution abilities.

Summary of PEPS-C Results for Jonathan and Robin

Jonathan

Jonathan's performance on the PEPS-C battery is summarized in Figure 11.3.

If, for whatever reason, Jonathan is unaware of the subtleties of intonational meaning, or how intonational meaning can combine with lexis and grammar, this could give rise to some misunderstandings on his part, and thence a failure to realize how he could be making use of intonational parameters in his own utterances to convey meaning effectively.

Name: Jonathan		INPUT	OUTPUT
Chunking	Function	×	×
	Form	×	××
Affect	Function	✓	✓✓
	Form	✓	×
Interaction	Function	×	×
	Form	✓	×
Focus	Function	✓	××
	Form	✓	✓

Key: × signifies a score of at least 1.5 SD below the mean compared to normally developing 8-year-olds. ×× signifies at least 2.5 SD below the mean. ✓ signifies a score between –1.5 and +1.5 SD, and a score ✓✓ of over +1.5 SD.

Figure 11.3: Jonathan's PEPS-C profile.

Jonathan's inability to use intonation appropriately in his own speech output, as measured by the Output Function tasks, is a major source of concern: he scored low on three out of these four tasks. This ties in with our impression of his conversational speech, illustrated at the beginning of the chapter. However, on the Affect task his performance was flawless. The result of the Affect task suggests that Jonathan is not incapable of using prosody deliberately to express his meaning, and it is significant that it was in this area that he made his only high score on an Input Function task, also near ceiling (15/16). The Affect result lends support to the notion that if Jonathan understands the potential of prosodic meaning he may be able to modify his own prosody so that it conveys meaning effectively.

Jonathan scored low on three of the four Output Form tasks, and near ceiling (22/24) on the fourth (Focus). It was noted during testing that Jonathan has a full range of tones, particularly the complex ones (rise–fall and fall–rise) which were the ones he used so appropriately in the Affect Function tasks. Although he was adept at using these tones on utterances that consisted of only the syllable 'mm', he succeeded less well in mapping the tones on to words. He seemed to have little appreciation of differences of pitch-height and range, but in the Focus task, where he scored highly, he was using differential pitch-height appropriately, if only to a limited extent.

Pervasively poor performance on the Output tasks suggests that Jonathan may have problems with output representation (motor programs) for some items in the intonation lexicon – but not all (cf Affect). He may also have low-level motor execution deficits.

The profile shows some differences in his performance according to communicative area. His performance is relatively strong on the Affect tasks. We have already noted that the stimuli are psycholinguistically somewhat simpler for Affect, since the stimuli and responses are short, and there is no requirement to integrate verbal with prosodic information. Given that some children with pragmatic and autistic-type difficulties are thought to have difficulties with affect in general, it is interesting to note that Jonathan appears to have an understanding of affective meaning, and some resources for expressing affect.

One relevant piece of information that we have withheld to this point is that Jonathan's parents are of West African origin. Although English is the first language of the family, informal observation suggested that their speech (including prosody) had characteristics of West African English (for a description of one such accent, see Criper-Friedman, 1990). It is quite likely that this accent background may be one factor in determining the prosodic patterns that Jonathan uses in his output, and it would certainly be relevant to any attempt to remediate his prosodic patterns. It may also be a factor in Jonathan's relatively poor performance on the Function Input tasks.

However, it would be a mistake to attribute all Jonathan's prosodic difficulties to the non-standard accent to which he is exposed. Many children growing up in London are exposed to varieties of West African or Afro-Caribbean English (the latter is prosodically quite similar to the former), yet these children do not have the bizarre prosodic patterns that characterize Jonathan's speech. Indeed, it was Jonathan's parents who were initially most distressed by his unusual prosody. Rather, it appears that Jonathan has a prosody learning problem, which may be compounded by the fact that he is exposed to different varieties of spoken English that have very different prosodic characteristics.

Robin

Robin's performance on the PEPS-C battery is summarized in Figure 11.4.

At the beginning of the chapter we noted that Robin's spontaneous speech did not show overtly atypical prosodic patterns. It is therefore quite surprising to discover that on the PEPS-C he had difficulties with both Input and Output. On Input Function, he scored below normal limits on all communicative areas except Chunking; in fact, he performed worse than Jonathan. Robin's difficulties with Input Function suggest that he has problems interpreting pragmatic aspects of prosody. This is likely to be one of the factors responsible for his difficulties with social interaction, and may therefore be a suitable area for intervention.

Robin was successful on three of the four Output Function tasks. This is somewhat paradoxical, given his failure on two of these (Affect,

Name: Robin		INPUT	OUTPUT
Chunking	Function	✓	✓✓
	Form	✓	××
Affect	Function	×	✓✓
	Form	✓✓	×
Interaction	Function	××	××
	Form	✓✓	✓
Focus	Function	×	✓
	Form	✓	××

Key: × signifies a score of at least 1.5 SD below the mean compared to normally developing 8-year-olds. ×× signifies at least 2.5 SD below the mean. ✓ signifies a score between −1.5 and +1.5 SD, and ✓✓ a score of over +1.5 SD.

Figure 11.4: Robin's PEPS-C profile.

Focus) on Input Function. It suggests that a child may be able to function passably, not sounding unusual in terms of his own prosody, yet still have problems making sense of intonation. This can be described as a covert prosodic deficit.

Robin scored low on three out of four Output Form tasks. Again, this is surprising, as he was within normal limits on the corresponding Output Function tasks. He seems to have problems with using intonation accurately when it is not generated from his own meaning system. One possibility is that the Output Form tasks bring intonation to the level of conscious awareness. Poor performance may thus be indicative of a child's lack of sensitivity to or awareness of intonational form.

Of the four communicative areas tested in PEPS-C, Robin had the strongest profile for Chunking. This is the most 'grammatical' area, as it involves the use of prosodic prominence to segment the utterance into different types of phrase. His success with Chunking may reflect the recent and dramatic improvements reported in Robin's language, as measured by standard language tests. The other three communicative areas, which caused Robin more difficulty, tap into more pragmatic aspects of meaning. This may reflect the current concern of his therapists and teachers, to work on Robin's social interaction skills.

A possible direction for intervention might therefore be to work on Robin's awareness of prosody as an important system for communicating meaning, particularly meaning in social interaction, as a precursor to working on his comprehension of specific aspects of intonation.

Conclusions

PEPS-C has shown up intonational difficulties in both Jonathan and Robin. Each has deficits in *comprehending* some functional aspects of prosody. This difficulty may to some extent account for Jonathan's unusual output: faulty representations of the semantic pragmatic or grammatical meaning of intonation contours in the lexicon might be expected to have an effect on the child's spoken output. For Robin, the deficit in prosodic comprehension may have a completely different effect: his output shows no overt prosodic peculiarities, but he presents with severe–moderate language disorder, both expressive and receptive.

The relatively strong performance of both boys on Input Form tasks suggests that their problems with functional comprehension of prosody cannot solely be attributed to perceptual deficits. The problem seems to be more to do with mapping intonational form on to linguistic meaning.

On the Output side, Jonathan's pattern of results suggests that comprehension problems may give rise to production difficulties. Conversely, the case of Robin suggests that apparently acceptable functional prosodic performance can coexist with prosodic comprehension deficits.

Interpreting the PEPS-C results of Jonathan and Robin within a psycholinguistic framework illustrates the diversity of profiles that can be found among children with speech and language difficulties. Prosody is, in this respect, no different from other aspects of speech processing, as illustrated by the cases presented in Book 1 and elsewhere in this volume. A psycholinguistic approach, using carefully constructed assessments and comparisons with normative data, enables us to identify the strengths and weaknesses of the individual child in their prosodic processing. The results can be useful for the therapist who wishes to work directly on overt prosodic problems, as in the case of Jonathan. Furthermore, the discovery of a covert prosodic deficit can open up a new perspective on the nature of the underlying difficulties of a particular child, as in the case of Robin. This in turn may lead the therapist or teacher to consider new approaches to intervention with that child.

Summary

- Though relatively neglected hitherto, prosody can play an important role in a child's speech and language difficulties.
- To identify underlying level of deficit in cases of atypical prosody, we need to tap different levels of processing.
- The PEPS-C battery has been developed as a tool for assessing intonation within the psycholinguistic framework.
- Intonation is not unitary: both Jonathan and Robin show differential

performance according to 'communicative area' and corresponding intonation subsystem.

- The PEPS-C profiles for Jonathan and Robin show that the relationship between prosodic input and output in children is not always simple or direct.
- In a case of overtly atypical intonation, such as Jonathan's, it is still important to investigate the child's comprehension of prosody: some of the output difficulties may derive from inaccurate intonational representations.
- Even in cases where there is no overt sign of a prosodic problem, it is valuable to investigate prosodic processing, since, as in the case of Robin, a covert prosodic deficit may be revealed.
- Identification of the underlying prosodic deficits is a necessary prerequisite to targeted intervention.

Key to Activity 11.1

Question B: Can the child discriminate speech sounds without reference to lexical representations?

Key to Activity 11.2

This corresponds to question E on the profile: Are the child's phonological representations accurate?

Key to Activity 11.3

In terms of the speech processing profile, the task addresses question G: Can the child access accurate motor programs? The programs here include both segmental and prosodic aspects.

Key to Activity 11.4

It addresses question I: Can the child articulate real words accurately? with the proviso that 'real words' should be modified to 'real utterances'.

Acknowledgements

The work reported here was supported through UK Economic and Social Research Council Awards R000236696 and R000222809. We are particularly grateful to the children who participated in this study, their parents, teachers and therapists.

Chapter 12
Identification and Intervention: Future Directions

Joy Stackhouse and Bill Wells

This book has applied the principles of psycholinguistic investigation presented in Book 1 (Stackhouse and Wells, 1997) to identification and intervention. It has shown how the psycholinguistic framework, comprising the speech processing profile and its theoretical models, has been extended and used in practice and research. This final chapter pulls together the main themes of the book and discusses further applications of the psycholinguistic approach.

Identification

Identifying children with actual and potential speech and literacy difficulties is a complicated process. Up to 60 per cent of children with speech or language delays will resolve their difficulties before 3 years of age (Law, Boyle, Harris, et al., 1998). However, this still leaves a significant number of children whose difficulties will persist through to the school years, and who are therefore at risk for associated educational difficulties. Chapter 1 of this volume stressed the importance of children having an intact speech processing system and well-developed spoken language skills when they start school. Certainly, children whose speech and language difficulties persist beyond CA 5;6 can experience quite significant literacy difficulties (Bishop and Adams, 1990; Stackhouse, Nathan, Goulandris, et al., 1999) and some will also have associated problems with numeracy (Donlan, 1998).

This is not surprising when the demands made by the school curriculum are analysed (see Chapters 1, 8 and 9, this volume). In the context of the National Curriculum for England and Wales, spoken language skills and phonological awareness need to be well developed during Key Stage 1 (age 5–7 years) if a child is going to cope with the increasing spoken and written language demands of Key Stage 2 (age 8–11 years). At Key Stage 2 children switch from using spoken language skills to develop literacy to using literacy to develop higher language skills and knowledge of their world. Language and literacy pervade all aspects of the curriculum and are necessary for developing not only concepts, for example in mathematics and science, but also accessing information and following instructions in all subjects (see Chapter 9, this volume). Follow-up studies have shown that children with a history of speech and language difficulties may not present with literacy problems until they are faced with the curriculum demands of Key Stage 2 at around 8 years of age (Dodd, Russell and Oerlemans, 1993). Others have shown that children's literacy difficulties may not be apparent until as late as at secondary school when the even more challenging curriculum precipitates their learning difficulties (Stothard, Snowling, Bishop, et al., 1998).

Identifying persisting speech and language difficulties is therefore not straightforward since not all children have obvious spoken difficulties throughout their school life. Many children have only 'illusory recovery' from their earlier, more obvious speech and language difficulties and their persisting problems go unnoticed until there are educational or behavioural problems. Further, there is not always a clear channel for communication about a child's speech and language difficulties between pre-school and school workers, so that teachers may not be aware that a child in their class is at risk for literacy problems because of earlier speech and language difficulties. This can be compounded if parents do not wish information about their child to be transferred between pre-school and school staff because they fear that a subsequent 'label' of difficulty would influence teachers' attitude toward their child and therefore affect his/her progress. This concern was expressed at a parent focus group conducted as part of an investigation of the training needs of early years workers (Wood, Wright and Stackhouse, in progress). Unless investigated specifically, a child's shaky foundation for literacy can remain unidentified until the child is failing with school work.

One of the advantages of the psycholinguistic approach is that it delves underneath the surface and uncovers the foundation of a child's literacy skills. This was the case for Luke in Chapter 8 of this volume. His spoken language difficulties appeared to have resolved but his subtle persisting auditory and speech difficulties militated against him developing phonological awareness skills and letter knowledge in line with his peer group. Similarly, the case of Richard presented in Chapter 5 of Book 1 illustrated how dyslexia can go unrecognized throughout primary school, particularly when the associated speech difficulties are manifested in more complex words and connected speech rather than at the single sound level.

Another advantage of the psycholinguistic framework is that it is not tied to a prescribed test battery in order to identify children with difficulties. Practitioners and researchers can slot into the framework their preferred means of assessing children depending on the age of the child and the purpose of the assessment. Neither is the framework fixed in time; new assessment procedures can be incorporated as they are published or designed. The key to psycholinguistic investigation and identification is that the assessments being used have been analysed appropriately (see Book 1, Chapters 2 and 3) so that a child's performance can be interpreted accurately.

Although there is now a wide range of assessment materials available, a child does not have to undergo a large test battery to complete a psycholinguistic investigation. This is particularly the case if there are opportunities to follow up a child over time. Even then, administering a large number of tests is not a requirement of a psycholinguistic investigation; available tests are merely one of the tools with which information might be sought. Observation of performance in teaching and therapy sessions is equally valid as a psycholinguistic assessment procedure:

> Fortunately, one of the advantages of working within the psycholinguistic framework is that pieces of information, which are gleaned by design or good fortune during investigative therapy, can be slotted into a child's profile.
>
> (Waters Chapter 6, this volume)

A psycholinguistic database for identification

However the information is collected, the speech processing profile (presented in Appendix 1) provides a means of collating children's assessment results in a systematic way. At the end of Book 1 (p.336) we suggested that if speech processing profiling sheets of individual cases were collected together, they would provide a useful database on the nature of children's speech processing difficulties and how they change over time. A database such as this could then be used to address issues such as the relationship between speech and literacy difficulties, early identification, and prognostic indicators. Since the publication of Book 1, a longitudinal study of children's speech and literacy development using the psycholinguistic framework has been completed (Stackhouse, Nathan, Goulandris, et al., 1999). Children in the age range of 4–7 years with pervasive speech processing problems involving both input and output sides of the profile were most likely to have associated language and literacy problems. The use of the speech processing profile also revealed which children had really resolved the difficulties that lay beneath the surface (Stackhouse, 2000). Further, by following through normally developing controls matched to the children with specific speech difficulties, the study has shown which are the most useful assessments for identifying and predicting speech and literacy problems and when to use them for maximum effect (see Chapter 1, this volume).

This is one of the few longitudinal studies to incorporate auditory processing tasks as well as phonological awareness and speech output tasks in the procedure. The lack of auditory investigations as a routine part of an assessment has also been evident in clinical practice (see Chapter 9, this volume). Certainly, feedback from users of the framework following training courses has been that by adopting the psycholinguistic approach their attention has been more focused on the input and representation aspects of the framework rather than only on the speech output side.

Extending the Assessment Framework

The psycholinguistic framework continues to be developed, in order to gain a deeper understanding of the nature of children's difficulties, as a basis for identification and, where appropriate, intervention. In this section we describe recent and ongoing research which, in different ways extends the scope of the assessment framework beyond the presentation in Book 1.

Speech disorders and working memory

The psycholinguistic framework has been used to disentangle the controversial relationship between speech processing skills and short-term memory (Vance, Donlan and Stackhouse, 1999). A range of published research findings have suggested that speech processing skills may be closely linked with short-term memory or working memory capacities (Adams and Gathercole, 2000). However, these studies have incorporated different tasks to measure memory span capacities, including nonword repetition, repeating a list of words heard, and pointing to pictures of words heard. Vance (1998) compared the differing speech processing demands of each of the tasks used and has applied a psycholinguistic methodology to the investigation of the speech processing skills of a group of normally developing children and individual children with speech and language difficulties. Preliminary findings from the speech processing profiles of the children with language impairments suggest that auditory discrimination skills may play a role in the development of short-term memory and in grammatical development. Children with speech and language impairments who have poorer short-term memory spans tended to have less well-developed speech production skills than those with better short-term memory spans. In terms of the speech processing model, these findings suggest that verbal working memory may not be conceptually distinguishable from the various components of the speech processing system (Snowling and Hulme, 1994). Further analysis of the data is currently being carried out to check and enlarge these initial findings.

Understanding unfamiliar accents

On the input side, the psycholinguistic framework is being used to investigate children's ability to understand speakers from different speech communities, whose accent is different from that of the child. This is an increasingly important functional skill for the child at school and, in general, in the world beyond the family. Unsurprisingly, it appears to be a skill that children get better at as they get older: Nathan, Wells and Donlan (1998) found that 7-year-old London children were significantly better than 4-year-old children on a task that involved defining and repeating single words presented in a Glaswegian accent. However, little is known about how children with speech and language difficulties cope with listening to different accents. The ability to understand accent variation may involve several processing routes, including both psycholinguistic processing (e.g. discrimination, categorization, mapping) and sociolinguistic awareness (e.g. detection of accent differences, awareness of one's own accent system).

Using an auditory lexical decision task, Nathan and Wells (1999) investigated the accent processing skills of 6-year-old children who had speech output difficulties, and compared them to normally developing controls. All the children were from London. The children with speech difficulties, but not the controls, had significantly greater difficulty in correctly identifying words spoken in a Glaswegian accent compared to words spoken in a London accent. In terms of the speech processing model, the results suggest that these children have deficits in phonological recognition and/or representation that impede the mapping of unusual variants of a word (i.e. a Glaswegian pronunciation) on to their stored lexical representation. This finding has implications for the management of children with speech processing difficulties, who will be exposed, like all children, to an increasing range of speech variability in their teachers, therapists and other key people with whom they communicate. Current work is pursuing both the theoretical and practical implications of this finding by investigating children with a range of difficulties (e.g. pragmatic language impairments as well as phonological impairments) and a larger number of normally developing controls between the ages of 4 and 7 years.

Word-finding difficulties

In Chapter 10 of this volume, Constable added to the original speech processing profile specific questions to be addressed in the investigation of children with word-finding difficulties. Designing specific procedures to tackle these questions has led to a better understanding of the complexity of children's lexical responses. Word-finding difficulties are not separate from the rest of a child's speech and language difficulties but can be a long-term consequence of speech processing difficulties. In terms of the speech processing model, the focus here is particularly on the lexical representations – the interconnections between the phonological representation, semantic representation and motor program (Constable, Stackhouse and Wells, 1997).

Diadochokinetic (DDK) tasks

Diadochokinesia has been defined as:

> study of motor control integrity in bodily functions through perform-ance in rapidly alternating movement ....In speech, the term has been extended to include syllable repetition at a maximum rate of utterance.
>
> (Fletcher, 1978)

Asking children to repeat such sequences as /p/ – /t/ – /k/ at speed, or repeat complex words like BUTTERCUP and HIPPOPOTAMUS three times quickly, have long been used by speech and language therapists and others to assess children's motor control of their articulators. However, there is surprisingly little normative data for such activities. Adopting the psycholinguistic approach to both the stimuli design (see Book 1, Chapter 11) and to the analysis of the results has revealed what young normally developing children can and cannot achieve on such tasks. Williams and Stackhouse (2000) described the performance of 30 normally developing children in the age range of 3–5 years on silent and spoken DDK tasks. Rate, accuracy and consistency measures of the children's performance were used to make comparisons with both the adult model presented and with each child's own speech sound system. The results show that, in general, accuracy and consistency of response are developmentally more sensitive DDK measures for pre-school children than the more commonly used rate of production.

This normative data were used to compare the performance of three children with specific speech difficulties (CA 4;4, 5;3 and 8;7). The three children were similar in terms of the severity of their speech diffi-culties, as measured by their Articulation Age (Williams and Stackhouse, 1998). The results showed that the children with specific speech diffi-culties performed differently from younger normally developing children who had been matched to them on Articulation Age. They also performed differently from one another: they presented with contrasting DDK profiles in psycholinguistic terms. One performed as might be expected of a child who has problems with motor program-ming; another performed like a child who has specific phonological delay as a result of inaccurately stored motor programs; and the third had a mixture of both motor programming and lower-level, motor execution difficulties. Thus, although the three children performed similarly on an articulation test, which provides a general measure of number of speech errors, their pattern of performance on the DDK tasks discriminated between them. Their DDK profiles suggested different aetiologies to their speech difficulties. This, in turn, influenced the approach taken in intervention.

Connected speech processes

While many of the speech processing assessments described in Book 1, and also the therapy tasks described in this volume, function principally at the level of single words, spoken language consists primarily of multiword utterances, which present additional challenges to the child's speech processing system. As briefly described in Book 1 (pp.226–228), segmental phonetic and phonological features specific to connected speech arise from the particular sequences that occur at the junction between the coda of one word and the onset of the next word. Some of these sequences give rise to predictable patterns of 'simplif-ication' in adult English, such as assimilation of alveolar stops to following bilabials or velars; elision of the middle of three consonants; and liaison of one vowel, by means of a glide, to a following vowel.

These connected speech processes occur with an adult-like frequency in children aged 4 to 7 years (Newton and Wells, 1999), suggesting that by this age normally developing children have already mastered them. Newton investigated the same processes in case studies of three 11-year-old children who had a history of severe speech and language difficulties, but whose segmental problems were by now largely resolved, at least in single word production (Newton, 1999). Acoustic analysis and electropalatography (EPG) (see Dent, this volume) were used to reveal details of the articulations used by the children in connected speech (Newton, Dent and Wells, 1999). It was found that each of the children was capable on some occasions of producing adult-like junctions. Sometimes, however, the children would produce a junction that was much simpler from an articulatory perspective, but atypical in terms of adult English and normal development, e.g. WATCHED TELEVISION → [wɒshɛəvɪzən].

Non adult-like patterns had also been found in a detailed case study of a normally developing boy, Christopher. From the very onset of multiword production, he would attempt to join adjacent words together phonetically, even though he did not yet have the phonetic skills to bring the junction off in an adult-like way (Newton, 1999). For example, at CA 2;4, Christopher realized LOST BERTIE as [lɒʔbɜti].

According to the model presented in Book 1, these connected speech processes occur at the motor planning stage of speech processing, where the motor programs for the individual words are assembled into a single plan for production, in accordance with the grammatical structure that the speaker has selected (Book 1, pp.272–273).

However, the possibility cannot be ruled out that input processing and phonological representations are also involved, since recent research has shown that there are age-related changes in children's processing of lexical items in connected speech environments such as assimilation (Loucas and Marslen-Wilson, 2000).

Like the case of Zoe presented in Chapters 9 and 10 of Book 1, Newton's three case studies demonstrate that connected speech poses particular challenges for children with speech difficulties, which are likely to affect the intelligibility of the entire utterance. Such features could become an important focus for intervention, particularly in the older child with a history of speech and language problems (Book 1, p.275) .

Prosodic processing

Another important aspect of connected speech, again little researched in relation to children with speech and language difficulties, is intonation. Wells and Peppé (Chapter 11, this volume) used the principles of the psycholinguistic framework presented in Book 1 to investigate the nature of prosodic difficulties in children with speech/language impairments. Their comparison of two cases reveals how the psycholinguistic approach can be used to identify both overt and covert prosodic problems. Just as with segmental phonology, the psycholinguistic approach highlights the importance of attending to both input and output sides of the model as well as the precision of the intonation representations. Children who have overt prosodic difficulties, i.e. on the output side, have been reported previously by therapists and researchers (Book 1, pp.222–226): the study of Jonathan in Chapter 11 of this volume suggests that such problems may arise not simply from output motor deficits, for example at the level of motor planning, but may, at least in part, derive from inaccurate phonological representations for intonation that the child has built up over the years. The implication for intervention is that ways have to be found of refining these intonational representations.

The case of Robin, a boy with receptive and expressive language difficulties who had no obvious output problems with intonation, is particularly intriguing. Testing within a psycholinguistic framework, reported in Chapter 11, revealed that he had problems understanding some fairly rudimentary prosodic distinctions. This suggests that prosodic processing may sometimes be implicated in receptive language difficulties. One implication for intervention with children who have comprehension difficulties is to give due consideration to prosody, including intonation, since it forms the basis on which grammatical structures ride in spoken language.

The relationship between prosodic processing and sentence processing is a central theme of a book by Shula Chiat, who pioneered case-based psycholinguistic analysis of children's speech and language disorders (Chiat, 2000). Through a series of case studies, this work highlights the relationships between speech processing on the one hand, and deficits in grammar, semantics and pragmatics on the other.

Extending the Clinical Range of the Psycholinguistic Framework

The wide scope of the psycholinguistic framework, in terms of its potential application to different types of speech and language disorder, was stressed in Book 1. The assessment framework can be used with normally developing children either as direct comparison with clinical groups or for the purposes of studying normal processes and development.

Although it originated in studies of children with specific phonological impairment and verbal dyspraxia, the psycholinguistic approach is not tied to a specific clinical entity. It can be used with almost any child whose communication difficulties may be related to underlying speech processing problems, e.g. children with Down's syndrome (Coffield, 1994) or acquired speech and language problems associated with epilepsy (Vance, 1997) or following road traffic accidents (Onslow, 1995), or with children with semantic pragmatic difficulties or autistic features (see Chapter 9, this volume). The speech processing profile can thus be used as a basis for intervention regardless of any medical diagnosis. Recently the clinical entities investigated have been extended to include cerebral palsy, hearing impairment and stuttering.

Cerebral palsy

Corkett (1997) investigated the auditory processing skills of two children, CA 9;10 and CA 10;9, with severe developmental dysarthria and cerebral palsy. The children's reading ability and letter knowledge was also assessed through tests and observation in the classroom situation. Both children had some input difficulties in addition to their very obvious speech output difficulties. Although their profiles of strengths and weaknesses on the auditory processing tasks were different, both children had difficulties with the accuracy and awareness of the internal structure of their phonological representations. The children's literacy skills were also different: the child with the more severe auditory processing difficulties had poorer literacy skills.

This study illustrates that the psycholinguistic framework can be adapted for children with severe mobility problems who are using alternative and augmentative communication, and can serve to uncover underlying and hitherto unsuspected processing difficulties. The study also emphasizes the individual variation between children with the same medical diagnosis, hence the importance of looking beyond the obvious presenting 'symptoms' when planning a child's intervention programme.

Hearing impairment

The psycholinguistic framework is being used by Rachel Rees and colleagues to investigate the speech processing and literacy problems of children with hearing impairments. A case study of TG, a 10-year-old girl with severe hearing impairment has shown how useful this might be (Ebbels, 2000). Systematic analysis of TG's input, representation and output skills revealed that her speech processing was breaking down at several levels, resulting in segmental errors and word retrieval difficulties. The application of the psycholinguistic framework confirmed clinical observations that TG had more speech and language difficulties than would be expected, given her hearing loss. Although TG's hearing impairment did affect her ability to hear the differences between some sound contrasts, she failed to contrast other sounds in her speech output which she could discriminate perfectly well. When planning intervention based on this information, Ebbels concluded that:

> For hearing-impaired children, words and contrasts that are not affected by lower level input processing skills may respond more quickly to therapy as children can use the auditory discrimination skills they do have to update phonological representations. Thus, the identification and treatment of these is invaluable in maximising intelligibility prior to working on those contrasts which the child cannot distinguish and will therefore require more intervention.
>
> (Ebbels, 2000)

As this case study shows, adopting the psycholinguistic framework helps to ensure that a child's intervention is specifically designed to meet his/her needs. The presence of a hearing impairment did not preclude the use of a psycholinguistic approach. The latter proved helpful in identifying the different levels of processing involved in the child's speech output errors and lexical retrieval difficulties.

Dysfluency

It is clear that the population of children who stutter is very heterogeneous in both presenting symptoms and possible underlying causes. Investigations of the rhyme skills in children who stammer have supported the view that some, but not all children, who stammer have associated speech processing difficulties (Forth, Stackhouse, Nicholas, et al., 1997).

Alison Nicholas, at the Michael Palin Centre for Stammering Children in London, has used the approach to identify children whose nonfluency may be accompanied by underlying speech processing difficulties (Nicholas, 1999). The long-term aim is to investigate how the speech processing difficulties might impact on a child's response to a therapy programme offered for dysfluency. The profiling of the children's speech processing skills in addition to the assessment of their nonfluency may help meet the need for more sophisticated measures to assess the linguistic skills of children who stutter (Bernstein-Ratner, 1997). Ten children who stutter (CA 4;7 to CA 5;10) were compared on a range of psycholinguistic tests to ten controls matched on age, gender and nonverbal ability. Taken as a group, the children who stuttered performed as well as the normally fluent controls on input processing tasks, phonological awareness tasks and the majority of speech output tasks. However, the results revealed considerable individual variation in the performance of the children who stuttered. This suggests that, as with other clinical entities (e.g. verbal dyspraxia or phonological impairment), group studies can mask the individual variation exhibited by children with communication difficulties. Poor performance on the psycholinguistic tasks was related not to the degree of severity of the stutter but rather to the presence or absence of additional language and/or speech problems.

There was one significant group difference between the children who stuttered and their controls. This was on speech rate during DDK tasks that involved, for instance, the multiple repetition of nonwords such as /kudɪgən/ (Nicholas, Stackhouse and Nathan, 2000). In terms of the speech processing model, this DDK task draws initially on the many levels required for nonword repetition (cf. Book 1, p.180), but for the subsequent repetitions taps mainly into motor planning and motor execution. This would appear to support the view of stuttering as a relatively low-level motor output deficit.

From Identification to Intervention

Psycholinguistic profiling of a child's processing skills is a necessary step in the identification of children in need of intervention and in identifying the areas that might be targeted in their intervention programmes:

> If we can understand a child's language deficit in terms of the psycholinguistic processes that are involved, we should be able to devise remedial approaches to facilitate language learning.
>
> (Bishop, 1997)

An advantage of the psycholinguistic approach when planning teaching or therapy is that it is not only deficit-centred. By definition, the completing of the speech processing profile ensures a systematic investigation of a range of skills, resulting in a full picture of a child's strengths as well as weaknesses. Comparing these strengths and weaknesses ensures appropriate aims and objectives are set (see Chapter 3, this volume) based on either targeting strengths or weaknesses or a combination of both. The case of Alan, presented by Daphne Waters in Chapter 6 of this volume, illustrates how time was well spent working on the input side of the model, a relative strength, prior to attempting to work on the output – the real weakness in Alan's processing skills. This targeting of input skills is also advocated by Hodson and Paden (1991) in *Targeting Intelligible Speech* and in the use of auditory bombardment techniques (see Chapter 2, this volume), particularly with younger children who do not always respond well to direct work on speech output.

A speech processing profile in itself, however, is not a sufficient basis on which to plan intervention. Other sources of information need to be used and fit well with the psycholinguistic data. In Chapter 1 of Book 1, we introduced the psycholinguistic perspective by comparing it with the contributions made by two other perspectives commonly taken on children with speech difficulties: the medical and linguistic. In this volume, other perspectives have been incorporated into the management of cases. Nathan and Simpson (Chapter 8, this volume) stressed the importance of including both the teacher and the parents in the intervention programme for Luke and how such programmes need to be based on multiple sources of information if a child's difficulties are to be viewed in context. Waters (Chapter 6, this volume) reminds us of the importance of acknowledging individual children's learning style as well as where they are at in their ability to take on board the challenges and practicalities of an intervention programme.

Even when all of this relevant information has been collected it can still be a daunting prospect to transform it into an intervention programme and work out 'what to do'. The journey from profile to programme was explained in Chapters 4 and 5 of this volume. Juliette Corrin's meticulous examination of the macro- and micro-stages of planning an intervention programme for Anna illustrates how time spent on the analysis is time well spent as it ensures that 'one is hitting the right targets from the start'.

Corrin also makes a very important point about the difference in nature between the tasks used for the purposes of identification and those used for intervention. When assessing a child, the tasks used should have minimal overlap in order to separate out the levels of processing (marked by the letters A–L) on the speech processing profile. For example, a task aimed at investigating auditory skills should not be contaminated by visual cueing. The aim of an assessment is to get a clear picture of a child's strengths and weaknesses in order to identify if s/he would benefit from intervention. In contrast, in an intervention programme the teacher/therapist is aiming to support the child as much as is necessary in order for a task to be completed successfully. It is desirable for activities to have maximal overlap in order to bridge between levels of processing so that intervention tasks scaffold the child's performance. In this case, for example, visual cueing to support an auditory task may be quite appropriate.

In order to fulfil this aim and to understand how to control and manipulate variables in an intervention programme, the teacher/therapist analyses intervention tasks in the same way as we analysed popular assessments in *What Do Tests Really Test?* in Book 1 (Chapters 2 and 3). Rachel Rees applied the same process to intervention tasks in this volume in *What Do Tasks Really Tap?* (Chapter 3, this volume) and posed a series of task analysis questions for us to follow.

By working with the formula:

Task = Materials + Procedure + Feedback ± Technique,

Rees illustrated how to identify and control the psycholinguistic properties of a task in order to achieve the aims and objectives that have been set for a particular child. When just one variable in this formula is manipulated, a task changes its nature and becomes more or less challenging. Maintaining control over the nature of the intervention tasks is a core aspect of the psycholinguistic approach to intervention. It is an important skill to develop not only in the teacher/therapist but also in the children themselves who can be taught to make tasks more accessible by introducing their favoured support strategies, e.g. self-cueing.

Thus, just as there is no one case of tests for psycholinguistic investigation, there is no one psycholinguistic intervention programme; nor is there a prescription for each type of speech processing profile. All materials have the potential to be used in a psycholinguistic way, since the approach is "in the head of the user" (Book 1, p.49). The psycholinguistic approach to intervention puts the emphasis first on the rationale behind the design and selection of tasks for the particular child; and second, on the order in which the tasks are to be presented to a child in order to exploit strengths and to support weaknesses. The approach tackles the issues of *what* to do *with whom, why, when* and *how*!

Tasks do not have to be novel to be used in this way. For example, the use of EPG as a psycholinguistic tool may be a novel application of this particular instrumental technique (see Chapter 7, this volume) but the underlying intervention rationale is reminiscent of Scripture's work of the 1920s, which encouraged the child to attend and consciously position the articulatory structures and control their movements (Scripture, 1923). Today we have technology to aid this approach. Similarly, the 'traditional' approach to articulation intervention that Van Riper developed between 1939 and 1978 is still alive and well (Van Riper, 1978). In fact the auditory bombardment aspects of this approach are undergoing a revival in the UK and have been promoted by Hodson (1997) and Lancaster and Pope (1989) and used by contributors to this volume (e.g. Rees and Waters).

Many current programmes cited in this volume have their origins in earlier work. The shifting of focus from sound to syllable level in speech therapy, for example, encapsulated in the *Nuffield Dyspraxia Programme* (*NDP*; Connery, 1992) was pioneered by McDonald (1964). The *NDP* was designed in the 1970s to address the speech difficulties of children presenting with developmental verbal dyspraxia. In keeping with the contemporary view of dyspraxia as an output difficulty, the programme advocated a 'bottom-up' approach helping the child to build up basic articulatory movements to single sounds, then words of increasing complexity, phrases and sentences. Some of the *NDP* tasks have been incorporated into activities in this volume (in the chapters by Corrin, for example), illustrating how established therapy materials can be used in a psycholinguistic way when analysed appropriately. The *NDP* is currently being revised by Pam Williams from the Nuffield Hearing and Speech Centre in London. The new version will make more explicit how the materials can be used for input as well as output activities. Task analysis of the activities will identify the processing demands being made and how to grade the tasks in terms of their complexity. The links with literacy will also be strengthened.

Although our definition and identification of children's difficulties may change, as do the political, social, educational and medical contexts in which we are expected to manage them, nothing is out of date when it comes to what to do. Fashions change as new programmes and approaches come on to the market but children's underlying difficulties are no different now to what they were 100 years ago. Intervention within the psycholinguistic approach involves selecting from the tasks available, then identifying their nature and properties, so that they can be adapted to meet the needs of individuals or groups of children. The rich legacy of resources devised by teachers and therapists over the years can thus be used effectively in our intervention programmes if their psycholinguistic properties and potential are identified. (See Weiss, Lillywhite and Gordon, 1980 for further discussion of approaches to speech intervention between 1920 and 1980; Hodson and Edwards, 1997 for a review of approaches to phonological therapy; and Howard 1998, Chapter 2, for a historical review of approaches to the analysis, classification and treatment of speech disorders.)

Intervention

There is little doubt that a psycholinguistic approach to intervention will result in a more targeted and principled intervention programme. Vance (1997) illustrated this in her intervention with a child who had acquired speech and language difficulties as a result of Landau–Kleffner syndrome. William was 10 years of age and had a marked auditory processing difficulty that resulted in multiple errors in his speech production. His completed speech processing profile revealed that the source of his speech errors lay in the inaccuracy of his phonological representations and the inaccurate motor programs for words that had been derived from these rather than at a lower articulatory level. His programme incorporated visual cueing to present phonological information and to update his representations. His intact articulatory skills were used in a bottom-up way to feed back phonological forms to the level of the motor program and to the phonological representation. Intelligibility and literacy skills improved in spite of persisting auditory processing problems into the teenage years (Vance, Dry and Rosen, 1999).

Intervention and the phase model

Several examples of principled intervention have been included in this volume. In planning and carrying out their intervention studies, the authors have drawn on the speech processing profile as a tool for systematic assessment and monitoring of change, and the box-and-arrow speech processing model as a tool for conceptualizing the locus of a child's deficits and strengths. The third main feature of the framework as presented in Book 1 is the developmental perspective: the notion that in the development of speech, and then literacy, the child needs to progress through a sequence of phases (Book 1, Chapters 7 and 8). These are illustrated in Figure 12.1

The concept of a sequence of developmental phases permits us to view intervention as a means of assisting the individual child to move on to the next phase. As an example, let us consider Alan, reported by Daphne Waters in Chapter 6. At the age of 5 years, prior to the psycholinguistically motivated intervention programme described in the chapter, Alan's speech output showed characteristics of the Whole Word Phase, described in Book 1, Chapter 7, pp.197–203. These included the use of a single place of articulation for all the consonants within a word, and the absence of any rule for predicting which place of consonant articulation Alan would adopt, from among the various places on offer within the target word. Thus, he pronounced BOAT as [bop] but BIN as [dɪn]. As Waters puts it, "the domain of contrast seemed to be the syllable, or possibly the word, and place of articulation seemed to be specified for onset + coda rather than for each separately". This is quite similar to the description of Zoe at CA 3;9 in Book 1, Chapter 9 (e.g. p.259).

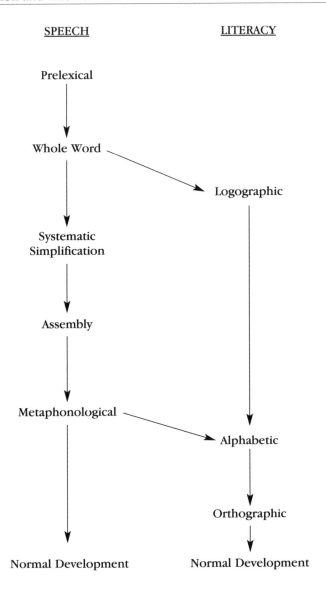

Figure 12.1: The relationship between the phases of speech and literacy development.

In contrast with his speech output, Alan's input skills proved to be at a more advanced stage of development. He was easily able to identify contrasts at specific places in the phonological structure, with nonwords as well as real words. This is typical of the Systematic Simplification Phase (Book 1, pp.203–204). He was also shown to have accurate phonological representations for lexical items, despite their aberrant pronunciations. Moreover, he soon learnt to demonstrate an awareness of the internal structure of phonological representations, in tasks that required him to match onsets or rhymes silently from pictures. His input and representational skills were thus more in line with the later Metaphonological Phase (Book 1, pp.228–232). From this perspective, the therapy programme that Daphne Waters devised for Alan can be seen as assisting him to bring his speech output skills forward from the Whole Word Phase to the Metaphonological Phase, so as to come into line with his input and representational skills. As Waters describes, the key to success was working on the relationship between the strong input and representational skills on the one hand, and the weak output skills on the other, to redress this developmental imbalance.

The study of Luke by Nathan and Simpson, reported in Chapter 8, illustrates the link between phases of speech processing development and phases of literacy development. The authors suggest that, as a result of a history of relatively subtle input and output deficits in speech processing, Luke at the age of 7 years did not yet have the accurate and fully structured phonological representations that characterize the Metaphonological Phase and which provide a platform for progression to the Alphabetic Stage of literacy development. In terms of his speech processing, he showed some relatively subtle deficits with input and in tasks that required the manipulation of phonological representations, particularly at the phonemic level. Luke's intervention programme targeted the skills that would allow him to progress fully to the Metaphonological Phase. Results showed that this was beginning to help him with literacy skills, in progressing to the Alphabetic Stage.

The other intervention studies reported in this book are equally susceptible to interpretation in terms of the Phase model, and the interested reader is encouraged to analyse them from this perspective.

Evaluating intervention outcomes

The success of the psycholinguistic approach to intervention may lie in the fact that it targets the underlying sources of difficulties rather than the symptoms alone. A recent therapy study of a Punjabi-English speaking child (Holm and Dodd, 1999) highlights the importance of identifying and targeting the deficit underlying the speech difficulties, which in this case were manifested in two languages. Intervention targeting these underlying difficulties proved to be more effective than correcting the surface errors specific to one of the languages; when this was done, subsequent improvement was seen only in the language targeted and there was no generalization of progress to the other non-targeted language.

However, there is still little information on how to measure the direct impact and outcome of intervention programmes. One of the problems is that children with developmental speech and literacy difficulties do not form a heterogeneous group and are subject to much individual variation. Children with similar scores on psychometric tests and with the same diagnostic label (e.g. dyspraxia or dyslexia) may have different speech processing profiles. Further, children with similar speech processing profiles can respond very differently to intervention tasks. Clearly, outcome of intervention is dependent on far more than a child's speech processing skills. Age, personality, motivation, social supports and expectations, family circumstances and cultural milieu all need to be taken into account (Goldstein and Gierut, 1998). Literacy outcome in particular is affected not only by a child's processing skills and attitude and the chosen teaching approach, but also by environmental factors such as maternal educational level, which may reflect not only child-rearing practices but also the linguistic environment of the home (Snowling, 2000).

When we bear in mind all of the above prognostic factors, as well as the fact that children are anyway constantly changing and developing, it is no wonder that Enderby and Emerson (1995) in their book *Does Speech and Language Therapy Work?* single out children with developmental speech and language disorders:

> ... there is no other client group... that demonstrates so many challenges to the researcher
>
> (Enderby and Emerson, 1995, p.35)

Perhaps this is why there were relatively few efficacy studies available to the authors of a recent systematic review of screening procedures for speech and language delay (Law, Boyle, Harris, et al., 1998). That said, on the basis of the studies available, the reviewers concluded that for children with specific speech difficulties direct work targeting the children's speech was most beneficial. In contrast to children with language delay, the children with specific speech difficulties did not benefit greatly from indirect intervention, e.g. intervention focusing on parent–child interaction. This is because children with specific speech difficulties are likely to have underlying processing problems that are not merely the result of environmental delay. Here the psycholinguistic approach comes into its own, since it uncovers these difficulties and bases intervention on an individual child's speech processing profile.

The intervention process

For the most part, psycholinguistically motivated intervention targeted at children's speech difficulties is carried out through spoken interactions between the child (alone or in a group) and the therapist or teacher. This is the case whether or not the intervention is specifically targeted at the correction or improvement of the child's spoken output.

It is therefore important to appreciate what pragmatic resources the child might bring to the particular type of social interaction that is 'speech therapy'. Speech disorders, since they give rise to reduced intelligibility, will have an impact on the child's ability to participate in everyday conversation, and thus affect the child's pragmatic functioning. At the same time, most children with speech disorders are pragmatically competent in many respects – for instance in turn-taking, establishing and developing a conversational topic, and, most importantly for the therapy session, in engaging in repair or correction behaviours. These pragmatic skills are strengths that can be exploited in intervention aimed at speech difficulties.

Although the child may be pragmatically competent, this does not mean that phonetic repair sequences in therapy sessions always pass off without pragmatic misunderstandings. Hilary Gardner, a speech and language therapist specializing in children's speech disorders, has made a detailed study of therapy sessions involving children with speech disorders, using the methodology of Conversation Analysis (Gardner, 1994, 1997, 1998). By considering some of her data and analyses, we can see how elements of the psycholinguistic approach can impact on the realities of moment-by-moment interaction in the therapy or teaching session.

The first extract to be considered is from a therapy session with Stuart, a 4-year-old boy who has speech difficulties that include the production of /s/ clusters in onset positions. The therapist's focus here is on the contrast between /sp/ and /p/. The target word, SPOTS, is presented in picture form and modelled by the therapist (line 1). Stuart attempts to imitate it (line 2), but his production is inaccurate. This gives rise to a repair sequence.

Stuart (St) and therapist (Th), second session. First presentation of /sp/ in SPOT (picture of spotty face)

1. Th:	s:pots	
2. St:	[pⁿts]	
	((looking at picture))	
3.Th:	pots?	
	[pʰɒts]?	
4. St:	[pⁿts]	
	((looking at therapist, then away))	
5. Th:	are they pots?	
	((St looks to therapist again))	
6. St:	((shakes head))	
7. Th:	let's hear the sammy snake sound at the beginning then	
	(.)	
8. Th:	.h s:pot	
9. St.	[pʰɒt]	

In line 3, the therapist attempts to initiate a repair from Stuart, by means of a request for clarification. This does not take the form of an exact repetition of Stuart's inaccurate production, which lacked an initial fricative but retained the *unaspirated* [p] from SPOTS. Instead, she produces, with rising intonation, an inaccurate 'redoing' of Stuart's production, with *aspirated* initial plosive. This constitutes the therapist's production as a different lexical item, POTS, since singleton voiceless plosives in stressed syllables are always aspirated in her accent of English. The therapist is thus using a kind of 'cognitive dissonance' strategy: confronting Stuart with the possibility that his original version of SPOTS in line 2 would be interpreted as POTS – a different lexical item. Although the therapist's overriding aim is to induce a phonetic repair from Stuart (this is explicit in line 7), in line 4 Stuart makes no attempt to modify the phonetic production from line 2. On the basis of this and similar examples, Gardner argues that the child is most unlikely to interpret a clarification request of the type found in line 3, as a request for *phonetic* repair. Unless the phonetic agenda is made explicit, the child will interpret repair initiations as being about lexical, rather than phonetic, matters. Thus here in line 4, by using his own pronunciation of SPOTS, Stuart is confirming that the word in question is indeed SPOTS, not POTS. It is only in lines 7–8 that the therapist asks explicitly for phonetic work from Stuart. Judging by Stuart's response in line 9, however, it appears that the therapist's earlier strategy of invoking a lexical minimal pair SPOTS ~ POTS has confused Stuart in his attempt to address the pronunciation issue: he now produces the target SPOT as POT (line 9), with the *aspirated* plosive at onset.

Drawing on Clare Tarplee's research on picture labelling sequences involving young children and adults (Tarplee, 1993, 1996), Gardner concludes that self-repair is a skill that is little required of young children in their everyday interactions with adults. Where repair *is* required of the child, it is initially concerned with 'factual' or lexical matters. On the basis of her own analyses, Gardner argues that "the child in therapy is having to cope with a blurring of the division between phonetic and lexical repair". This means that the therapist has to do specific work to make his/her phonetic agenda explicit.

Let us now consider the SPOTS extract in terms of the speech processing demands on the child. The therapist presents a picture, which encourages Stuart to access his motor program for SPOTS. The therapist also presents a spoken model of the target word. By exaggerating the initial /s/, (line 1) she is drawing attention to a particular aspect of the phonological representation of the word so that Stuart will be particularly aware of it during his input processing of her production. This might then be expected to lead to Stuart revising his own motor program of the word, to incorporate the initial /s/. However, in line 2 we see that Stuart is still unable to produce a completely accurate motor program: he omits the initial /s/.

The therapist's 'redoing' in line 3 takes the form of an accurate motor program for a *different* word, POTS. To make sense of the therapist's turn in line 3, Stuart needs to access his lexical representation (including semantic and phonological aspects) for POTS as well as for SPOTS. In order to come up with a correct response, i.e. one that will satisfy the therapist's agenda of phonetic correction, Stuart then needs to:

(i)   compare the phonological representations for POTS and SPOTS, and realize that they are different;
(ii) conclude that the two lexical items, if they have different phonological representations, should also have different motor programs;
(iii) note that his own motor program for SPOTS is similar to or even identical to the motor program for POTS;
(iv) revise his motor program for SPOTS so as to differentiate it from POTS;
(v)   plan and execute a production of SPOTS that demonstrates to the therapist that he has achieved the previous four steps.

This is a complex series of steps for Stuart to carry out without explicit guidance. Stuart's response in line 4 can be interpreted as indicating that he has accomplished steps (i) and (ii), since he reaffirms, albeit in his own pronunciation, that the word is not POTS but SPOTS. However, there is no evidence that he appreciates level (iii), i.e. that the unaspirated and aspirated pronunciations of /p/ might be confusable; or that he sees any need for (iv), to revise his motor program for SPOTS. Even if he does appreciate the need for (iv), there is no evidence that he has the articulatory skill needed for (v).

The therapist's turn in line 5 indicates to Stuart that there is still a problem somewhere, but does not give him any more explicit guidance as to which step or level of processing is involved. Given the range of levels of processing that are implicit in the therapist's approach to this therapy task, it is perhaps not surprising that little progress is made.

Gardner observes in her data that phonetic repair sequences are more likely to be successful if, when 'redoing' the child's erroneous form, the therapist imitates it *accurately*, rather than producing an alternative but phonetically similar candidate word (like POTS in the above extract). This can be seen in the following extract, where Elizabeth (E; CA 4;0) is with her therapist (Th):

Target FEET (picture)

1. Th: feet
2. E: erf (.) two
3. Th: yeh. two what?
4. E: two [dit]
5. Th: two [dit]?
6. E: feet
7. Th: oh yeah, nearly thought you said it wrong then!

In line 5, the therapist makes an accurate redoing of the child's erroneous try from line 4, and formulates it as a clarification request by using rising pitch. There is no alternative referent for [dit] (unlike POTS in the previous example), so the child has no occasion to make a lexical correction: instead, she makes a phonetic correction in line 6.

In speech processing terms, by using a picture the therapist encourages Elizabeth to access her own motor program for FEET. By modelling FEET (line 1) she encourages Elizabeth to compare her own phonological representation with the phonological representation that is implicit in the therapist's pronunciation. In line 5, the therapist makes an accurate redoing of Elizabeth's erroneous pronunciation. The child has to check [dit] against her own phonological presentation for FEET (which had been refreshed in line 1). On correctly concluding that [dit] does not match the phonological representation, she has to modify her own motor program for FEET, so that it is compatible with her phonological representation. She then has to plan and execute a production of FEET based on that newly revised motor program. As line 6 shows, she is able to do this. As [dit] does not correspond to another lexical item (thence another phonological representation and motor program) the processing puzzle for the child is much less complicated than in the SPOTS extract.

In the final extract, we return to Stuart. As in the FEET example with Elizabeth, the therapist produces as a clarification request (in line 3) an accurate redoing of the child's erroneous production from line 2. However, whereas in the FEET example, the therapist had already modelled the correct form of the target word, in this example the therapist does not model the correct form of NURSE – the target word for pronunciation work here.

Stuart and therapist, second session. Presentation of /s/ in NURSE (picture of NURSE)

1. Th: And who's this? She helps you when you go to hospital
2. St: nurt
          [nɜt]
3. Th: The nurt?
          (.)
4.   What, what should it be?
          (.)
5.   not the nurt, the:
6. St: Doctor.
7. Th: No; you were right but you said it wrong. You forgot the snakey sound at the end.
8. St: snurt
          [snɜt]

The therapist's turn at line 3 seems to put Stuart in a difficult position. Her next utterance (line 4) makes it clear to him that something about his original turn in line 2 is inappropriate, and the longer he withholds his response, the more the therapist makes this point (line 5). When put on the spot, Stuart effects a lexical, rather than a phonetic repair: 'doctor' (line 6). In the absence of specific direction from the therapist, Stuart opts to repair at the level of the word, rather than the phonetic segment. When the therapist eventually draws his attention to phonetic matters explicitly (line 7), he finally attempts phonetic correction – albeit erroneous.

In speech processing terms, the picture of a NURSE serves to help Stuart access his motor program for NURSE. However, unlike the previous two extracts, the therapist does not model the target word, so there is no opportunity for Stuart to check the accuracy of his phonological representation for NURSE, as a basis for revising his motor program. That revision is needed is suggested by line 2, where Stuart's production indicates that he may well have an inaccurate motor program for NURSE. In line 3, the therapist does not address explicitly the need for Stuart to revise his motor program: her accurate redoing of his inaccurate production can be interpreted in a variety of ways, as we have seen. One possibility is that Stuart considers [nɜt] to be an acceptable variant of NURSE: that his phonological representation for NURSE will accommodate this pronunciation, and will licence /nɜt/ as a motor program. This interpretation is made more plausible by the fact that at no point does the therapist offer a model pronunciation of NURSE; and by the fact that there is no alternative lexical item NURT with which NURSE could be confused. This would explain why Stuart does not attempt a phonetic correction at line 6, even though the therapist is clearly pressing for some kind of repair work (lines 3–5). Stuart's response in line 8 to the therapist's eventual indication that phonetic work is needed (line 7) is also revealing: he attaches the [s] to the onset of the word, instead of using it as the coda. This suggests that he has a quite imprecise or indistinct phonological representation for NURSE.

Consideration of these three extracts has shown that the inter-actional structure of intervention sessions can impact hugely on the sense that the child makes of what the session is about, in speech processing terms; and so can influence the success or otherwise of the intervention. Traditional therapy techniques, such as working with minimal pairs, may pose particular difficulties if the requirements are not made explicit. Gardner (1998) concludes:

> Therapists must be aware of the complexity of skills such as that labelled 'metalinguistic awareness' and the need to control the inter-actional aspects of therapy as well as the cognitive ones becomes clear. Specifically, for instance, these findings bring requests for self-repair into question as techniques for gaining phonetic repair except as a carefully directed target behaviour at a specific stage in therapy.

A realistic expectation of the child's metalinguistic awareness is important for therapists and teachers, whether working at the phono-logical or at the grammatical level. Recent research by Rhonwen Shaw has provided much needed developmental data on the emergence of normally developing children's awareness of words and of grammar, and on the type of difficulties encountered by children with specific language impairments (Shaw, 1997). Her assessment materials make a valuable test battery for the developmental therapist or teacher (Shaw, 2000).

Groups and collaboration

Much of the intervention for children with speech difficulties is trad-itionally carried out in a one-to-one setting, as in Hilary Gardner's data. Within the psycholinguistic approach to assessment, too, there is an emphasis on the individual child, with a possibly unique profile of strengths and weaknesses. However, this emphasis on individual children does not in the least preclude intervention being carried out through group work – although the psycholinguistic approach may influence how children are selected to such groups (see Chapter 9 this volume). Group work offers many opportunities for the children and their teachers/therapists. Backus and Beasley (1951) developed a group approach to children with speech difficulties because they believed that an emphasis on speech drills and ear training alone did not carry over to social situations in everyday life. The group setting allowed them to teach speech skills through interactions within the group. Backus

(1957) also noted that children with different types of speech difficulties could perform in a similar way in these groups and that children with similar speech difficulties could be quite different. The use of labels for speech disorders as a basis for intervention was therefore queried long before the publication of Book 1! Backus did not believe that there could be a prescribed intervention programme for a specific speech disorder. This captures not only the philosophy of the psycholinguistic approach to intervention but is also a reminder of the history of current approaches and the wealth of resources available to us.

This 'real life' approach to intervention is being put into practice in innovative residential group work for older children with cleft lip and palate whose speech communication and psychosocial adjustment have plateaued (Stengelhofen, Nash, Toombs, et al., 2000). All of the members of the group were individually assessed and some received specific speech correction work if appropriate (e.g. using EPG). However, in addition the programme aims to change the children's perceptions of themselves as communicators by using the group situation to develop their communication and psychosocial skills. In particular, it focuses on how to manage the listener and others when the speaker is unintelligible because of persisting speech difficulties which may not fully resolve. The children on the course became more willing to talk because they felt valued by the group.

The group approach to intervention emphasizes the value of communication among children with speech difficulties. A corollary of this philosophy is to emphasize the value of communication among the professionals involved with children who have speech and literacy diffi-culties – a recurrent theme in this volume. Juliette Corrin reported that adopting the psycholinguistic framework provided a 'clinical shorthand for team communication' between speech and language therapists within a specialist centre (Chapter 5). Jill Popple and Wendy Wellington described how use of the framework facilitated collabor-ation between teachers and speech and language therapists within a school setting (Chapter 9). The subsequent joint development and monitoring of individual educational plans for children with speech and literacy diffi-culties has ensured that intervention is meaningful to the children's learning and is more likely to carry over from one context to another (see also Chapter 8, this volume).

Conclusion

In this final chapter, we have seen how the psycholinguistic framework is being extended into new areas for assessment purposes, and how it provides a theoretical structure for thinking about intervention. As presented in Book 1, the framework consists of three parts: the speech processing profile, the box-and-arrow speech processing model and the developmental phase model.

The profile is a flexible tool, into which ongoing assessment results can be incorporated. There is no set battery of tests that has to be carried out: each question on the profile can be addressed through a variety of assessment procedures, formal or informal, the exact nature of which will be determined by the age of the child and by practical circumstances. By summarizing the assessments in a systematic way, the profile can provide a basis for structured and psycholinguistically motivated intervention. It also provides a tool for assessing the effects of intervention and identifying remaining areas that need to be targeted: the profile can be completed again once the therapy programme is over, and compared to the original; and then for subsequent monitoring to check that the child's processing difficulties have truly resolved.

The box-and-arrow speech processing model is a tool for identifying with some precision the levels in the speech processing system that are giving rise to the child's difficulties – though it does not necessarily follow that intervention should target these deficits directly (cf. Marshall, 1997). Furthermore, as Chapter 6 of Book 1 shows, the model provides a disciplined approach to the analysis of tasks that are to be used in assessment: it enables one to pose, and answer, the question: which levels of processing are involved in this particular assessment activity? The model can be used in just the same way to think about the tasks used for intervention, as has been illustrated by the authors of several chapters in this volume. The model is thus a tool for bringing greater clarity to the planning of intervention.

The phase model of speech processing and literacy, presented in Chapters 7 and 8 of Book 1, provides a developmental perspective on intervention. We can use the phase model to step back from the immediate details of the child's deficits in speech processing and literacy, to consider the important broader questions. Where is this child at now, in developmental terms? Where would we realistically expect a child of this age to be? How can we devise an intervention programme that will accelerate this child's progress along the developmental trajectory? The phase model provides a theoretical structure in which to answer the first two questions. The answers can then inform the setting of realistic, achievable and developmentally coherent aims for intervention.

In these ways, the psycholinguistic framework helps to make the process of intervention more transparent and explicit. By promoting the setting of realistic aims and quantifiable objectives, it also makes a contribution to the measurement of the efficacy of intervention. Finally, the aggregation of intervention case studies within this common framework will result in a body of knowledge upon which a theory of intervention can be built.

Summary

* The collection of speech processing profiles from a range of children will constitute an important database on the nature of speech, language and literacy difficulties.
* The psycholinguistic framework has been extended to include new aspects of speech processing, including prosody and word finding, and to incorporate techniques such as EPG.
* The psycholinguistic framework is currently being extended to other aspects of speech processing, including the role of working memory, understanding unfamiliar accents, the comprehension and production of connected speech and motor control in DDK tasks.
* The psycholinguistic framework is also being extended to investigate a wider range of clinical populations, including children with cerebral palsy, children who stammer, children with hearing impairments and children with acquired language disorders.
* There is no prescribed intervention programme for a particular category of speech disorder.
* There is no one-to-one match between speech processing profile and intervention programme. Children with similar speech processing profiles can respond differently to intervention tasks, so it is necessary to take account of extrinsic factors.
* The psycholinguistic approach does not focus exclusively on deficits; it reveals strengths as well, which can be built on in intervention.
* The essence of the psycholinguistic approach to intervention lies in the rationale for the design and selection of particular tasks and for the order in which they are presented.
* One way of conceptualizing intervention within the psycholinguistic framework is that it aims to help a child move on to the next phase of speech processing or literacy development.
* The psycholinguistic approach to intervention targets underlying sources of difficulty as well as presenting symptoms.
* Psycholinguistically motivated intervention is generally carried out in face-to-face interactions between the child and the therapist or teacher.
* The way in which the interaction unfolds (for example in the handling of repair) strongly influences the child's understanding of what a session or task is about, and thus the ultimate success of the intervention.
* Controlling the interactional aspects of the session is therefore as important as designing psycholinguistically appropriate tasks.
* Tasks focusing on speech drills and ear training, if presented in isolation, are unlikely to carry over to everyday communication.

- Conversely, interaction with the child that does not include intervention targeted at speech is unlikely to improve intelligibility.
- The psycholinguistic framework, as an approach to assessment and intervention, can facilitate collaboration among professionals working with children who have speech and literacy difficulties.

Appendix 1
For Photocopying

SPEECH PROCESSING PROFILE

SPEECH PROCESSING PROFILE

Name: Comments:

Age: d.o.b:

Date:

Profiler:

INPUT

F

Is the child aware of the internal structure of phonological representations?

E

Are the child's phonological representations accurate?

D

Can the child discriminate between real words?

C

Does the child have language-specific representations of word structures?

B

Can the child discriminate speech sounds without reference to lexical representations?

A

Does the child have adequate auditory perception?

OUTPUT

G

Can the child access accurate motor programs?

H

Can the child manipulate phonological units?

I

Can the child articulate real words accurately?

J

Can the child articulate speech without reference to lexical representations?

K

Does the child have adequate sound production skills?

L

Does the child reject his/her own erroneous forms?

Appendix 2
For Photocopying

SPEECH PROCESSING MODEL

SPEECH PROCESSING MODEL

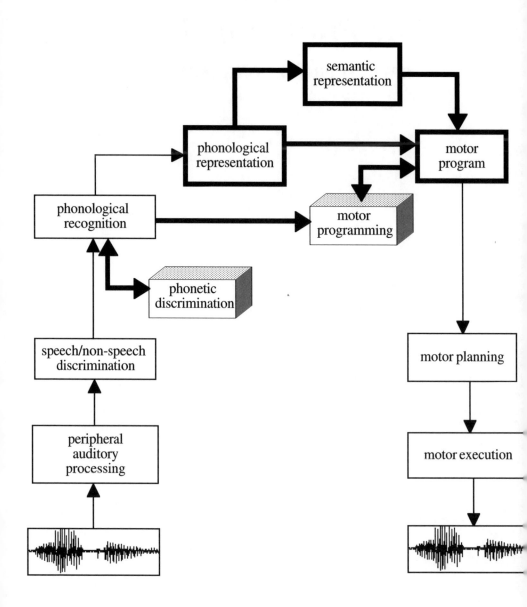

References

Abberton, E., Hu, X., Fourcin, A. (1998) Real-time speech pattern element displays for interactive therapy. *International Journal of Language and Communication Disorders, Supplement – Proceedings of the RCSLT 1998 Conference* **33**: 292–297.

Adams, A.M., Gathercole, S.E. (2000) Limitations in working memory: Implications for language development. *International Journal of Language and Communication Disorders* **35 (1)**: 95–116

Anthony, A., Bogle, D., Ingram, T.T.S.I., McIsaac, M.W. (1971) *The Edinburgh Articulation Test*. Edinburgh: Churchill Livingstone.

Backus, O. (1957) Group structure in speech therapy. In Travis, L. (Ed.) *Handbook of Speech Pathology and Audiology*. New York: Appleton-Century-Crofts.

Backus, O and Beasley, J. (1951) *Speech Therapy with Children*. Boston, MA: Houghton Mifflin.

Badian, N. (1995) Predicting reading ability over the long term: The changing roles of letter naming, phonological awareness and orthographic processing. *Annals of Dyslexia* **45**: 79–96.

Baltaxe, C., Simmons, J. (1985) Prosodic development in normal and autistic children. In Schopler, E. and Mesibov, G. (Eds) *Communication Problems in Autism*, pp.95–125. New York: Plenum.

Beery, K.E., Buktenica, N.A. (1997) *Beery Buktenica Developmental Test of Visual-Motor Integration*. Parsippany, NJ: Modern Curriculum Press.

Bernhardt, B., Gilbert, J. (1992) Applying linguistic theory to speech–language pathology: the case for non-linear phonology. *Clinical Linguistics and Phonetics* **6**: 123–145.

Bernstein-Ratner, N. (1997) Stuttering: A psycholinguistic perspective. In Curlee, R., Siegel, G. (Eds) *Nature and Treatment of Stuttering: New Directions*. 2nd Edition. Boston, MA: Allyn and Bacon.

Bielby, N. (1994) *Making Sense of Reading: The New Phonics and its Practical Implications*. Leamington Spa: Scholastic Publications.

Bigland, S., Speake, J. (1992) *Semantic Links*. Ponteland, Northumberland: STASS publications.

Bird, J., Bishop D.V.M., Freeman, N.H. (1995) Phonological awareness and literacy development in children with expressive phonological impairments. *Journal of Speech and Hearing Research* **38**: 446–462.

Bishop, D.V.M. (1989) *Test for Reception of Grammar*. 2nd Edition. Manchester: Department of Psychology, University of Manchester.

Bishop, D.V.M. (1997) *Uncommon Understanding: Development and Disorders of Language Comprehension in Children*. Hove: Psychology Press.

Bishop, D.V.M., Adams, C. (1990) A prospective study of the relationship between specific language impairment, phonological disorders and reading retardation. *Journal of Child Psychology and Psychiatry* **31**: 1027–1050.

Blachowicz, C.L.Z. (1994) Problem-solving strategies for academic success. In Wallach, G.P., Butler, K. (Eds) *Language Learning Disabilities in School-age Children and Adolescents: Some Principles and Applications*. New York: Macmillan College Publishing Company.

Bradley, L., Bryant, P. E. (1983) Categorising sounds and learning to read – a causal connection. *Nature* **301** (3) February, 419–421.

Brand, V. (1984) *Spelling Made Easy*. Royston: Egon Publishers.

Bray, M., Ross, A. Todd, C. (1999) *Speech and Language: Clinical Process and Practice*. London: Whurr Publishers.

Bridgeman, E., Snowling, M. (1988) The perception of phoneme sequence: A comparison of dyspraxic and normal children. *British Journal of Disorders of Communication* **23** (3): 245–252.

British Psychological Society (1999) *Dyslexia, Literacy and Psychological Assessment*. Leicester: The British Psychological Society.

Broom, Y.M., Doctor, E.A. (1995) Developmental phonological dyslexia: A case study of the efficacy of a remediation programme. *Cognitive Neuropsychology* **12** (7): 725–766.

Broomfield, H., Combley, M. (1997) *Overcoming Dyslexia: A Practical Handbook for the Classroom*. London: Whurr Publishers.

Bruck, M., Treiman, R. (1990) Phonological awareness and spelling in normal children and dyslexics: The case of initial consonant clusters. *Journal of Experimental Child Psychology*. **50**: 156–178.

Bryan, A., Howard, D. (1992) Frozen phonology thawed: The analysis and remediation of a developmental disorder of real word phonology. *European Journal of Disorders of Communication* **27**: 343–365.

Bryant, P. (1998) Sensitivity to onset and rhyme does predict young children's reading : A comment on Muter, Hulme, Snowling and Taylor. *Journal of Experimental Child Psychology* **71**: 29–37.

Buzan, T. (1974) *Use Your Head*. London: BBC Books.

Byng, S (1995) What is aphasia therapy? In Code, C., Müller, D. (Eds) *Treatment of Aphasia: From Theory to Practice*. London: Whurr Publishers.

Caramazza, A. (1988) Some aspects of language processing revealed through the analysis of acquired aphasia: The lexical system. *Annual Review of Neurosciences* **11**: 395–421.

Carver, C. (1970) *Word Recognition Test*. London: Hodder & Stoughton.

Catts, H.W. (1993) The relationship between speech–language impairments and reading disabilities. *Journal of Speech and Hearing Research* **36**: 948–958.

Chiat, S., (1994) A psycholinguistic approach. In Law, J. (Ed.) *Before School: A Handbook of Approaches to Intervention with Preschool Language Impaired Children*. London: AFASIC.

Chiat, S. (1997) Making new connections: In whose interests? In Chiat, S., Law, J., Marshall, J. (Eds) *Language Disorders in Children and Adults: Psycholinguistic Approaches to Therapy.* London: Whurr Publishers.

Chiat, S. (2000) *Understanding Children with Language Problems.* Cambridge: Cambridge University Press.

Chiat, S., Hunt, J. (1993) Connections between phonology and semantics: an exploration of lexical processing in a language impaired child. *Child Language Teaching and Therapy* **9**: 200–213.

Clarke-Klein, S., Hodson, B. (1995) A phonologically based analysis of misspellings by third graders with disordered-phonology histories. *Journal of Speech and Hearing Research* **38**: 839–849.

Coffield, C. (1994) *An Investigation into the Speech Output of Four Down's Syndrome Adolescents.* MSc Thesis. National Hospital's College of Speech Sciences/Institute of Neurology, London.

Connery, V. (1992) *Nuffield Centre Dyspraxia Programme.* London: Nuffield Hearing and Speech Centre, Royal National Throat, Nose and Ear Hospital.

Constable, A. (1993) *Investigating Word-finding Difficulties in Children.* Unpublished MSc thesis, College of Speech Sciences, National Hospital, University College London.

Constable, A., Stackhouse, J., Wells, B. (1997) Developmental word finding difficulties and phonological processing: the case of the missing handcuffs. *Applied Psycholinguistics* **18**: 507–536.

Cootes, C., Simpson, S. (1996) Teaching spelling to children with specific learning difficulties. In: Snowling, M., Stackhouse, J. (Eds) *Dyslexia, Speech and Language: A Practitioner's Handbook.* London: Whurr Publishers.

Corkett, R. (1997) *Auditory Processing Skills in Children with Severe Developmental Dysarthria: Two Case Studies.* BSc (Hons) project. Department of Human Communication Science, University College London.

Courtright, J.A., Courtright, I.C. (1983) The perception of non-verbal vocal cues of emotional meaning by language-disordered children. *Journal of Speech and Hearing Research* **26**: 412–417.

Crawford, R. (1995) Teaching voiced velar stops to profoundly deaf children, using EPG: two case studies. *Clinical Linguistics and Phonetics* **9**: 255–269.

Criper-Friedman, L. (1990) The tone system of West African coastal English. *World Englishes* **9**: 63–77.

Cruttenden, A. (1985) Intonation comprehension in 10 year olds. *Journal of Child Language* **12**: 643–661.

Crystal, D. (1987) Teaching vocabulary: the case for a semantic curriculum. *Child Language Teaching and Therapy* **3**: 40–56.

Crystal, D. (1998) Sense: the final frontier. *Child Language Teaching and Therapy* **14** (1): 1–28.

Cutler, A., Swinney, D. (1987) Prosody and the development of comprehension. *Journal of Child Language* **14**: 145–167.

Dean, E.C., Howell, J., Hill, A., Waters, D. (1990) *Metaphon Resource Pack.* Windsor: NFER-Nelson.

Dean, E.C., Howell, J., Waters, D., Reid, J. (1995) Metaphon: A metalinguistic approach to the treatment of phonological disorders in children. *Clinical Linguistics and Phonetics* **9**: 1–19.

Denckla, M.B., Rudel, R.G. (1976) Naming of object-drawings by dyslexic and other learning disabled children. *Brain and Language* **3**: 1–15.

Dent, H., Gibbon, F., Hardcastle, W. (1992) Inhibiting an abnormal lingual pattern in a cleft palate child using electropalatography. In Leahy, M., Kallen, J. (Eds) *Interdisciplinary Perspectives in Speech and Language Pathology*. Dublin: School of Clinical Speech and Language Studies.

Dent, H., Gibbon, F., Hardcastle, W. (1995) The application of electropalatography (EPG) to the remediation of speech disorders in school-aged children and young adults. *European Journal of Disorders of Communication* **30**: 264–277.

Department for Education (1994) *Code of Practice on the Identification and Assessment of Special Educational Needs*. London: HMSO.

Department for Education (1995a) *The Revised National Curriculum*. London: Central Office of Information.

Department for Education (1995b) *English in the National Curriculum*. London: HMSO.

Department for Education (1995c) *Key Stages 1 and 2 of the National Curriculum*. London: HMSO.

Department for Education and Employment (1998) *The National Literacy Strategy*. London: Central Office of Information.

Dodd, B., Russell, T., Oerlemans, M. (1993) Does a past history of speech disorder predict literacy difficulties? In Joshi, R.M. Leong, C.K. (Eds) *Reading Disabilities: Diagnosis and Component Processes*, pp.199–212. Amsterdam: Kluwer Academic Publishers.

Dollaghan, C. (1987). Fast mapping in normal and language-impaired children. *Journal of Speech and Hearing Disorders* **52**: 218–222.

Donlan, C. (1998) Number without language? Studies of children with specific language impairment. In Donlan, C. (Ed.) *The Development of Mathematical Skills*. Hove: Psychology Press.

Dunn, L.M., Dunn, L.M., Whetton, C., Pintillie, D. (1982) *The British Picture Vocabulary Scales*. Windsor: NFER-Nelson.

Dunn, L.M., Dunn, L.M., Whetton, C., Burley, J. (1997) *The British Picture Vocabulary Scales*. 2nd Edition. Windsor: NFER-Nelson.

Easton, C., Sheach, S., Easton, S. (1997) Teaching vocabulary to children with word-finding difficulties using a combined semantic and phonological approach: an efficacy study. *Child Language Teaching and Therapy* **13** (2): 125–142.

Ebbels, S. (2000) Psycholinguistic profiling of a hearing-impaired child. *Child Language Teaching and Therapy* **16** (1): 3–22.

Ehri, L.E. (1992) Reconceptualizing the development of sight word reading and its relationship to recoding. In Gough, P., Ehri, L.C. Treiman, R. (Eds) *Reading Acquisition*. Hillsdale, NJ: Erlbaum.

Ehri, L.E. (1995) Phases of development in learning to read words by sight. *Journal of Research in Reading* **18**: 116–125.

Ehri, L., Robbins, C. (1992) Beginners need some decoding skill to read words by analogy. *Reading Research Quarterly*, **27** (1): 13–26.

Elliott, C.D. (1992) *British Ability Spelling Scales*. Windsor: NFER-Nelson.

Elliott, C.D., Murray, D.J., Pearson, L.S. (1983) *British Ability Scales*. Windsor: NFER-Nelson.

Elliott, C.D., Smith, P., McCulloch, K. (1996) *British Ability Scales-II (BAS-II)*. Windsor: NFER-Nelson.

Enderby, P., Emerson, J. (1995) *Does Speech and Language Therapy Work?* London: Whurr Publishers.

Fletcher, S.A. (1978) *The Fletcher Time-by-count Test of Diadochokinetic Syllable Rate*. Tigard OR: C.C. Publications.

Flynn, L., Lancaster, G. (1996) *Children's Phonology Sourcebook*. Bicester: Winslow Press.

Foorman, B., Francis, D., Novy, D., Liberman, D. (1991) How letter–sound instruction mediates progress in first grade reading and spelling. *Journal of Educational Psychology,* **84** (4): 456–469.

Forth, T., Stackhouse, J., Nicholas, A., Cook, F. (1997) *An Investigation of Rhyme Skills in Children who Stammer.* Proceedings of the International Dysfluency Conference, Oxford, July 1996.

Fowler, A.E. (1991) How early phonological development might set the stage for phoneme awareness. In Brady, S.A. Shankweiler, D.P. (Eds) *Phonological Processes in Literacy: A Tribute to Isabelle Liberman.* Hillsdale, NJ: Erlbaum.

Francis, H. (1982) *Learning to Read: Literate Behaviour and Orthographic Knowledge*. London: Unwin.

Frederickson, N., Frith, U., Reason, R. (1997) *Phonological Assessment Battery*. Windsor: NFER-Nelson.

Frith, U. (1985) Beneath the surface of developmental dyslexia. In Patterson, K. Marshall, J,. Coltheart, M. (Eds) *Surface Dyslexia.* London: Routledge & Kegan Paul.

Gardner, H. (1994) *Doing talk about speech: A study of speech/language therapists and Phonologically Disordered Children Working Together.* PhD thesis, University of York.

Gardner, H. (1997) Are your minimal pairs too neat? The dangers of phonemicisation in phonology therapy. *European Journal of Disorders of Communication* **32**, 2 (special issue) pp.167–175.

Gardner, H. (1998) Social and cognitive competences in learning: which is which? In Hutchby, I., Moran-Ellis, J. (Eds) *Children and Social Competence.* London: Falmer Press.

Gathercole, S., Baddeley, A. (1990). Phonological memory deficits in language disordered children: is there a causal connection? *Journal of Memory and Language* **29**: 339–360.

German, D. (1989) *Test of Word Finding.* Leicester: Taskmaster.

Gibbon, F. (1990) Lingual activity in two speech-disordered children's attempts to produce velar and alveolar stop consonants: evidence from electropalatographic (EPG) data. *British Journal of Disorders of Communication* **25**: 329–340.

Gibbon, F.E. (1999) Undifferentiated lingual gestures in children with articulation/phonological disorders. *Journal of Speech, Language and Hearing Research* **42**: 382–397.

Gibbon, F., Dent, H., Hardcastle, W. (1993) Diagnosis and therapy of abnormal alveolar stops in a speech-disordered child using EPG. *Clinical Linguistics and Phonetics* **7**, 247–268.

Gibbon, F., Hardcastle, W., Dent, H., Nixon, F. (1996) Types of deviant sibilant production in a group of school-aged children, and their response to treatment using EPG. In Ball, M., Duckworth, M. (Eds) *Advances in Clinical Phonetics.* Amsterdam: John Benjamins.

Gillon, G., Dodd, B. (1997) Enhancing the phonological processing skills of children with specific reading disability. *European Journal of Disorders of Communication* **32**: 2. (Special Issue): 67–90.

Goldstein, H, Gierut, J. (1998) Outcomes measurement in child language and phonological disorders. In Frattali, M. (Ed.) *Measuring Outcomes in Speech-Language Pathology.* New York: Thiene.

Goswami, U. (1993) Towards an interactive analogy model of reading development: decoding vowel graphemes in beginning readers. *Journal of Experimental Child Psychology* **56**: 443–475.

Goswami, U. (1994) The role of analogies in reading development. *Support for Learning* **9**: 22–25.

Goswami, U. (1996) *Rhyme and Analogy: A Teacher's Guide.* Oxford: Oxford University Press.

Goswami, U. (1999) Causal connections in beginning reading: The importance of rhyme. *Journal of Research in Reading* **22**: 217–240.

Goswami, U., Bryant, B. (1990) *Phonological Skills and Learning to Read.* Hillsdale, NJ: Erlbaum.

Grieve, R. (1990) Children's awareness. In Grieve, R., Hughes, M. (Eds) *Understanding Children.* Oxford: Basil Blackwell.

Grundy, K. (1995) Clinical forum: Metaphon: unique and effective? *Clinical Linguistics and Phonetics.* **9**: 20–24.

Grunwell, P. (1985) *Phonological Assessment of Child Speech (PACS).* Windsor: NFER-Nelson.

Grunwell, P. (1992) Principled decision making in the remediation of children with phonological disability. In Fletcher, P., Hall, D. (Eds) *Specific Speech and Language Disorders in Children.* London: Whurr Publishers.

Hardcastle, W., Gibbon, F. and Jones, W. (1991) Visual display of tongue–palate contact: Electropalatography in the assessment and remediation of speech disorders. *British Journal of Disorders of Communication* **26**: 41–74.

Hardcastle, W., Gibbon, F., Dent, H. (1993) Assessment and remediation of intractable articulation disorders using EPG. *Research Institute of Logopedics and Phoniatrics Annual Bulletin, University of Tokyo* **27**: 159–170.

Hardwick, A., Walter, P. (1994) *Making the Alphabet Work.* Brocton, Staffs: Crossbow Publishers.

Hargrove, P., Sheran, C. (1989) The use of stress by language-impaired children *Journal of Communication Disorders* **22**: 361–373.

Hatcher, P. (1994) *Sound Linkage: An Integrated Programme for Overcoming Reading Difficulties.* London: Whurr Publishers.

Hatcher, P. (1996) Practising sound links in reading intervention with the school-age child. In Snowling, M., Stackhouse, J. (Eds) *Dyslexia, Speech and Language: A Practitioner's Handbook.* London: Whurr Publishers.

Hatcher, P.J., Hulme, C. (1999) Phonemes, rhymes, and intelligence as predictors of children's responsiveness to remedial reading instruction: Evidence from a longitudinal intervention study. *Journal of Experimental Child Psychology* **72**: 130–153.

Hatcher, P.J., Hulme, C., Ellis, A.W. (1994) Ameliorating early reading failure by integrating the teaching of reading and phonological skills: The phonological linkage hypothesis. *Child Development* **65**: 41–57.

Haynes, C. (1992) Vocabulary deficit – one problem or many? *Child Language Teaching and Therapy* **8** (1): 1–17.

Heselwood, B., Bray, M., Crookston, I. (1995) Juncture, rhythm and planning in the speech of an adult with Down's syndrome. *Clinical Linguistics and Phonetics* **9** (2): 121–137.

Hewitt, A. (1996) From spoken to written language disorder? A follow-up study of language unit children. *Royal College of Speech and Language Therapists Bulletin* January, 8–9.

Highnam, C., Morris, V. (1987) Linguistic stress judgements of language learning disabled students. *Journal of Communication Disorders* **20**: 93–103.

Hodson, B W. (1997) Disordered phonologies: What have we learned about assessment and treatment? In Hodson, B.W. and Edwards, M.L. (Eds) *Perspectives in Applied Phonology*. Gaithersburg, Maryland: Aspen Publishers, Inc.

Hodson, B.W., Paden, E. (1991) *Targeting Intelligible Speech: A Phonological Approach to Remediation*. 2nd Edition. Austin, TX: Pro-Ed.

Hodson, B., Edwards, M.L. (1997) *Perspectives in Applied Phonology*. Gaithersburg, MD: Aspen.

Hoien T., Lundberg, I., Stanovich, K.E., Bjaalid, I.K. (1995) Components of phonological awareness. *Reading and Writing: An Interdisciplinary Journal* **7**: 171–188.

Holm, A., Dodd, B. (1999) An intervention case study of a bilingual child with phonological disorder. *Child Language Teaching and Therapy* **15** (2): 139–158.

Howard, D., Patterson, K. (1992) *The Pyramids and Palm Trees Test*. Bury St Edmunds: Thames Valley Test Company.

Howard, S. (1998) *Phonetic Constraints on Phonological Systems: Combining Perceptual and Instrumental Analysis in the Investigation of Speech Disorders*. PhD thesis, University of Sheffield.

Howell, J., Dean, E. (1994) *Treating Phonological Disorders in Children: Metaphon – Theory to Practice*. London: Whurr Publishers.

Hulme, C., Quinlan, P., Bolt, G., Snowling, M. (1995) Building phonological knowledge into a connectionist model of word naming. *Language and Cognitive Processes* **10**: 387–391.

Hyde Wright, S., Gorrie, B., Haynes, C., Shipman, A. (1993) What's in a name? Comparative therapy for word-finding difficulties using semantic and phonological approaches. *Child Language Teaching and Therapy* **9** (3): 214–229.

Ingram, D. (1986) Explanation and phonological remediation. *Child Language Teaching and Therapy* **2**: 1–29.

Kail, R., Hale, C.A., Leonard, L.B., Nippold, M.A. (1984). Lexical storage and retrieval in language-impaired children. *Applied Psycholinguistics* **5**: 37–49.

Kirk, S.A., McCarthy, J.J., Kirk, W.D. (1968) *Illinois Test of Psycholinguistic Abilities*. Revised Edition. Illinois: Board of Trustees of the University of Illinois.

Lancaster, G., Pope, L. (1989) *Working with Children's Phonology*. Bicester: Winslow Press.

Landells, J. (1995) Assessment of semantics. In Grundy, K. (Ed). *Linguistics in Clinical Practice*. 2nd Edition. London: Whurr Publishers.

Lane, S. (1993) *Stages in the Development of Rhyme Production Skills.* Unpublished BSc thesis. College of Speech Sciences, National Hospital, University College London.

Larrivee, L.S., Catts, H.W. (1999) Early reading achievement in children with expressive phonological disorders. *American Journal of Speech–Language Pathology* 8: 118–128.

Law, J., Boyle, J., Harris, F., Harkness, A., Nye, C. (1998) Screening for speech and language delay: A systematic review of the literature. *Health Technology Assessment* 2, 9.

Layton, L., Deeney, K., Upton, G. (1997) *Sound Practice: Phonological Awareness in the Classroom.* London: David Fulton.

Leitao, S. Hogben, J., Fletcher, J. (1997) Phonological processing skills in speech and language impaired children. *European Journal of Disorders of Communication* 32 (2) 91–113.

Leonard, L.B., Nippold, M.A., Kail, R., Hale, C.A. (1983) Picture naming in language impaired children. *Journal of Speech and Hearing Research* 26: 609–615.

Letterland: Further information from: Letterland Ltd, Barton, Cambridge CB3 7AY.

Liberman, I.Y., Shankweiler, D., Fischer, F.W., Carter, B. (1974) Explicit syllable and phoneme segmentation in the young child. *Journal of Experimental Child Psychology* 18: 201–212.

Lindamood, P., Bell, N., Lindamood, P. (1997) Achieving competence in language and literacy by training in phonemic awareness, concept imagery, and comparator function. In: Hulme, C., Snowling, M. (Eds) *Dyslexia: Biology, Cognition and Intervention.* London: Whurr Publishers.

Lloyd, S. (1992) *The Phonics Handbook.* Chigwell: Jolly Learning.

Local, J., Wootton, T. (1995) Interactional and phonetic aspects of immediate echolalia in autism. *Clinical Linguistics and Phonetics* 9: 155–184.

Locke, J. (1980) The inference of speech perception in the phonologically disordered child. Part II: Some clinically novel procedures, their use, some findings. *Journal of Speech and Hearing Disorders* 45: 445–468.

Loucas, T., Marslen-Wilson, W. (2000) An experimental and computational exploration of developmental patterns in lexical access and representation. In Perkins, M., Howard, S. (Eds) *New Directions in Language Development and Disorders.* New York: Kluwer/Plenum.

McDonald, E. (1964) *Articulation Testing and Treatment: A Sensory-Motor Approach.* Pittsburgh, PA: Stanwix House.

MacDonald, G.W., Cornwall, A. (1995) The relationship between phonological awareness and reading and spelling achievement eleven years later. *Journal of Learning Disabilities* 28: 523–527.

Magnusson, E., Naucler, K. (1990) Reading and spelling in language disordered children – linguistic and metalinguistic prerequisites: report on a longitudinal study. *Clinical Linguistics and Phonetics* 4 (1): 49–61.

Marshall, J. (1997) Psycholinguistic applications to language therapy. In Chiat, S., Law, L., Marshall, J. (Eds) *Language Disorders in Children and Adults: Psycholinguistic Approaches to Therapy.* London: Whurr Publishers.

Martin, D., Miller, C. (1996) *Speech and Language Difficulties in the Classroom.* London: David Fulton Publishers.

McCormick, M. (1995) The relationship between the phonological processes in early speech development and later spelling strategies. In Dodd, B. (Ed.) *Differential Diagnosis and Treatment of Children with Speech Disorder*. London: Whurr Publishers.

McGregor, K.K. (1994) Use of phonological information in a word-finding treatment for children. *Journal of Speech and Hearing Research* **37**: 1381–1393.

McGregor, K.K. (1997) The nature of word finding errors of pre-schoolers with and without word finding deficits. *Journal of Speech and Hearing Research* **40**: 1232–1244.

McGregor, K.K., Waxman, S.R. (1998) Object naming at multiple hierarchical levels: a comparison of preschoolers with and without word-finding deficits. *Journal of Child Language* **25** (2): 419–430.

Merritt, D.D., Culatta, B. (1998) *Language Intervention in the Classroom*. London: Singular Publishing.

Meyer, M.S., Wood, F.B., Hart, L.A., Felton, R.H. (1998) Selective predictive value of rapid automatized naming in poor readers. *Journal of Learning Disabilities* **31** (2): 106–117.

Mody, M., Studdert-Kennedy, M., Brady, S. (1997) Speech perception deficits in poor readers: auditory processing or phonological coding? *Journal of Experimental Child Psychology* **64**: 199–231.

Morgan, J., Demuth, K. (1996) *Signal to Syntax: Bootstrapping from Speech to Grammar in Early Acquisition*. Hillsdale, NJ: Erlbaum.

MorganBarry, R. (1988) *The Auditory Discrimination and Attention Test*. Windsor: NFER-Nelson.

MorganBarry, R. (1995a) EPG treatment of a child with the Worster-Drought syndrome. *European Journal of Disorders of Communication* **30**: 256–263.

MorganBarry, R. (1995b) The relationship between dysarthria and verbal dyspraxia in children: a comparative study using profiling and instrumental analyses. *Clinical Linguistics and Phonetics* **9**: 277–309.

Moss, H., Reason, R. (1998) Interactive group work with young children needing additional help in learning to read. *Support for Learning*, **13** (1): 32–37.

Muter, V. (1996) Predicting children's reading and spelling difficulties. In Snowling, M., Stackhouse, J. (Eds) *Dyslexia, Speech and Language: A Practitioner's Handbook*. London: Whurr Publishers.

Muter, V., Hulme, C., Snowling, M. (1997) *Phonological Abilities Test*. London: The Psychological Corporation.

Muter, V., Hulme, C., Snowling, M., Taylor, S. (1998) Segmentation, not rhyming, predicts early progress in learning to read. *Journal of Experimental Child Psychology* **71**: 3–27.

Naresmore, R.C., Densmore, A.E., Harman, D.R. (1995) *Language Intervention with School-aged Children: Conversation, Narrative, and Text*. London: Singular Publishing.

Nathan, L., Stackhouse, J., Goulandris, N. (1998) Speech processing abilities in children with speech vs speech and language difficulties. *International Journal of Language and Communication Disorders* **33**: 457–462.

Nathan, L., Stackhouse, J., Goulandris, N. (1999) *Literacy Outcome of Children with Specific Speech and Language Difficulties*. Poster presented at the *AFASIC* 3rd Symposium: Speech and Language Impairments: From Theory to Practice, York.

Nathan, L., Wells, B., Donlan, C. (1998) Children's comprehension of unfamiliar regional accents: A preliminary investigation. *Journal of Child Language* **25**: 343–365.

Nathan, L., Wells, B. (1999) *Cross-speaker Variability and Phonological Impairment: How Do Children with Speech Disorders Process Accent Variation?* Poster presented at the 7th International Clinical Phonetics and Linguistics Association Symposium, Montreal Canada.

Neale, M. (1989) *Neale Analysis of Reading Ability*, Revised British Edition. Windsor, Berks: NFER-Nelson.

Nation, K., Hulme, C. (1997) Phonemic segmentation, not onset-rime segmentation, predicts early reading and spelling skill. *Reading Research Quarterly* **32** (2): 154–167.

Newton, C (1999) *Connected Speech Processes in Phonological Development.* PhD thesis, University College London.

Newton C., Wells, B. (1999) The development of between-word processes in the connected speech of children aged between three and seven. In Maassen, B., Groenen, P. (Eds) *Pathologies of Speech and Language: Advances in Clinical Phonetics and Linguistics*, pp.67–75. London: Whurr Publishers.

Newton, C., Dent, H., Wells, B. (1999) *The Effects of Speech Difficulties on the Production of Between-word Processes.* Poster presented at 3rd International AFASIC Symposium: Speech and Language Impairments from Theory to Practice, York.

Nicholas, A. (1999) *A Study of Speech Processing Skills in Young Children who Stammer.* MSc project, Department of Human Communication Science, University College London.

Nicholas, A., Stackhouse, J., Nathan, L. (2000) *A Study of Speech Processing Skills in Children Who Stutter.* Proceedings of the 3rd World Congress on Fluency Disorders, Nyborg, Denmark.

Nimmo, E. (1998) *Speech Processing and Literacy Skills in Children Whose Speech Difficulties Appear to Have Resolved.* Unpublished MSc thesis, Department of Human Communication Science, University College London.

North, C., Parker, M. (1993) *Phonological Awareness Assessment.* Downside Cottage, Summerhill, Althorne, Essex CM3 6BY.

Onslow, D. (1995) *Investigating Word Finding Difficulties in Children with Developmental and Acquired Language Disorders.* MSc thesis, Department of Human Communication Science, University College.

Parker, A., Rose, H. (1990) Deaf children's phonological development. In Grunwell P. (Ed.) *Developmental Speech Disorders.* London: Whurr Publishers.

Passy, J. (1993a) *Cued Articulation.* Ponteland, Northumberland: STASS Publications.

Passy, J. (1993b) *Cued Vowels:* Ponteland, Northumberland: STASS Publications

Peppé, S. (1998) *Investigating Linguistic Prosodic Ability in Adult Speakers of English.* Unpublished PhD thesis, University College London.

Peppé, S., Maxim, J., Wells, B. (in press) Prosodic variation in southern British English. *Language and Speech.*

Perfetti, C.A., Beck, I, Bell, I. C., Hughes, C. (1987) Phonemic knowledge and learning to read are reciprocal: A longitudinal study of first grade children. *Merrill Palmer Quarterly* **33**: 283–319.

Plaut, D.C., McClelland, J.L., Seidenberg, M.S., Patterson, K. (1996) Understanding normal and impaired word reading: Computational principles in quasi-regular domains. *Psychological Review* **103**: 56–115.

Qualifications and Curriculum Authority (1997) *The Baseline Assessment Information Pack*. London: Qualifications and Curriculum Authority Publications.

Rack, J., Hulme, C., Snowling, M., Wightman, J. (1994) The role of phonology in young children learning to read words; the direct mapping hypothesis. *Journal of Experimental Child Psychology* **57**: 42–71.

Raven, J.C. (1984) *The Coloured Progressive Matrices*. London: H.K. Lewis.

Read, C. (1978) Children's awareness of language with emphasis on sound systems. In Sinclair, A., Jarvella, R. J., Levelt, W.J. (Eds) *The Child's Conception of Language*. Berlin: Springer.

Reason, R. (1998) Effective academic interventions in the United Kingdom: does the 'specific' in specific learning difficulties (disabilities) now make a difference to the way we teach? *Educational and Child Psychology* **15** (1): 71–83.

Reason, R., Boote, R. (1994) *Helping Children with Reading and Spelling: A Special Needs Manual*. London: Routledge.

Rebus symbols (1997) *The Symbol Collection* (software for PC or Acorn) Widgit Software, 102 Redford Road, Leamington Spa CV31 1LF.

Reid, J. (1987) *Sunnybank Colour Coding Scheme*. Unpublished therapy scheme developed at the Sunnybank School Language Unit, Aberdeen.

Renfrew, C.E.(1972) *Word-finding Vocabulary Scale*. Bicester: Winslow Press.

Renfrew, C.E. (1989) *Renfrew Action Picture Test*. 3rd Edition. Bicester: Winslow Press.

Renfrew, C.E. (1991) *The Bus Story: A Test of Continuous Speech*. Bicester: Winslow Press.

Renfrew, C.E. (1995) *Word-finding Vocabulary Test*. Bicester: Winslow Press.

Reynell, J., Huntley, M. (1985) *Reynell Developmental Language Scales*. 2nd Edition. Windsor: NFER-Nelson.

Royal College of Speech and Language Therapists (1996) *Communicating Quality 2: Professional Standards for Speech and Language Therapists*. London: Royal College of Speech and Language Therapists.

Scobbie, J.M., Gibbon, F., Hardcastle, W.J., Fletcher,P. (1998) Covert contrasts and the acquisition of phonetics and phonology. In Ziegler, W., Deger, K. (Eds) *Clinical Phonetics and Linguistics*. London: Whurr Publishers.

Scripture, E. (1923) *Stuttering, Lisping and Correction of Speech of the Deaf*. New York: Macmillan Publishing Co. Inc.

Semel, E., Wiig, E., Secord, W. (1987) *Clinical Evaluation of Language Fundamentals* – Revised. London: The Psychological Corporation.

Share, D.L. (1995) Phonological recoding and self-teaching: sine qua non of reading acquisition. *Cognition* **55**: 151–217.

Shaw, R.E. (1997) *Word Awareness and Grammatical Awareness in Normally Developing Children and Children with Specific Language Impairment*. PhD thesis, Manchester Metropolitan University.

Shaw, R.E. (2000) *Test of Word and Grammatical Awareness (TOWGA)*. Windsor: NFER-Nelson.

Shriberg, L., Aram, D., Kwiatowski J. (1997) Developmental apraxia of speech III: A subtype marked by inappropriate stress. *Journal of Speech, Language and Hearing Research* **40**: 313–337.

Simpson, S. (2000) Dyslexia: A developmental language disorder. *Child: Care, Health, and Development.*

Snow, D. (1998) Prosodic markers of synactic boundaries in the speech of 4-year-old children with normal and disordered language development. *Journal of Speech, Language and Hearing Research* **41**: 1158–1170.

Snowling, M. J. (1996) Annotation: Contemporary approaches to the teaching of reading. *Journal of Child Psychology and Psychiatry* **37** (2): 139–148.

Snowling, M. J. (1998) Reading development and its difficulties. *Educational Psychology in Practice* **15** (2): 44–58.

Snowling, M. (2000) Language and literacy skills: Who is at risk and why? In Bishop, D.V.M., Leonard, L. (Eds) *Speech and Language Impairments in Children: Causes, Characteristics, Intervention and Outcome.* Hove: Psychology Press.

Snowling, M., Hulme, C. (1994) A longitudinal case study of developmental phonological dyslexia. *Cognitive Neuropsychology* **6**: 379–401.

Snowling, M. J, Hulme, C., Smith, A., Thomas, J. (1994) The effects of phonetic similarity and list length on children's sound categorization performance. *Journal of Experimental Child Psychology* **58**: 160–180.

Snowling, M.J., Stothard, S., McClean, J. (1996) *Graded Nonword Reading Test.* Bury St Edmunds: Thames Valley Test Company.

Snowling, M. J, Stothard, SE (unpublished) *Graded Naming Test.*

Snowling, M., Stackhouse, J. Rack, J. (1986) Phonological dyslexia and dysgraphia — a developmental analysis. *Cognitive Neuropsychology* **3** (3): 309–340.

Snowling, M., Stackhouse, J. (Eds) (1996) *Dyslexia, Speech and Language: A Practitioner's Handbook.* London: Whurr Publishers.

Snowling, M. van Wagtendonk, B., Stafford, C. (1988) Object naming deficits in developmental dyslexia. *Journal of Research in Reading* **11**: 67–85.

Stackhouse, J. (1984) Phonological therapy: A case and some thoughts. *The College of Speech Therapists Bulletin* **381**: 10–11.

Stackhouse, J. (1993) Phonological disorder and lexical development: two case studies. *Child Language, Teaching and Therapy* **9**(3): 230–241.

Stackhouse, J. (1996) Speech, spelling and reading: Who is at risk and why? In Snowling, M., Stackhouse, J. (Eds) *Dyslexia, Speech and Language: A Practitioner's Handbook.* London: Whurr Publishers.

Stackhouse, J. (1997) Phonological awareness: Connecting speech and literacy problems. In Hodson, B., Edwards, M.L. (Eds) *Perspectives in Applied Phonology.* Gaithersburg, MD: Aspen.

Stackhouse, J. (2000) Barriers to literacy development in children with speech and language difficulties. In Bishop, D.V.M., Leonard, L. (Eds) *Speech and Language Impairments in Children: Causes, Characteristics, Intervention and Outcome.* Hove: Psychology Press.

Stackhouse J., Wells B. (1993) Psycholinguistic assessment of developmental speech disorders. *European Journal of Disorders of Communication* **28**: 331–348.

Stackhouse, J., Nathan, L., Goulandris, N., Snowling, M. (1999) *The Relationship Between Speech Disorders and Literacy Problems: Identification of the At Risk Child. Report on a 4 Year Longitudinal Study.* Department of Human Communication Science, University College London.

Stackhouse, J., Nathan, L., Goulandris, N. (1999) Speech processing, language and emerging literacy skills in 4 year old children with specific speech difficulties. *Journal of Clinical Speech and Language Studies* 9: 11–34.

Stackhouse J., Wells B. (1997) *Children' s Speech and Literacy Difficulties, Book 1, A Psycholinguistic Framework*. London: Whurr Publishers.

Stengelhofen, J., Nash, P., Toombs, L., Kellow, B., Brown, J. (2000) *A Residential Intervention Programme for Children aged 8–14 with Persisting Communication Problems Associated with Cleft Palate*. Paper presented at the Spring 2000 Meeting of the Craniofacial Society of Great Britain and Ireland.

Stothard, S.E., Snowling, M., Bishop, D.V.M., Chipchase, B.B, Kaplan, C.A. (1998) Language-impaired preschoolers: A follow-up into adolescence. *Journal of Speech, language and Hearing Research* 41: 407–418.

Swan, D., Goswami, U. (1997) Phonological awareness deficits in developmental dyslexia and the phonological representations hypothesis. *Journal of Experimental Child Psychology* 66: 18–41.

Tarplee, C. (1993) *Working on Talk: The Collaborative Shaping of Linguistic Skills Within Child–Adult Interaction*. PhD thesis, University of York.

Tarplee, C. (1996) Working on young children's utterances: Prosodic aspects of repetition during picture labelling. In Couper-Kuhlen, E., Selting, M. (Eds) *Prosody in Conversation: Interactional Studies*. Cambridge: Cambridge University Press.

Thomas, E., Senechal, M. (1998) Articulation and phoneme awareness of 3-year-old children. *Applied Psycholinguistics* 19: 363–391.

Thurston, A. (1999) *An Investigation into the Link between Speech Processing Abilities, Language Skills and Literacy Development: A Follow-up Study of Children Whose Speech Difficulties Appeared to Have Resolved*. Unpublished MSc thesis, Department of Human Communication Science, University College London.

Tod, J., Blamires, M. (1999) *Individual Education Plans: Speech and Language*. London: David Fulton.

Topping, K. (1995) *Paired Reading, Spelling and Writing*. London: Cassell.

Treiman, R. (1993) *Beginning to Spell. A Study of First Grade Children*. New York: Oxford University Press.

Treiman, R. Broderick, V, Tincoff, R., Rodriguez, K. (1998a) Children's phonological awareness: confusions between phonemes that differ only in voicing. *Journal of Experimental Child Psychology* 68: 3–21.

Treiman, R., Tincoff, R., Rodriguez, K., Mouzaki, A., Francis, D. (1998b) The foundations of literacy: Learning the sounds of letters. *Child Development* 69 (6): 1524–1540.

Vance, M. (1997) Christopher Lumpship: Developing phonological representations in a child with an auditory processing deficit. In Chiat, S.W., Law, J., Marshall, J. (Eds) *Language Disorders in Children and Adults*. London: Whurr Publishers.

Vance, M. (1998) Why Can't Speech and Language Impaired Children Remember? The Relationship Between Short-term Memory and Speech Processing Skills. In *Language Impairment: Theory and Practice. Proceedings of the 1998 NAPLIC Conference*. Cheerful Publications: St Catherine's School, Ventnor, Isle of Wight PO38 1TT.

Vance, M., Donlan, C., Stackhouse, J. (1999) Speech processing limitations on nonword repetition in children. In Garman, M., Letts, C., Richards, B.,

Schelleter, C., Edwards, S. (Eds) *Issues in Normal and Disordered Child Language: From Phonology to Narrative.* The New Bulmershe Papers, University of Reading.

Vance, M., Dry, S., Rosen, S. (1999) Auditory processing deficits in a teenager with Landau-Kleffner syndrome. *Neurocase* **5**: 545–554.

Vance, M., Stackhouse, J., Wells, B. (1994) 'Sock the wock the pit-pat-pock' — Children's responses to measures of rhyming ability, 3–7 years. Department of Human Communication Sciences, University College London: *Work in Progress* **4**: 171–185.

Vance, M., Stackhouse, J., Wells, B. (1995) The relationship between naming and word repetition skills in children age 3–7 years. Department of Human Communication Sciences, University College London: *Work in Progress* **5**: 127–133.

Van Riper, C. (1978) *Speech Correction Principles and Methods.* 6th Edition. Engelwood Cliffs, NJ: Prentice-Hall.

Vincent, D., de la Mare, M. (1990) *The Individual Reading Analysis.* Windsor: NFER-Nelson.

Wagner, R.K., Torgesen, J.K., Rashotte, C.A., Hecht, S.A., Barker, T.A., Burgess, S.R., Donahue, J., Garon, T. (1997) Changing relations between phonological processing abilities and word level reading as children develop from beginning to skilled readers: A 5-year longitudinal study. *Developmental Psychology* **33**: 408–479.

Walton, M. (1998) *Teaching Reading and Spelling to Dyslexic Children.* London: David Fulton Publishers.

Webster, P.E., Plante, A.S. (1992) Effects of phonological impairment on word, syllable, and phoneme sequentation and reading. *Language, Speech and Hearing Services in Schools* **23**: 176–182.

Wechsler, D. (1992) *Wechsler Intelligence Scale for Children.* 3rd Edition. London: The Psychological Corporation.

Weiner, F. (1981) Treatment of phonological disability using the method of meaningful minimal contrast: two case studies. *Journal of Speech and Hearing Disorders* **46**: 97–103.

Weiss, C., Lillywhite, H.S., Gordon, M.E. (1980) *Clinical Management of Articulation Disorders.* St Louis, MO: Mosby.

Wells, B. (1994) Junction in developmental speech disorder: a case study. *Clinical Linguistics and Phonetics* **5**: 1–25.

Wells, B., Local. J. (1993) The sense of an ending: a case of prosodic delay. *Clinical Linguistics and Phonetics* **4**: 59–73.

Wells, B., Peppé S (1998) *The Prosodic Abilities of School-age Children: A Developmental Study.* ESRC End of Award Report, R000236696.

Wells, B., Peppé S (1999) *Prosodic Ability in Children with Speech and Language Difficulties.* ESRC End of Award Report, R000222809.

Wells, B, Peppé S., Vance, M. (1995) Linguistic assessment of prosody. In Grundy, K. (Ed.) *Linguistics in Clinical Practice.* 2nd Edition. London: Whurr Publishers.

Williams, P., Stackhouse, J. (1998) Diadochokinetic skills: Normal and atypical performance in children aged 3–5 years. *International Journal of Language and Communication Disorders* **33**: 481–486.

Williams, P., Stackhouse, J. (2000) Rate, accuracy and consistency: diadochokinetic performance of young normally developing children. *Clinical Linguistics and Phonetics.* **14** 4: 267–293.

Wilson, J. (1993) *Phonological Awareness Training: A New Approach to Phonics*. Aylesbury: The County Psychological Service.

Wilson, J. (1993–96) *Phonological Awareness Training (PAT) Programme. Levels 1,2, and 3*. Aylesbury: County Psychological Service.

Wing, C.S. (1990) A preliminary investigation of generalisation to untrained words following two treatments of children's word-finding problems. *Language Speech and Hearing Services in Schools* 21:151–156.

Wittman, S. (1996) A case study in word finding. *Child Language Teaching and Therapy* 12 (3): 300–313.

Wolf, M. (1991). Naming speed and reading: The contribution of the cognitive neurosciences. *Reading Research Quarterly,* 26 (2): 123–141.

Wood, S. (1995) An electropalatographic analysis of stutterers' speech. *European Journal of Disorders of Communication* 30: 226–236.

Wood, J., Wright, J., Stackhouse, J. (1999) Language and literacy in the early years: Professionals' training needs. Poster presented at AFASIC 3rd International Symposium, 1999. University of York. UK. 21–25 March.

Wood, J., Wright, J., Stackhouse, J. (in progress) *Language and Literacy: Early Years Training Project*. Department of Human Communication Science, University College London in collaboration with the British Dyslexia Association and AFASIC.

Wright, J., Kersner, M. (1998) *Supporting Children with Communication Problems: Sharing the workload*. London: David Fulton Publishers Ltd.

Index